Platelets and Megakaryocytes

METHODS IN MOLECULAR BIOLOGY™

John M. Walker, SERIES EDITOR

METHODS IN MOLECULAR BIOLOGY™

Platelets and Megakaryocytes

Volume 1
Functional Assays

Edited by

Jonathan M. Gibbins

School of Animal and Microbial Sciences,
The University of Reading, Reading, UK

Martyn P. Mahaut-Smith

Department of Physiology,
University of Cambridge, Cambridge, UK

HUMANA PRESS ✳ TOTOWA, NEW JERSEY

© 2004 Humana Press Inc.
999 Riverview Drive, Suite 208
Totowa, New Jersey 07512

www.humanapress.com

This publication is printed on acid-free paper. ∞
ANSI Z39.48-1984 (American Standards Institute)

Permanence of Paper for Printed Library Materials.

Production Editor: Mark J. Breaugh.

Cover design by: Patricia F. Cleary.

Cover Illustrations: Background: Scanning electron microscopic images of human platelets at rest (upper panel) and after ADP-evoked aggregation (lower panel). See Fig. 2 on p. 21. Inset: Thrombus formation studied in vivo using fluorescently labeled platelets (left panel). See Fig. 3 on p. 195. Proplatelet-forming megakaryocyte grown in culture (right panel). See Fig. 1 on p. 288.

For additional copies, pricing for bulk purchases, and/or information about other Humana titles, contact Humana at the above address or at any of the following numbers: Tel.: 973-256-1699; Fax: 973-256-8341; E-mail: humana@humanapr.com; or visit our Website: www.humanapress.com

Printed in the United States of America. 10 9 8 7 6 5 4 3 2 1

E-ISBN: 1-59259-782-3

ISSN: 1064-3745

Library of Congress Cataloging in Publication Data

Platelets and megakaryocytes / edited by Jonathan M. Gibbins, Martyn P. Mahaut-Smith.

  p. ; cm. -- (Methods in molecular biology ; 272-273)

 Includes bibliographical references and index.

 ISBN 1-58829-101-4 (v. 1 : alk. paper) -- ISBN 1-58829-011-5 (v. 2 : alk. paper)

 1. Blood platelets--Laboratory manuals. 2. Megakaryocytes--Laboratory manuals.

 [DNLM: 1. Blood Platelets--physiology. 2. Histological Techniques. 3. Megakaryocytes--physiology. WH 300 P71788 2004] I. Gibbins, Jonathan M. II. Mahaut-Smith, Martyn P. III. Methods in molecular biology (Clifton, N.J.) ; v. 272-273.

 QP97.P568 2004

 612.1'17--dc22

2004002112

Preface

The average human body has in the order of 10^{12} circulating platelets. They are crucial for hemostasis, and yet excessive platelet activation is a major cause of morbidity and mortality in western societies. It is therefore not surprising that platelets have become one of the most extensively investigated biological cell types. We are, however, far from understanding precisely how platelets become activated under physiological and pathophysiological conditions. In addition, there are large gaps in our knowledge of platelet production from their giant precursor cell, the megakaryocyte. Understanding megakaryocyte biology will be crucial for the development of platelet gene targeting. The aim of *Platelets and Megakaryocytes* is therefore to bring together established and recently developed techniques to provide a comprehensive guide to the study of both the platelet and the megakaryocyte. It consists of five sections split between two volumes. The more functional assays appear in Volume 1, whereas Volume 2 includes signaling techniques, postgenomic methods, and a number of key perspectives chapters.

Part I of Volume 1, *Platelets and Megakaryocytes: Functional Assays*, describes many well established approaches to the study of platelet function, including aggregometry, secretion, arachidonic acid metabolism, procoagulant responses, platelet adhesion under static or flow conditions, flow cytometry, and production of microparticles. Although one would ideally wish to perform experiments with human platelets, studies within the circulation using intravital microscopy require the use of animal models, which are described in Chapter 16, vol. 1. These approaches are becoming increasingly important in our understanding of how platelet responses contribute to the complex formation of thrombi within the circulation. Although naturally occurring genetic mutations can indicate the importance of specific proteins, these are limited in frequency and scope and thus many laboratories are using transgenic animals to delete or upregulate individual gene products (*see* Chapter 2, vol. 2). Consequently, the application of platelet techniques to murine models has become a focus of many labs in recent years (e.g., Chapters 2, 16, 20, vol. 1). In addition to basic and advanced approaches to study platelet function, several chapters in this section (particularly 1 and 2, vol. 1) focus on the long-standing issue of the effects of different anticoagulants and procedures to prepare platelets. The experimenter has a choice of studying platelets within the blood, in plasma, or in an artificial medium. In whole blood, potential interactions with other cell types and plasma proteins are included, which is in many ways the most physiological in vitro approach (*see* Chapter 6, vol. 1), however this is a complex situation and interpretation can be difficult. In studies within plasma, other cells are removed, but the clotting cascade is retained (*see* Chapter 5, vol. 1). Frequently, however, platelets are studied in isolation from other cells and plasma following their resuspension in an artificial medium. The preparation of platelets from human and other species is not a trivial matter and great care is required to ensure that the method of preparation does not adversely affect subsequent analysis (see Chapter 2, vol. 1).

Part II of Volume 1 focuses on approaches used to study megakaryocyte function, including the development of specialized structures for future production of platelets (e.g., the demarcation membrane system), the appearance of platelet-specific surface receptors, and the increase in ploidy. The source of megakaryocytes is often a complex issue facing many researchers owing to the extremely low density (<1%) of this cell type in its primary location, the marrow. Techniques to purify megakaryocytes from marrow based on their unique size and surface markers are described in Chapter 22, vol. 1, along with approaches to maintain these cells in culture and monitor formation of platelet-generating proplatelet structures. An alternative approach to generating megakaryocytes is to grow them in culture from precursor cells as detailed in Chapter 23, vol. 1. This requires the presence of thrombopoietin (Chapter 26, vol. 1) acting through its receptor, c-Mpl, and normally other cytokines. The availability of systems to generate megakaryocytes in vitro provides a promising avenue to generate genetically modified platelets. Although there is no doubt that continuous megakaryocyte cell lines are useful for some studies of signaling in these cells, they have their limitations and the pros and cons are discussed in Chapter 27, vol. 1.

Many basic and advanced techniques for the general study of cell signaling have been applied in studies to characterize the mechanisms of regulation of platelet function. These include ligand binding assays, the study of protein and lipid kinases and phosphatases, the analysis of lipid rafts in the regulation of cell signaling, the measurement of intracellular calcium levels, electrophysiological techniques, nitric oxide signaling, the use of venom proteins, and the internalization of proteins into platelets through permeabilization. These techniques and more are presented in Part II of Volume 2. In many respects the megakaryocyte is a giant platelet. Differences do occur in the arrangement of cellular organelles and cytoskeleton in the two cells, however megakaryocytes respond to platelet agonists such as ADP with full downstream functional responses (discussed in Chapters 1 and 16, vol. 2). Therefore, despite differences in ultrastructure, the megakaryocyte has earned its place as a sufficient, if not comparable model of platelet signaling. Many of the signaling techniques are therefore beginning to be applied to the megakaryocyte which, because of its size, is proving to be an extremely interesting model for platelet signaling, particularly using single cell approaches such as imaging and electrophysiology (*see* Chapters 16 and 17, vol. 2).

Part III of Volume 2 is dedicated to recent advances in molecular techniques and post-genomic techniques and how they may be applied to the study of platelets and megakaryocytes. This section includes descriptions of how retroviruses may be used to express genes in primary megakaryocytes, the use of GFP-fusion proteins to study signaling in live cells, two-dimensional electrophoresis for platelet proteomics, the production of platelet cDNA libraries and the use of gene array technology.

Although the main aim of the book is to include practical approaches to the study of platelets and megakaryocytes, a series of perspectives chapters are included (Part I, vol. 2). These chapters review the current understanding of platelet and megakaryocyte biology in addition to their discussions of important new developments and experimental strategies. Many of the methods chapters also include further discussion and background on specific techniques.

This book has only been made possible by the efforts of many international experts in the field. We are grateful to them for their willingness to contribute their knowledge, in particular their tricks of the trade, which have resulted from many years of dedicated hands-on work. We also wish to thank our colleagues within the Department of Physiology at Cambridge and the School of Animal and Microbial Sciences at Reading for helpful discussion during the course of the editing work, in particular Peter Wooding on electron microscopy and Gwen Tolhurst on molecular techniques. We are also grateful to Margaret Bardy and Karen Parr for considerable secretarial assistance. We are also grateful to the following companies for supporting the cost of color reproduction: Eli Lilly and Company, Cairn Research Ltd., Bio Rad Laboratories Ltd., and Sysmex UK Ltd.

Jonathan M. Gibbins
Martyn P. Mahaut-Smith

Contents of Volume 1

Functional Assays

CONTENTS OF THE COMPANION VOLUME

Volume 2: Perspectives and Techniques

xiii

Contributors

WARREN S. ALEXANDER • *The Walter and Eliza Hall Institute of Medical Research, Royal Melbourne Hospital, Victoria, Australia*

GULIE ALIMARDANI • *Départment d'Hématologie, Institut Cochin Paris, and Faculté de Médecine d'Amiens, Amiens, France*

JACKIE APPLEBY • *Department of Cardiovascular Sciences, University of Leicester, Glenfield Hospital, Leicester, UK*

WOLFGANG BERGMEIER • *The Center for Blood Research, Harvard Medical School, Boston, MA*

EDOUARD M. BEVERS • *Department of Biochemistry, CARIM, Maastricht University, The Netherlands*

CAROL BRIGGS • *Department of Haematology, University College London Hospitals, London, UK*

DOMINIQUE CASSEL • *INSERM U.311, Etablissement Français du Sang-Alsace, Strasbourg, France*

JEAN-PIERRE CAZENAVE • *INSERM U.311, Etablissement Français du Sang-Alsace, Strasbourg, France*

ALESSANDRO CELI • *Center for Hemostasis and Thrombosis Research, Beth Israel Deaconess Medical Center and Harvard Medical School, Boston, MA*

PAUL COMFURIUS • *Department of Biochemistry, CARIM, Maastricht University, The Netherlands*

ELISABETH M. CRAMER • *Départment d'Hématologie, Institut Cochin Paris, Service d'hématologie et d'immunologie, Faculté de Médecine Paris, Paris, France*

DAVID CROSBY • *Department of Pharmacology, University of Bristol, Bristol, UK*

NAJET DEBILI • *Institut Gustave Roussy, Institut Fédératif de Recherche, Villejuif, France*

JOANNA L. DIETRICH • *Department of Biochemistry, University of Cambridge, Cambridge, UK*

SACHA M. DOPHEIDE • *Australian Centre for Blood Diseases, Department of Medicine, Monash University, Clayton, Victoria, Australia*

ARNAUD DROUIN • *Départment d'Hématologie, Institut Cochin Paris, Service d'hématologie et d'immunologie, Faculté de Médecine Paris, Paris, France*

ANITA ECKLY • *INSERM U.311, Etablissement Français du Sang-Alsace, Strasbourg, France*

JORGE D. ERUSALIMSKY • *The Wolfson Institute for Biomedical Research, University College London, London, UK*

SHAHROKH FALATI • *Center for Hemostasis & Thrombosis Research, Beth Israel Deaconess Medical Center and Harvard Medical School, Boston, MA*

RICHARD W. FARNDALE • *Department of Biochemistry, University of Cambridge, Cambridge, UK*

MARION A. H. FEIJGE • *Department of Biochemistry, CARIM, Maastricht University, The Netherlands*

ROBERT FLAUMENHAFT • *Center for Hemostasis and Thrombosis Research, Beth Israel Deaconess Medical Center and Harvard Medical School, Boston, MA*

SHIROU FUKUHARA • *The First Department of Internal Medicine, Kansai Medical School, Osaka, Japan*

BARBARA C. FURIE • *Center for Hemostasis and Thrombosis Research, Beth Israel Deaconess Medical Center and Harvard Medical School, Boston, MA*

BRUCE FURIE • *Center for Hemostasis and Thrombosis Research, Beth Israel Deaconess Medical Center and Harvard Medical School, Boston, MA*

CHRISTIAN GACHET • *INSERM U.311, Etablissement Français du Sang-Alsace, Strasbourg, France*

ADRIAN R. L. GEAR • *Department of Biochemistry and Molecular Genetics, University of Virginia, Charlottesville, VA*

JONATHAN M. GIBBINS • *School of Animal and Microbial Sciences, The University of Reading, Reading, Berkshire, UK*

ALISON H. GOODALL • *Department of Cardiovascular Sciences, University of Leicester, Glenfield Hospital, Leicester, UK*

PETER L. GROSS • *Center for Hemostasis & Thrombosis Research, Beth Israel Deaconess Medical Center and Harvard Medical School, Boston, MA*

IAN S. HARPER • *Australian Centre for Blood Diseases, The Microscopy & Imaging Research Facility, Monash University, Clayton, Victoria, Australia*

PAUL HARRISON • *Oxford Haemophila Centre and Thrombosis Unit, Churchill Hospital, Oxford, UK*

PHILIP G. HARGREAVES • *Department of Biochemistry, University of Cambridge, UK*

M. FRED HEATH • *Department of Clinical Veterinary Medicine, University of Cambridge, Cambridge, UK*

BÉATRICE HECHLER • *INSERM U.311, Etablissement Français du Sang-Alsace, Strasbourg, France*

JOHAN W. M. HEEMSKERK • *Department of Biochemistry, CARIM, Maastricht University, The Netherlands*

LARS HENNING • *Medizinische Klinik IV, Charite-Campus Benjamin Franklin, Berlin, Germany*

STANLEY HEPTINSTALL • *Cardiovascular Medicine, Queen's Medical Centre, Nottingham, UK*

YING HONG • *The Wolfson Institute for Biomedical Research, University College London, London, UK*

SASCHA C. HUGHAN • *Australian Centre for Blood Diseases, Department of Medicine, Monash University, Clayton, Victoria, Australia*

CRAIG HYLAND • *The Walter & Eliza Hall Institute of Medical Research, Royal Melbourne Hospital, Melbourne, Victoria, Australia*

SHAUN P. JACKSON • *Australian Centre for Blood Diseases, Department of Medicine, Monash University, Clayton, Victoria, Australia*

JOACHIM JANKOWSKI • *Medizinische Klinik IV, Charite-Campus Benjamin Franklin, Berlin, Germany*

GAVIN E. JARVIS • *Department of Biochemistry, University of Cambridge, Cambridge, UK*

ROSEMARY J. KEOGH • *Department of Biochemistry, University of Cambridge, Cambridge, UK*

NORIO KOMATSU • *Division of Hematology, Department of Medicine, Jichi Medical School, Tochigi-ken, Japan*

SUHASINI KULKARNI • *Australian Centre for Blood Diseases, Department of Medicine, Monash University, Clayton, Victoria, Australia*

ROBERT M. LEVEN • *Department of Anatomy & Cell Biology, Rush Medical College, Chicago, IL*

FAWZIA LOUACHE • *INSERM U362, Institut Gustave Roussy, Institut Fédératif de Recherche, Villejuif, France*

SAMUEL J. MACHIN • *Department of Haematology, University College London Hospitals, London, UK*

MARTYN P. MAHAUT-SMITH • *Department of Physiology, University of Cambridge, UK*

ANTHONY MATHUR • *Queen Mary's School of Medicine and Dentistry, University of London, UK*

JANE A. MAY • *Cardiovascular Medicine, Queen's Medical Centre, Nottingham, UK*

GLENN MERRILL-SKOLOFF • *Center for Hemostasis & Thrombosis Research, Beth Israel Deaconess Medical Center and Harvard Medical School, Boston, MA*

GERARD B. NASH • *Department of Physiology, The University of Birmingham Medical School, Birmingham, UK*

WARWICK S. NESBITT • *Australian Centre for Blood Diseases, Monash University, Clayton, Victoria, Australia*

BERNHARD NIESWANDT • *Department of Vascular Biology, Rudolf Virchow Centre for Experimental Biomedicine, University of Wuerzberg, Wuerzberg, Germany*

SHOSAKU NOMURA • *The First Department of Internal Medicine, Kansai Medical University, Osaka, Japan*

PHILIPPE OHLMANN • *INSERM U.311, Etablissement Français du Sang-Alsace, Strasbourg, France*

RENATA POLANOWSKA-GRABOWSKA • *Department of Biochemistry and Molecular Genetics, University of Virginia Health System, Charlottesville, VA*

ALASTAIR W. POOLE • *Department of Pharmacology, School of Medical Sciences, University of Bristol, Bristol , UK*

TARA W. RUTLEDGE • *Department of Molecular and Cellular Biochemistry, University of Kentucky College of Medicine, Lexington, KY*

HARTMUT SCHLÜTER • *Medizinische Klinik IV, Charite-Campus Benjamin Franklin, Berlin, Germany*

VALERIE SCHULTE • *Department of Vascular Biology, Rudolf Virchow Centre for Experimental Biomedicine, University of Wuerzberg, Wuerzberg, Germany*

DEREK SIM • *Center for Hemostasis & Thrombosis Research, Beth Israel Deaconess Medical Center and Harvard Medical School, Boston, MA*

JOANNE M. STEVENS • *School of Animal and Microbial Sciences, University of Reading, Reading, UK*

WILLIAM VAINCHENKER • *INSERM U362, Institut Gustave Roussy, Institut Fédératif de Recherche, Villejuif, France*

GUOSU WANG • *The Wolfson Institute for Biomedical Research, University College London, London, UK*

JAMES G. WHITE • *Departments of Pediatrics, Laboratory Medicine and Pathology, University of Minnesota School of Medicine, Minneapolis, MN*

SIDNEY W. WHITEHEART • *Department of Molecular and Cellular Biochemistry, University of Kentucky College of Medicine, Lexington, KY*

Color Plates

Color Plates 1–7 appear as an insert following p. 44.

PLATE 1   An example of a scattergram produced by the Sysmex XE-2100 hematology analyzer in both cartoon and dot plot formats. (See full caption on p. 38, Chapter 3.)

PLATE 2   Schematic representation of intravital setup for evaluation of real-time thrombus formation. (See full caption on p. 190, Chapter 16.)

PLATE 3   Time course of thrombus formation in vivo and fluorescent labeling of venous thrombus components. (See full caption on p. 195, Chapter 16.)

PLATE 4   Cross-section of cartridge showing the principle of the PFA-100 test. (See full caption on p. 217, Chapter 18.)

PLATE 5   Cross-section of a cartridge before and after performing the PFA-100 test. (See full caption on p. 217, Chapter 18.)

PLATE 6   Light microscopic appearance of MKs from a normal bone marrow smear, stained by the Romanovski technique. (See full caption on p. 331, Chapter 25.)

PLATE 7   Human normal bone marrow biopsy immunostained for fibrinogen by the APAAP technique. (See full caption on p. 332, Chapter 25.)

I

Platelet Functional Assays

1

Effects of Anticoagulants Used During Blood Collection on Human Platelet Function

Jane A. May and Stanley Heptinstall

1. Introduction

Nearly all the chapters in this book involve some sort of study of platelets (and megakaryocytes) in vitro with a view to gaining insight into the true behaviour of these cells in the circulation. But a word of warning is required. Studies performed in vitro can only approximate the true situation in vivo. If, for example, we choose to study platelets in platelet-rich plasma (PRP), we are studying them in the absence of other blood cells that may well influence the way platelets behave. Even if studies are performed in whole blood, platelets are being studied in the absence of vascular endothelial cells, which contribute to the inhibition of their activity within the vasculature.

For practical purposes, in vitro studies of platelet function in both whole blood and PRP are virtually always performed after adding something to prevent the blood and PRP from clotting. A solution that contains citrate is often used for this purpose. Without addition of such an anticoagulating solution, freshly drawn blood will clot within a few minutes of collection. However, it should always be remembered that this creates a wholly unsatisfactory nonphysiological environment. Typically, citrate addition reduces the level of ionized calcium in the blood plasma from about 1.2 mM to about 0.1 mM. It also reduces the levels of ionized magnesium. Other types of anticoagulants (e.g., heparin or hirudin) can be used that maintain Ca^{2+} at physiological levels, but these also have their own drawbacks which will be explained in more detail later.

There may not be a lot we can do about all this, except to be continually aware of the potential dangers involved in extrapolating from data obtained in vitro to the true in vivo situation. In student lectures we sometimes use the following analogy to emphasize the dangers involved: "Studies of platelet function in vitro as a means of gaining information on true platelet function in vivo may be considered to be analogous to attempts to gain information on the physiology of a herring through the study of a kipper on a plate."

From: *Methods in Molecular Biology, vol. 272:*
Platelets and Megakaryocytes, Vol. 1: Functional Assays
Edited by: J. M. Gibbins and M. P. Mahaut-Smith © Humana Press Inc., Totowa, NJ

In this chapter we will be looking at anticoagulation and its effects on platelet function. We will present data that demonstrate the different results that can be obtained in studies of platelet aggregation, simply as a consequence of the choice of anticoagulant that is used. We will draw heavily on our own platelet research experience.

2. Materials

2.1. Anticoagulant Solutions

Our main experience has been with citrate, heparin, and hirudin anticoagulants:

1. Citrate, 3.13% (w/v): 3.13 g trisodium citrate dihydrate in 100 mL water. Store at 4°C. Transfer 1 mL to a 10-mL graduated polystyrene tube and use to anticoagulate 9 mL blood (*see* **Note 1**).
2. Heparin: This is obtained commercially. We currently use Monoparin (Heparin Injection BP, Heparin Sodium [Mucous] from CP Pharmaceuticals Ltd, Wrexham, UK) which is supplied at a concentration of 1000 U/mL. Transfer 100 μL to a 10-mL graduated polystyrene tube and use to anticoagulate 9.9 mL blood (*see* **Note 2**).
3. Hirudin: We use recombinant hirudin (Revasc®), supplied in solid form by Novartis. Dissolve 15 mg in 3 mL NaCl saline (item 4, below) and store frozen. Just prior to use, thaw this solution and transfer 100 μL to a 10-mL graduated polystyrene tube and use to anticoagulate 9.9 mL blood (*see* **Note 3**).
4. NaCl saline: We use a commercial preparation (Code B1323) that is supplied for intravenous infusion by Baxter Healthcare (Thetford, UK). It contains 150 mM NaCl, which is 0.9% (w/v) sodium chloride in water. Other commercial preparations are available.

2.2. Other Materials and Equipment

1. 19-g sterile needles and polypropylene syringes from the Terumo Corporation.
2. 10-mL graduated polystyrene tubes and caps from Sarstedt Ltd., Leicester, UK (parts nos. 62.492 and 65.793, respectively).
3. PAP-4 Platelet Aggregation Profiler (Bio-Data Corp, Horsham, PA) for measurements of platelet aggregation in PRP by light absorbance.
4. Multi-Sample Agitator, (Medical Engineering Unit, University of Nottingham) for measurements of platelet aggregation in whole blood by platelet counting under conditions of standard agitation (equivalent to 1000 rpm).
5. Phosphate-buffered saline (PBS): 4.5 mM Na$_2$HPO$_4$, 1.6 mM KH$_2$PO$_4$, and 150 mM NaCl (pH 7.4).
6. Fixative solution: for PBS plus 4.6 mM Na$_2$EDTA and 0.16% w/v formaldehyde. Store at 4°C. This is used to fix single platelets and aggregates prior to aggregation measurements by platelet counting.
7. Sysmex KX21 Hematology Analyzer (TOA Medical Electronics Co. Ltd., Kobe, Japan) or a Becton Dickinson FACScan Flow Cytometer (BD Biosciences, San Jose, CA) for platelet counting.
8. Platelet agonists (ADP, ATP) are prepared by dissolving the solid, obtained commercially from the Sigma Chemical Co., cat. nos. A6646 (ADP) and A7699 (ATP), in 150 mM NaCl saline (Baxter Healthcare).

3. Methods

3.1. Blood Collection and Procedures Post-Anticoagulation

1. Blood collection (*see* **Note 4**): In all our experiments, blood is obtained by venepuncture using a 19-g needle (*see* **Note 5**) attached to a polypropylene syringe, using as little pulling pressure as possible. The needle is then discarded and blood transferred to polystyrene tubes with the chosen anticoagulant, filling up to the 10-mL mark. The tubes are then capped and blood and anticoagulant mixed by inverting the tube gently three times (*see* **Note 6**).

2. Platelet preparation for aggregation studies in whole blood: To measure aggregation in whole blood in as reproducible a way as possible, we initially maintain the blood at 37°C (using a water bath or other means of temperature control) for 30 min. This (1) allows the platelets to "recover" from the insult of being mixed with a foreign solution, and (2) enables standardization of the procedure in the case of samples transferred to the laboratory from distant hospital wards and the like. The aggregation studies are performed immediately after this standard 30-min incubation.

3. Platelet preparation for aggregation studies in PRP: Immediately after blood collection, centrifuge the blood at 180*g* for 10 min at room temperature. Then gently transfer the PRP (the upper layer) to another polystyrene tube using a plastic pipet and cap the tube. Recentrifuge the residual blood at 1500*g* for 10 min to prepare platelet-poor plasma (PPP); this is used to (1) adjust the platelet count in the PRP to 300,000/μL and (2) set up the aggregometer (*see* Chapter 5). All this takes about 30 min. At this point, platelet aggregation studies are commenced. The PRP is kept at room temperature throughout, but aliquots are always warmed to 37°C (this takes 2 min) before the response of the platelets to an agonist is investigated.

3.2. Platelet Aggregation

We will not describe here the exact procedures that are employed, as these are described elsewhere in this book (*see* Chapters 5 and 6, vol. 1). Most of our platelet aggregation measurements in whole blood involve stirring blood samples under carefully controlled conditions (e.g., using the Multi-Sample Agitator) followed by fixation and use of a platelet-counting technique to determine the degree of aggregation that occurs (e.g., using a dedicated whole blood platelet counter such as a Sysmex KX21, or a flow cytometer) with aggregation expressed as the percent fall in platelet count. Platelet aggregation in PRP is assessed by light absorbance using a conventional aggregometer (e.g., a PAP-4 Platelet Aggregation Profiler) and/or by platelet counting.

3.3. Examples of the Influence of the Anticoagulant Used

3.3.1. Effect of Citrate on ADP-Induced Aggregation

Perhaps the most well-known effect of an anticoagulant on platelet aggregation is the ability of citrate to enhance platelet responses to ADP. In PRP prepared from citrated anticoagulated blood in which the aggregation is measured by light absorbance, ADP produces both primary and secondary waves of aggregation; the latter is a result of the ADP-induced formation of thromboxane A_2 (TXA_2) and an associated release

reaction involving secreted ADP (*see* Chapters 2, 7, and 11 of this book for further discussion). However, in anticoagulants that maintain physiological divalent cation concentrations (e.g., hirudin or heparin), TXA_2 formation and release is minimal and
primary aggregation predominates (*1–3*). The effect of the citrate was demonstrated to
be via the reduced concentration of Ca^{2+} in the plasma (*4–6*).

3.3.2. Enhanced Spontaneous Aggregation in Whole Blood During Pregnancy

Stirring whole blood can cause some "spontaneous" platelet aggregation, as measured using platelet counting, and probably involves small amounts of ADP liberated
from red cells in the blood (*7–10*). During normal pregnancy there is an increased
platelet sensitivity to ADP and other aggregating agents that becomes evident from
16 weeks gestation and returns to normal postpartum. We discovered that this increased
platelet sensitivity resulted in a clear enhancement of spontaneous platelet aggregation
in whole blood collected into heparin, but not into citrate (*11*, **Fig. 1**). It may well be
that the presence of the heparin serves to accentuate the increased sensitivity to ADP
during pregnancy (*see* **Subheading 3.3.3.**).

3.3.3. Heparin (But Not Hirudin) Enhances Platelet Responses to ADP

In a hitherto unpublished study in which we measured platelet aggregation in whole
blood using platelet counting, we compared directly the influence of three different
anticoagulants (heparin, hirudin and citrate) on ADP-induced aggregation (**Fig. 2**).
In this study we clearly observed potentiation of platelet responses by heparin in
comparison with the other anticoagulants.

3.3.4. Citrate and Heparin (But Not Hirudin) Reduce the Degree of Inhibition of ADP-Induced Aggregation by $P2Y_{12}$-Receptor Antagonist

There is a great deal of interest in pharmacological inhibitors of platelet function that
may be developed as antithrombotic agents. This includes antagonists of ADP-activated
$P2Y_{12}$ purinergic receptors on platelets (*12,13*). In assessing one $P2Y_{12}$ antagonist,
AR-C69931, we compared the ability of the drug to inhibit ADP-induced aggregation in
blood containing different anticoagulants. We found that the degree of inhibition of
aggregation was greater in blood anticoagulated with hirudin compared with blood anticoagulated with citrate or heparin (**Fig. 3**).

3.3.5. Citrate Enhances the Degree of Inhibition of Platelet Aggregation by GPIIb/IIIa Antagonist

Studies with the GPIIb/IIIa antagonist integrilin (eptifibatide) performed both in
whole blood (platelet counting) and PRP (light absorbance) showed markedly reduced
IC_{50} values for inhibition of both ADP- and collagen-induced aggregation when citrate
was used as the anticoagulant. Compared with hirudin, citrate enhanced the potency of
eptifibatide by up to fourfold in both PRP and whole blood (*14*). This study from our
own group followed from the initial findings of Phillips et al. (*15*); the results are
explained by an increase in affinity of the drug for its receptor under conditions of low

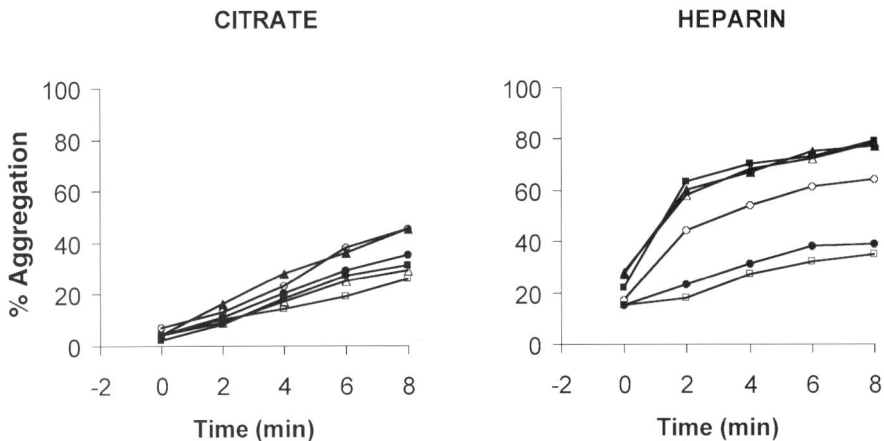

Fig. 1. Effect of anticoagulant on spontaneous platelet aggregation in stirred whole blood during pregnancy. The blood was anticoagulated with either citrate or heparin. Aggregation was measured by platelet counting at 16 (○), 24 (▲), 32 (△), and 36 (■) wk gestation, and at 6 wk post-natal (□). Also shown are results obtained for nonpregnant female controls (●) (Reproduced with permission from **ref. 11**).

Ca^{2+}. Extrapolation of data obtained from findings in the presence of citrate led to a gross underestimation of the amount of drug required to effectively inhibit platelet aggregation under physiological conditions.

3.3.6. Citrate Masks a Pro-Aggregatory Effect of Some Radiographic Contrast Media

Radiographic contrast media of various types are now used routinely for cardiac imaging; however, concerns have been expressed about their possible prothrombotic effects. In investigating the effects of three different radiographic contrast media on platelet aggregation in whole blood anticoagulated with hirudin, we observed potentiation of aggregation by two of these agents and inhibition by the third *(16)*. Similar results were also seen in fresh non-anticoagulated blood. Interestingly, in blood anticoagulated with citrate, all three agents inhibited platelet aggregation. **Figure 4** illustrates data obtained using PAF as the platelet agonist in whole blood collected using hirudin or citrate. Very similar data were obtained with ADP. The intensity of the potentiation of aggregation by iopamidol in the presence of hirudin was such that it induced aggregation directly in stirred whole blood (*see* **ref. 16**). Thus, once again, the nature of the anticoagulant selected for in vitro investigation was found to markedly affect the results that were obtained.

3.3.7. ATP Induces Platelet Aggregation in Whole Blood But Not in PRP Anticoagulated With Hirudin (Platelet Counting)

Compared to our considerable knowledge of the actions of ADP on platelets, very little is known about the effects of ATP. We recently showed *(17)* that ATP can, in fact,

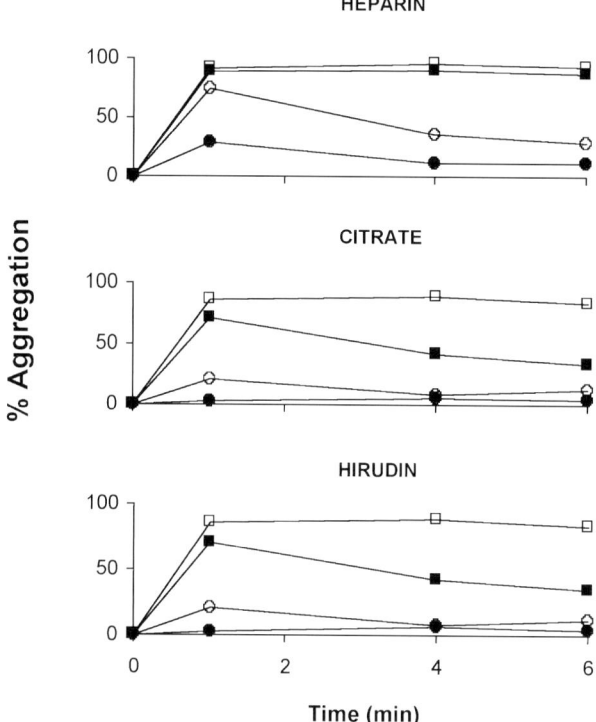

Fig. 2. Potentiation of platelet responses by heparin compared to other anticoagulants. Aggregation induced in whole blood by a range of concentrations of ADP, 0.1 (●), 0.3 (○), 1.0 (■), and 3.0 μ*M* (□). The blood was anticoagulated with heparin, citrate, or hirudin and parallel determinations performed using platelet counting. Results are the means of data obtained from six different volunteers.

cause platelet aggregation in whole blood containing hirudin as the anticoagulant, but not in PRP. The aggregation that occurs in whole blood appears to be a consequence of the ATP being converted into ADP by ecto-ATPases on leukocytes and of removal of any adenosine that is also generated (which might otherwise inhibit the aggregation) via uptake into erythrocytes. ATP-induced aggregation in whole blood that contained citrate as the anticoagulant appeared to be less extensive than when hirudin was used as the anticoagulant, and this may reflect the cation dependence of the leukocyte ATPases.

3.3.8. Conclusion

It is very clear that the nature of the anticoagulant added at the point of blood collection can markedly affect platelet function. It is therefore important that a possible effect of a particular anticoagulant be anticipated, tested, and its effect assessed before extrapolating findings obtained in vitro to the real situation in the circulation.

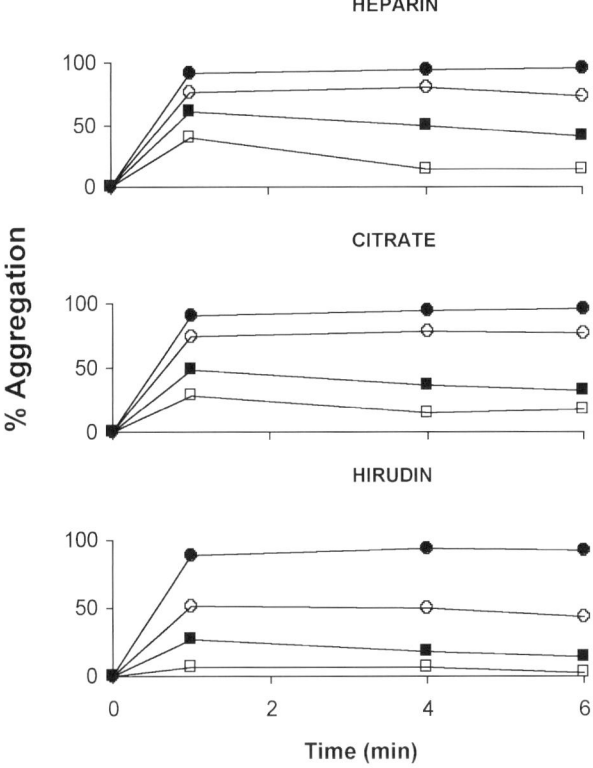

Fig. 3. Comparison of the inhibitory action of a P2Y$_{12}$ receptor antagonist in different anticoagulants. Aggregation induced in whole blood by ADP (10 µM) and the effects of AR-C69931, 0 (●), 10 (○), 30 (■), and 100 nM (□). The blood was anticoagulated with heparin, citrate, or hirudin and parallel determinations performed using platelet counting. Results are the means of data obtained from six different volunteers.

4. Notes

1. We routinely use 3.13% (w/v) trisodium citrate dihydrate in water as our anticoagulant solution; we believe that this is fairly common. Some investigators choose to use 3.8% (w/v) trisodium citrate dihydrate in water. We do not use the latter because it slightly increases the osmolality of the blood. We also note that some investigators use ACD (acid-citrate-dextrose). This reduces the pH of the blood and is another complicating factor that should be borne in mind, as platelet responses are pH-dependent.

2. The heparin that we use is unfractionated heparin; it is possible that other forms (e.g., low-molecular-weight heparin) would give different results. This is an area that requires further investigation.

3. The availability of hirudin for in vitro studies of platelet function is a real problem. We were fortunate in obtaining a gift of hirudin from Novartis but we understand that no further supplies of Revasc® are available. Hirudin is available from other sources but it is

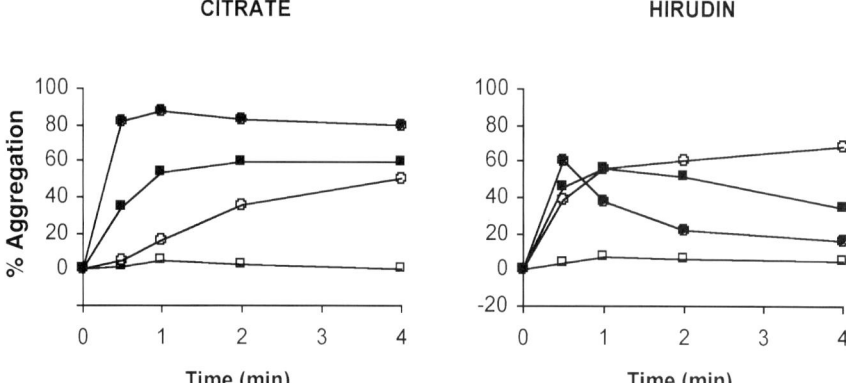

Fig. 4. Effect of anticoagulant type on the modulation of platelet aggregation by radiographic contrast media. Platelet aggregation induced by 0.3 μM PAF in whole blood without added contrast media (●), and in blood containing iopamidol (○), iodixanol (■), or ioxaglate (□). The blood was anticoagulated with either citrate or hirudin and aggregation monitored by platelet counting. (Reproduced with permission from **ref. *16*.**)

very expensive. An alternative thrombin inhibitor that we have sometimes used is PPACK. This is readily available from a number of commercial sources and we found that it is effective as an anticoagulant at a final concentration of 40 μM in blood.

4. The first stage in working on human blood is to get the permission of the appropriate ethics committee to draw the blood. This may seem either obvious or trivial but it is very important. Ethics committees are concerned that some groups of people (e.g., laboratory staff employed by the researcher) are not put under undue pressure to act as "controls" or as "normal volunteers." Everyone (volunteers and patients) needs to be fully informed of the reasons for requesting that a sample of blood be taken.

5. We believe that insufficient attention may sometimes be given to the possibility of inadvertent activation of platelets and other blood cells during blood collection. Use of needles with a smaller diameter than 19 g (e.g., 21 g) or exertion of a high vacuum during blood collection should be avoided.

6. Years ago, before plastic became readily available, blood was collected routinely into glass tubes that had been coated with a layer of silicon. Presumably the use of ordinary glass sometimes led to activation of the blood cells. We find that the use of plastic (polypropylene or polystyrene) syringes, tubes, and pipets provides a satisfactory means of handling blood samples, but we do try to keep handling artifacts to a minimum by avoiding vigorous mixing or stirring until the point at which platelet aggregation (or other) studies are to be performed.

References

1. Macfarlane, D. E, Walsh, P. N., Mills, D. C. B., Holmsen, H., and Day, H. J. (1975) The role of thrombin in ADP-induced platelet aggregation and release: a critical evaluation. *Brit. J. Haematol.* **30,** 457–463.

2. Mustard, J. F., Perry, D. W., Kinlough-Rathbone, R. L., and Packham, M. A. (1975) Factors responsible for ADP-induced release reaction of human platelets. *Amer. J. Physiol.* **228,** 1757–1765.

3. Heptinstall, S. and Mulley, G. P. (1977) Adenosine diphosphate-induced platelet aggregation and release reaction in heparinized platelet rich plasma and the influence of added citrate. *Brit. J. Haematol.* **36,** 565–571.

4. Heptinstall, S. and Taylor, P. M. (1979) The effects of citrate and extracellular calcium ions on the platelet release reaction induced by adenosine diphosphate and collagen. *Thromb. Haemost.* **42,** 778–793.

5. Lages, B. and Weiss, H. J. (1981) Dependence of human platelet functional responses on divalent cations: aggregation, and secretion in heparin- and hirudin-anticoagulated platelet-rich plasma and the effects of chelating agents. *Thromb. Haemost.* **45,** 173–179.

6. Packham, M., Bryant, N., Guccione, M., Kinough-Rathbone, R., and Mustard, J. (1989) Effect of concentration of Ca^{2+} in the suspending medium on the responses of human and rabbit platelets to aggregating agents. *Thromb. Haemost.* **62,** 968–976.

7. Fox, S. C., Burgess-Wilson, M., Heptinstall, S., and Mitchell, J. R. A. (1982) Platelet aggregation in whole blood determined using the Ultra-Flo 100 Whole Blood Platelet Counter. *Thromb. Haemost.* **48,** 327–329.

8. Saniabadi, A. R., Lowe, G. D. O., Barbenel, J. C., and Forbes, C. D. (1984) A comparison of spontaneous platelet aggregation in whole blood with platelet rich plasma: additional evidence for the role of ADP. *Thromb. Haemost.* **51,** 115–118.

9. Hendra, T. J. and Yudkin, J. S. (1990) Whole blood platelet aggregation based on cell counting perocedures. *Platelets* **1,** 57–66.

10. Armstrong, R., May, J. A., Lösche, W., and Heptinstall, S. (1995) Factors that contribute to spontaneous platelet aggregation and streptokinase-induced aggregation in whole blood. *Thromb. Haemost.* **73,** 297–303.

11. Burgess-Wilson, M. E., Morrison, R., and Heptinstall, S. (1986) Spontaneous platelet aggregation in heparinized blood during pregnancy. *Thromb. Res.* **41,** 385–393.

12. Gachet, C. (2001) ADP receptors of platelets and their inhibition. *Thromb. Haemost.* **86,** 222–232.

13. Storey, R.F. (2001) The $P2Y_{12}$ receptor as a therapeutic target in cardiovascular disease. *Platelets* **12,** 197–209.

14. Storey, R. F., Wilcox, R. G., and Heptinstall, S. (1998) Differential effects of glycoprotein IIb/IIIa antagonists on platelet microaggregate and macro aggregate formation and effect of anticoagulant on antagonist efficacy: implications for assay methodology and comparison of different antagonists. *Circulation* 1998; **98,** 1616–1621.

15. Phillips, D. R., Teng, W., Arfsten, A., Nannizzi-Alaimo, L., White, M. M., Longhurst, C., et al. (1997) Effects of Ca^{2+} on GP IIb-IIIa interactions with integrilin: enhanced GP IIb-IIIa binding and inhibition of platelet aggregation by reductions in the concentration of ionized calcium in plasma anticoagulated with citrate. *Circulation* **95,** 860–867.

16. Heptinstall, S., White, A., Edwards, N., Pascoe, J., Sanderson, H. M., Fox, S. C., et al. (1998) Differential effects of three radiographic contrast media on platelet aggregation and degranulation: implications for clinical practice? *Br. J. Haematol.* **103,** 1023–1030.

17. Stafford, N. P., Pink, A. E., White, A. E., Glenn, J. R., and Heptinstall, S. (2003) Mechanisms involved in adenosine triphosphate-induced platelet aggregation in whole blood. *Arterioscler. Thromb. Vasc. Biol.* **23,** 1928–1933.

2

Preparation of Washed Platelet Suspensions From Human and Rodent Blood

Jean-Pierre Cazenave, Philippe Ohlmann, Dominique Cassel, Anita Eckly, Béatrice Hechler, and Christian Gachet

1. Introduction

Citrate is the preferred anticoagulant for blood collection, as EDTA damages platelets and heparin modifies their function *(1)*. Citrate allows the rapid generation of platelet-rich plasma (PRP), with a high yield of platelets; however, this method has certain disadvantages. In particular, the PRP preparation has a limited stability (no longer than 2 h) and contains plasma proteins, including enzymes. In addition, human platelet-rich plasma (PRP) prepared from blood collected into trisodium citrate (3.8% w/v) has a depressed ionic calcium concentration, which can cause platelet aggregation and release of substances during centrifugation *(2)*. To overcome these different problems, a centrifugation technique has been developed for the isolation and washing of platelets from human or rodent blood anticoagulated with acid-citrate-dextrose (ACD). The cells are resuspended in a physiological buffer under well-defined conditions, notably the presence of plasmatic ionic calcium concentrations (2 mM) and the absence of coagulation factors or other plasma components.

The method for isolation of human platelets by centrifugation and washing described by Cazenave et al. *(3)* is derived directly from the technique of Mustard et al. *(4)*. Blood collected into ACD is used to prepare PRP, from which the platelets are isolated by successive centrifugation steps and resuspended in Tyrode's buffer, an iso-osmotic phosphate buffer at pH 7.35 containing glucose (0.1%, w/v), human serum albumin (HSA) (0.35%, w/v), calcium (2 mM), and magnesium (1 mM). Prostacyclin (PGI$_2$) is used to prevent transitory platelet activation during the preparation. Addition of apyrase (adenosine 5'-triphosphate diphosphohydrolase, EC 3.6.1.5) to the final suspending medium prevents the cells from becoming refractory to ADP and maintains their discoid shape *(5)*. Suspensions of washed platelets prepared by this method are stable for 5–8 h at 37°C, compared with citrated PRP preparations, which are stable for no more than 2 h.

From: *Methods in Molecular Biology, vol. 272:*
Platelets and Megakaryocytes, Vol. 1: Functional Assays
Edited by: J. M. Gibbins and M. P. Mahaut-Smith © Humana Press Inc., Totowa, NJ

Suspending platelets in an artificial medium presents two main advantages: (1) plasma enzymes (e.g., thrombin generated during the collection and preparation process) are excluded and (2) it is possible to manipulate the inorganic ions, proteins, and other constituents in the suspension. When such a medium is employed, the pH should lie in the physiological range (7.2–7.4) to avoid affecting platelet functions *(6)*. The solution should be iso-osmotic and contain glucose as a source of metabolic energy and physiological concentrations of divalent cations *(7)*. In addition, the platelets can be labeled with radioisotopes (^{51}Cr, ^{111}In-oxine, ^{14}C- or ^{3}H-serotonin) and used either in vitro to study platelet secretion or accumulation on artificial and natural surfaces, or in vivo to follow platelet survival and detect sites of sequestration or thrombus formation in humans and animals.

2. Materials

2.1. Equipment

A Sorvall RC3BP centrifuge (Kendro Laboratory Products, Newton, CT) is used with an H6000A-HBB6 rotor and 15- or 50-mL conical-bottom polypropylene centrifuge tubes. Wide-bore plastic Pasteur pipets (Pastettes, Biolyon, Dardilly, France) are employed to transfer anticoagulated blood, PRP, and washed platelet suspensions, which must be kept in plastic tubes (polypropylene, ref. 430291, Corning Inc., Corning, NY) or siliconized glass containers to prevent platelet activation and blood coagulation. Human blood is collected with a 16-gauge needle mounted on a short length (10–20 cm) of plastic tubing (ref. HC-15R, Nissho Nipro Europe N.V., Zaventem, Belgium). Rat and mouse blood are collected with 18-gauge and 25-gauge needles, respectively. Platelets are counted in an automatic hematology analyzer for human blood (Sysmex K-1000, Merck, Darmstadt, Germany) or rodent blood (Coulter, Miami, FL).

2.2. Reagents for Blood Collection and Washed Platelet Preparation

All chemicals from commercial sources (Prolabo, Paris, France; Merck, Darmstadt, Germany; Sigma-Aldrich-Fluka, Saint-Quentin Fallavier, France) should be of analytical grade.

1. Acid-citrate-dextrose (ACD) anticoagulant solution (*see* **Note 1**): Prepare this anticoagulant by dissolving 25 g of trisodium citrate dihydrate, 14 g of citric acid monohydrate, and 20 g of anhydrous D(+)glucose in a final volume of 1 L of distilled water. The final concentrations are, respectively, 85 mM, 66.6 mM, and 111 mM; the solution has an osmolarity of 450 mOsm/L and a pH of about 4.5. One volume of anticoagulant is required for six volumes of blood.
2. Stock solutions for Tyrode's buffer (*see* **Note 2**):
   Stock I: 160 g 2.73 M NaCl, 4 g (53.6 mM) KCl, 20 g (238 mM) NaHCO$_3$, and (1.16 g) 8.6 mM NaH$_2$PO$_4$, H$_2$O made up to 1 L in distilled water and stored at 4°C.
   Stock II: 20.33 g (0.1 M) MgCl$_2$•6H$_2$O made up to 1 L.
   Stock III: 21.9 g (0.1 M) CaCl$_2$•6H$_2$O made up to 1 L.
   HEPES stock: 0.5 M (*N*-[2-hydroxyethyl]piperazine-*N'*-[2-ethanesulfonic acid]) sodium salt (119 g) made up to 1 L (*see* **Note 3**).

Human serum albumin (HSA) stock: 200 g/L pasteurized human serum albumin for intravenous injection (Etablessement Français du Sang-Alsace, Strasbourg, France) (purity > 98%).

3. Tyrode's albumin buffer *(0.35% albumin)* (*see* **Note 4**): 5 mL stock I, 1 mL stock II, 2 mL stock III, 1 mL HEPES stock, 1.75 mL HSA stock, and 0.1 g anhydrous D(+)glucose in a final volume of 100 mL of distilled water. Adjust the pH to 7.35 with HCl and the osmolarity to 295 mOsm/L with 30% NaCl or distilled water.

4. Tyrode's buffer: 50 mL of stock I and 950 mL of distilled water, pH 7.35 with HCl.

5. Washing salines for platelet preparation

    First wash: Tyrode's albumin buffer containing 10 U/mL heparin (Roche, Neuilly-sur-Seine, France).

    Second wash: Tyrode's albumin buffer.

    Final suspension: Tyrode's albumin buffer containing 2 µL/mL apyrase (preparation described below).

6. Apyrase preparation: Apyrase (adenosine 5′-triphosphate diphosphohydrolase, EC 3.6.1.5) is an ADP scavenger that is added to the final suspension at 0.02 U/mL, a concentration sufficient to prevent the desensitization of platelet ADP receptors during storage at 37°C. The enzyme can be purchased (e.g., type VII apyrase, Sigma). However, we use apyrase prepared by a modification of the method of Molnar and Lorand *(8)* in a two-stage procedure at 4°C:

    Stage I: Peel, wash, and slice 10 kg of potatoes (preferably white potatoes, at least 6 mo old), homogenize in a Waring blender with 1 L of distilled water, and then mix for 30 min. Centrifuge the suspension at 900*g* for 10 min, filter the supernatant fluid through multiple layers of cheesecloth, and measure the volume of the effluent.

    Stage II: Add 0.1 *M* $CaCl_2$ to the supernatant to bring the solution to a final $CaCl_2$ concentration of 0.025 *M*, stir for 15 min, allow to settle for 60 min, and centrifuge for 20 min at 3500*g*. Resuspend the precipitate in 1 *M* $CaCl_2$ (1/10 of the original volume of effluent), stir for 60 min, and centrifuge for 20 min at 3500*g*. Dialyze the supernatant using a regenerated cellulose membrane tubing, diameter depending on the volume to be used (molecular weight cut-off (MWCO): 10,000 Daltons, Spectra/Por, American Pacific, CA) for 24 h against 0.1 *M* KCl (20 L for 10 kg of potatoes) and then centrifuge for 20 min at 3500*g*. Add to the supernatant fluid 30.4 g of $(NH_4)_2SO_4$ for every 100 mL of fluid; after dissolving (10 min), stir for 40 min and centrifuge for 15 min at 3500*g*. Discard the precipitate and add again to the supernatant 30.4 g of $(NH_4)_2SO_4$ to 100 mL of fluid; after dissolving, stir for 40 min and centrifuge for 15 min at 3500*g*. Discard the supernatant and dissolve the precipitate in a minimum of distilled water (precipitate obtained from 10 kg of potatoes is dissolved in 150 mL of distilled water) and dialyze with same tubing (MWCO: 10,000) against several changes of 0.154 *M* (0.9% w/v) NaCl.

    Determine the protein concentration with the bicinchoninic acid (BCA) protein assay system (Pierce, Rockford, IL) and dilute to 3 mg/mL with 0.154 *M* NaCl. Store the concentrate (brown solution) in small aliquots (2 mL) at –20°C. Before use, centrifuge the concentrate for 5 min at 12,000*g*, dilute the supernatant 5- to 10-fold in modified Tyrode's buffer, aliquot in 1-mL quantities and store at –20°C (*see* **Note 5**). This apyrase stock is for use at a final activity of 0.02 U/mL (or higher, at 0.9 U/mL, if $P2X_1$ receptors are being studied). The optimal concentration of diluted apyrase to prevent ADP receptor desensitization should be determined empirically, since the amount required will vary with different enzyme preparations (*see* **Note 5**). The nucleotidase activity of the apyrase preparation can be determined by measuring the rate at which it degrades ADP and ATP. Incubate 2 µL of apyrase (0.3 mg/mL) with 20 µL of 1 mM ADP or ATP in 1 mL of Tyrode's albumin buffer for various times (0, 1, 3, 4, and 5 min) at 37°C. At each time point, stop the reaction by adding 100 µL of ice-cold 6 N perchloric acid (HClO$_4$). Centrifuge the samples at 12,000g for 5 min at 4°C and extract the non-degraded nucleotides from the supernatant in 2 mL of freon/trioctylamine (1/1), mix the samples for 10 min and centrifuge as before. The nucleotides (AMP, ADP, ATP) are separated by HPLC on an anionic exchange column (P10SAX-25QS, Interchim, Montluçon, France). The specific ADPase or ATPase activity is about 10–100 U/mg of apyrase, depending on the preparation (*see* **Note 5**).

7. Heparin, 5000 U/mL: Standard heparin (Sanofi-Synthélabo, Toulouse, France) is a solution ready to use at 5000 U/mL and can be stored at 4°C for several weeks. Heparin (2 µL of the stock solution) is added in the first step of the platelet-washing procedure at a final concentration of 10 U/mL in the platelet suspension (*see* **Note 6**).

8. Prostacylin (PGI$_2$), 1 mM: Prostacyclin (sodium salt, ref P-6188, Sigma) is prepared as a 1 mM stock solution in ice-cold buffer (50 mM Tris-HCl, pH 8.8) and stored in 100-µL aliquots at –20°C. PGI$_2$ is used at each step of the platelet washing procedure (*see* **Subheading 3.**) at a final concentration of 0.5 µM (0.5 µL of the stock solution for 1 mL of platelet suspension) (*see* **Note 7**).

3. Methods

3.1. Preparation of Washed Human Platelets

3.1.1. Blood Collection (see **Note 8**)

Collect blood from a forearm vein, using a wide-bore (16-gauge) needle mounted on a short length (10–20 cm) of plastic tubing, directly into a conical 50-mL centrifuge tube containing 1 volume of ACD anticoagulant for 6 volumes of blood (final pH 6.5 and citrate concentration 22 mM). After discarding the first few milliliters, which are contaminated with tissue factor (TF) and containing trace amounts of thrombin, allow the blood to flow down the tube wall in order to minimize air contact or bubble formation. Immediately after collection, close the tubes, mix the blood gently with the anticoagulant, and place the tubes in a water bath at 37°C for a maximum storage period of 15 min.

3.1.2. Washed Platelet Preparation

1. Prewarm the Sorvall centrifuge to 37°C and centrifuge the anticoagulated blood at 250g for a period of time depending on the quantity of blood (*see* **Table 1**) to obtain platelet-rich plasma (PRP) (*see* **Fig. 1**).

2. Carefully collect the PRP with a 10-mL syringe and transfer to a new conical 50-mL centrifuge tube.

3. After 10 min incubation at 37°C, centrifuge the PRP at 2200g for a period of time depending on the quantity of plasma (*see* **Table 1**).

4. Discard the supernatant consisting of platelet-poor plasma (PPP) using a Pasteur pipet connected to a vacuum pump, taking care to remove all traces of plasma from the tube walls or near the platelet pellet to avoid generation of thrombin during the subsequent washing steps (*see* **Note 9**).

Table 1
Centrifugation Time and Relative Centrifugal Force (RCF) Used
for Platelet Isolation and the Different Washing Steps

	Volume of fluid (mL)					
	15-mL tube	50-mL tube	RCF *(g)*	RPM	Time (min)	Brake
Human blood	15	50	250	926	16	no
	10	40	250	926	15	no
	6	25	250	926	13	no
Human PRP	10	40	2200	2749	16	yes
	9	35	2200	2749	15	yes
	8	30	2200	2749	14	yes
	6.5	25	2200	2749	13	yes
	5	20	2200	2749	12	yes
	4.5	15	2200	2749	10	yes
Washing steps	10	40	1900	2254	8	yes
	8	30	1900	2254	8	yes

Centrifugation times depend on the volume of fluid; the time and relative centrifugal force *(g)* are given here for the Sorvall RC3BP centrifuge with an H600A-HBB6 rotor.

5. Gently resuspend the platelet pellet in Tyrode's albumin solution containing 10 U/mL heparin and 0.5 μM PGI$_2$ (*see* **Note 10**). A wash volume of 10 mL is normally required for the platelet pellet from 50–100 mL of blood.
6. After 10 min incubation at 37°C, add 0.5 μM PGI$_2$ to the first wash and centrifuge at 1900g for 8 min (for 30–40 mL of platelet suspension).
7. Resuspend the platelet pellet in Tyrode's albumin solution containing PGI$_2$ (0.5 μM).
8. Remove 120 μL of platelet suspension with a pipet and count the platelets in an automatic analyzer. After 10 min incubation at 37°C, add 0.5 μM PGI$_2$ to the second wash and centrifuge at 1900g for 8 min (for 30–40 mL of suspension).
9. Resuspend the platelet pellet in Tyrode's albumin buffer containing 0.02 U/mL apyrase and adjust the cell count in the final suspension to 300,000/μL with the same buffer (*see* **Note 11**).

3.2. Preparation of Washed Rodent Platelets

3.2.1. Blood Collection

Local and national regulations for animal care, anesthesia, and removal of blood should be followed at all times. In our laboratory, rats weighing 250–300 g are anaesthetised by injection of a mixture (1/4: v/v) of 2% xylazine and 10% ketamine (1 mL/kg of body weight). Mice 8 wk old and weighing about 20 g are anesthetized by injection of a mixture of 0.2% xylazine base and 1% ketamine in physiological saline (50 μL/10 g of body weight). Blood is then collected from the abdominal aorta using an 18-gauge (rat) or 25-gauge needle (mouse) mounted on a syringe containing 1 volume of ACD for 6 volumes of blood. The quantity of blood obtained from a rat weighing 200 g is about 10 mL, while the volume drawn from a mouse weighing 20 g is about 1 mL.

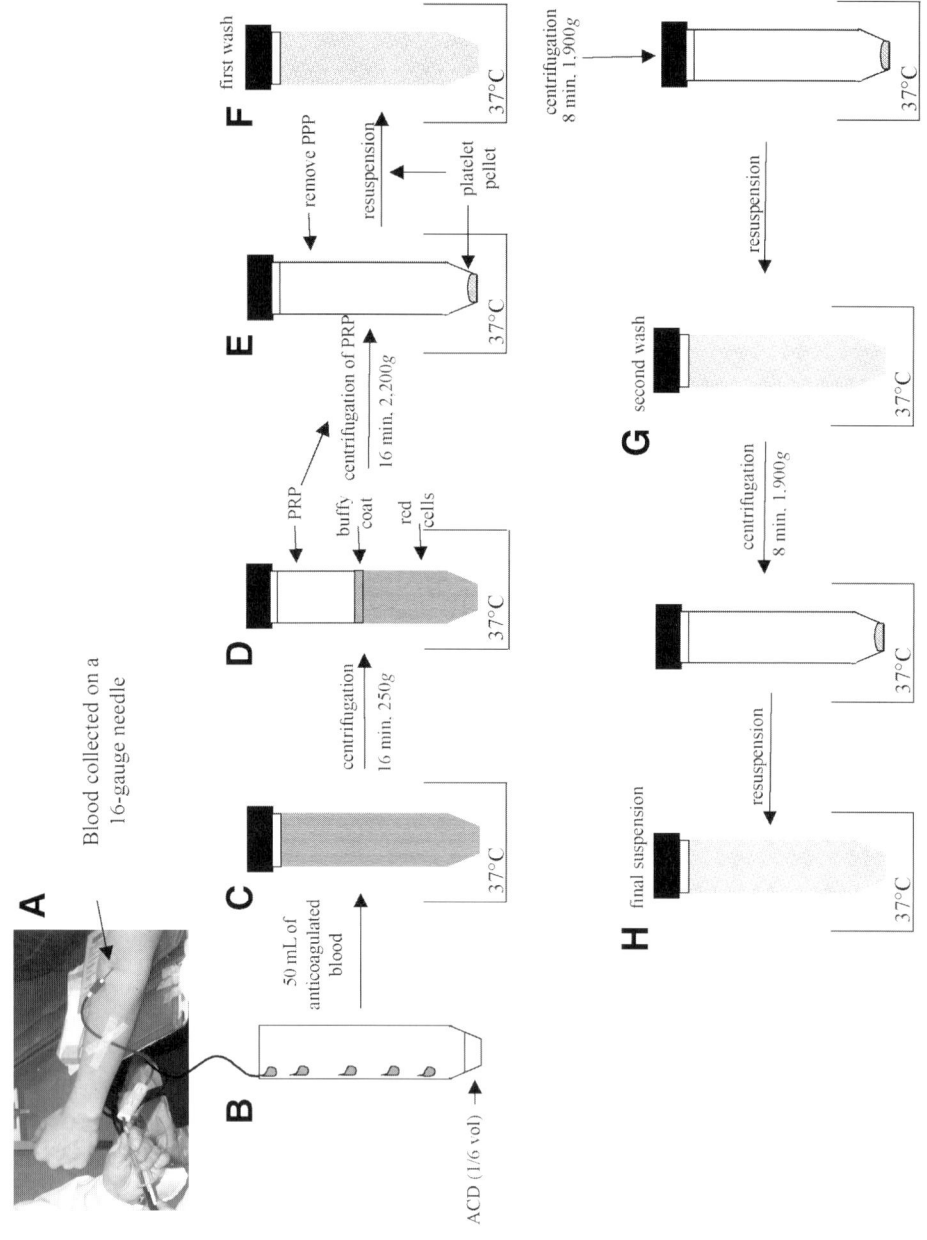

A

Blood collected on a
16-gauge needle

B ACD (1/6 vol)

50 mL of
anticoagulated
blood

C 37°C

centrifugation
16 min, 250g

D 37°C

PRP

buffy
coat

red
cells

centrifugation of PRP
16 min, 2,200g

E 37°C

remove PPP

resuspension

platelet
pellet

F first wash 37°C

centrifugation
8 min, 1,900g

37°C

resuspension

G second wash 37°C

centrifugation
8 min, 1,900g

37°C

resuspension

H final suspension 37°C

18

3.2.2. Washed Platelet Preparation

1. Rodent blood is centrifuged at a higher force (2300*g*) than human blood to obtain PRP. Centrifugation time depends on the volume (10 s per mL).
2. Collect the PRP and centrifuge at 2200*g* for a period of time depending on the volume of plasma: in a 15-mL centrifuge tube, 4 min for 1 mL of PRP, 5 min for 2 mL, 6 min for 3 mL, 8 min for 4 mL, and 10 min for 5 mL.
3. Discard the supernatant PPP using a Pasteur pipet connected to a vacuum pump, taking care to remove all traces of plasma from the tube walls or near the platelet pellet to avoid generation of thrombin during the subsequent washing steps.
4. Resuspend the platelets in Tyrode's albumin buffer containing heparin (10 U/mL) and PGI_2 (0.5 μ*M*). After incubation for 10 min at 37°C, add PGI_2 (0.5 μ*M*) and centrifuge at 1900*g* for a period of time depending on the suspension volume: in a 15-mL centrifuge tube, 3 min for 2–3 mL, 4 min for 4–5 mL, 5 min for 6–7 mL, 6 min for 8–9 mL, and 7 min for 10 mL.
5. Resuspend the platelets in Tyrode's albumin buffer containing 0.5 μ*M* PGI_2. After incubation for 10 min at 37°C, add 0.5 μ*M* PGI_2 and centrifuge as in **step 4**.
6. The platelets are finally resuspended at approx 100,000 to 300,000/μL in Tyrode's albumin buffer containing 0.02 U/mL apyrase. A blood volume of 10 mL from one rat yields 10 mL of washed platelets at 300,000/μL. A mouse blood volume of 5 mL (pool from five mice with 1 mL/mouse) gives 30 mL of washed platelets at 100,000/μL. In this case, working below 5 mL of blood does not give a good yield.

3.3. Results and Discussion of Platelet Responses to Agonists

3.3.1. Human Platelets

Use of washed human platelets separated from their plasma environment and in the absence of anticoagulants is essential for the study of intrinsic platelet properties. The results reported by Mustard et al. *(4)* and Cazenave et al. *(3)* demonstrate that human

---

Fig. 1. *(see opposite page)* Preparation of washed human platelets. **(A)** Blood is collected from a forearm vein using a 16-gauge needle **(B)** into a conical 50-mL tube containing 1 volume of ACD for 6 volumes of blood. **(C)** Each 50 mL of anticoagulated blood is centrifuged at 37°C for 16 min at 250*g* (*see* **Table 1** for centrifugation details of other volumes). **(D)** The upper phase (PRP) is carefully collected while the lower phase (red cells) and the interface (buffy coat containing mainly leukocytes and a few platelets) are discarded. **(E)** The pooled PRP (30 mL obtained from 100 mL of anticoagulated blood) is centrifuged for 16 min at 2200*g* and the PPP is removed. **(F)** The platelet pellet is gently resuspended in the first washing solution (Tyrode's albumin buffer containing 10 U/mL heparin and 5 μ*M* PGI_2). After 10 min, a further 5 μ*M* PGI_2 is added and the platelets are centrifuged at 1900*g* for 8 min. **(G)** The platelet pellet is resuspended in the second washing solution (Tyrode's albumin buffer with 5 μ*M* PGI_2). **(H)** After a second centrifugation, the platelets are adjusted to 300,000/μL in the final suspending medium (Tyrode's albumin buffer containing 0.02 U/mL apyrase without PGI_2) and stored at 37°C.

platelets isolated by a centrifugation technique and resuspended in Tyrode's albumin buffer containing apyrase retain their physiological properties and their ability to respond to agents inducing aggregation and release equally as well as platelets in citrated PRP *(5)*. The platelet suspensions are stable for 5–8 h at 37°C. Scanning electron microscopy **(Fig. 2A)** confirms the discoid shape of the cells and the absence of pseudopods, while transmission electron microscopy **(Fig. 3)** shows the presence of normal dense and α-granules *(9)*.

In Tyrode's albumin containing calcium (2 m*M*) and magnesium (1 m*M*), the platelets aggregate in response to ADP (5 μ*M*), but only in the presence of added human fibrinogen (0.25 g/L) (*see* **Note 12**). The platelets then spontaneously disaggregate rather than show a second wave of aggregation, which is observed in ADP-stimulated citrated PRP and is due to granule secretion and thromboxane A$_2$ formation **(Fig. 2, Fig. 4A1**; percentage 5HT release from the dense granules is shown beside each figure) *(7)*. It is well known that the lack of a secondary aggregation phase in washed platelets is due to the presence of millimolar concentrations of calcium. If magnesium is omitted from the Tyrode's albumin, only a slight modification is observed (a more rapid disaggregation) **(Fig. 4A2)**. In contrast, if calcium is omitted from the external medium, a second wave of aggregation occurs **(Fig. 4A3)** *(7)*. This second wave of aggregation requires thromboxane A$_2$ synthesis, as it is inhibited by aspirin (either in washed platelets or in citrated PRP; data not shown). When external calcium is further lowered by chelation with EDTA or EGTA, ADP fails to induce primary or secondary aggregation, although shape change is still observed *(7)*. This effect is due to the absolute requirement of external calcium for fibrinogen binding to the IIbIIIa receptor *(10)*. Sufficient calcium is present in the experiments conducted in nominally Ca^{2+}-free Tyrode's albumin for fibrinogen binding; however, the chelators lower Ca^{2+} to levels that do not support fibrinogen binding and thus aggregation.

In the absence of added external fibrinogen, the "weak" agonist ADP only induces shape change whereas thrombin does not require added fibrinogen to induce full aggregation and granule secretion **(Fig. 4B1,2)**. After addition of collagen, arachidonic acid, or ionophore A23187, the platelets aggregate and secrete their granule contents, while in response to PAF they aggregate without secretion (not shown). Adrenaline per se does not induce shape change or aggregation of washed platelets in the presence or absence of fibrinogen **(Fig. 4B3)**, but potentiates the effects of traces of any other aggregating agent (not shown) *(11)*. Addition of ristocetin (0.05–0.1 g/mL) in the pres-

---

Fig. 2. *(see facing page)* Morphological changes of washed platelets during ADP-induced aggregation. An aggregation response was obtained by stimulating platelets with 5 μ*M* ADP (arrow). The platelets were fixed at different time points and their surface features were visualized by scanning electron microscopy (SEM). **(A)** Discoid cells in the resting state. **(B)** Formation of early pseudopods (7 s). **(C)** Full shape change and first platelet-platelet interactions (20 s). **(D)** Large platelet aggregates (45 s). **(E)** Isolated platelets after disaggregation (3 min). Bars = 1 μm.

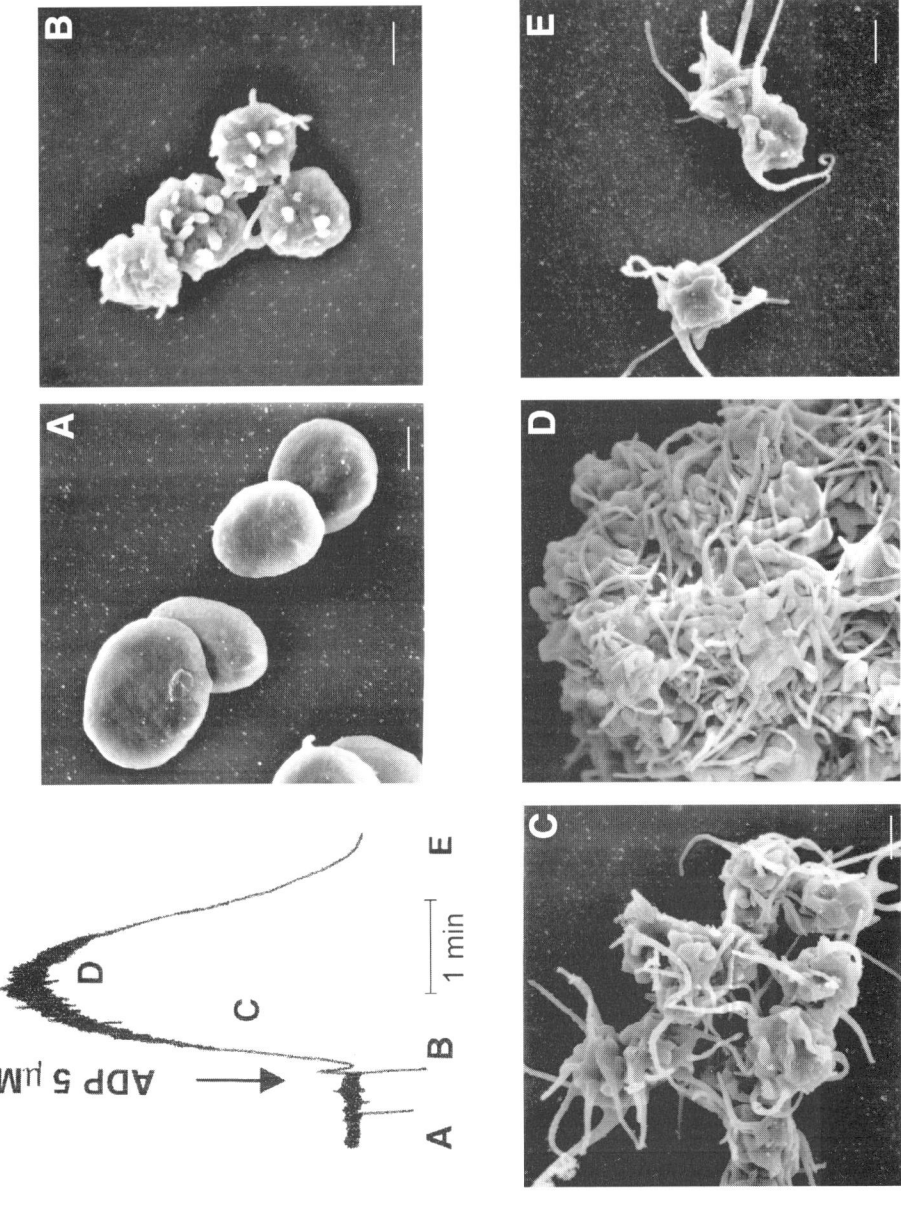

21

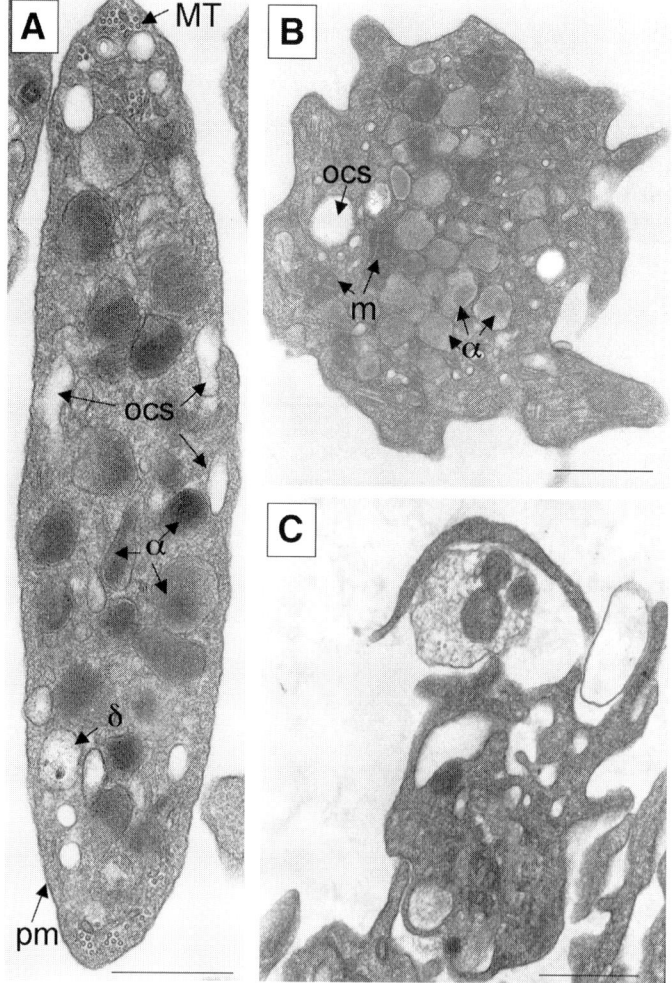

Fig. 3. Ultrastructure of washed human platelets visualized by transmission electron microscopy (TEM). (**A**) The characteristic discoid shape of a resting platelet in cross-section. (**B**) ADP-stimulated platelet showing a spherical shape and centralisation of granules. (**C**) Degranulated platelets after stimulation with thrombin. Abbreviations: Structures labeled by arrows are plasma membrane (pm), open canalicular system (OCS), microtubules (MT), alpha granules (α), dense granules (δ), mitochondrion (m). Bars = 500 nm.

ence of EDTA (10 m*M*) and platelet-poor plasma gives rise to a single wave of irreversible agglutination (not shown).

One important point is the requirement of apyrase, an ATP- and ADP-degrading enzyme, to the final platelet suspension in order to preserve platelet responsiveness to

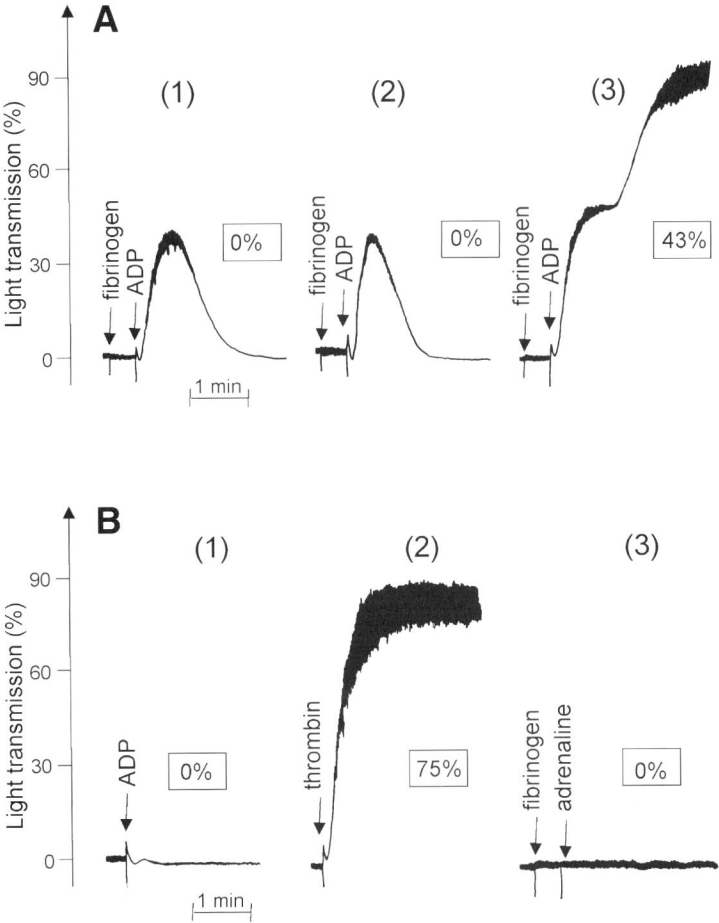

Fig. 4. Platelet responses to a weak agonist (ADP) and a strong agonist (thrombin). **(A)** Effect of calcium and/or magnesium on the aggregation induced by ADP (5 μM) in washed platelets that have also been labeled with tritiated serotonin to allow parallel studies of percentage serotonin release. The platelets were resuspended in modified Tyrode's albumin buffer containing apyrase and DiFP-treated fibrinogen (final concentration 0.25 mg/mL) was added before addition of the agonist (*see* **Note 12**). **(1)** Platelet suspension containing calcium (2 mM) and magnesium (1 mM); **(2)** suspension without magnesium; **(3)** suspension without added calcium. **(B)** Responses to various agonists in the absence of fibrinogen; **(1)** ADP (5 μM); **(2)** thrombin (1 U/mL), or **(3)** adrenaline (100 μM) in the presence of fibrinogen. The percentage release of radioactivity into the supernatant was measured 3 min after addition of the agonist and is indicated beside each aggregation curve.

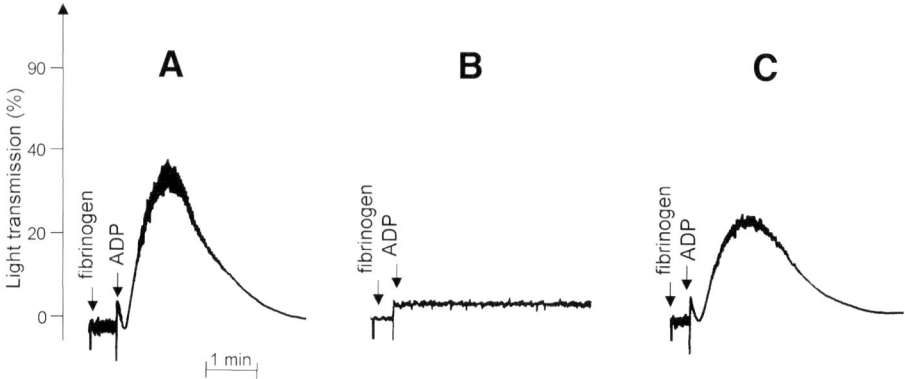

Fig. 5. Effect of apyrase on the platelet aggregation induced by ADP. Platelets were resuspended in Tyrode's albumin buffer and aggregation was induced by addition of ADP (5 μ*M*) in the presence of fibrinogen (0.25 mg/mL). Platelets were resuspended in buffer **(A)** containing apyrase (0.02 U/mL), **(B)** without apyrase, or **(C)** initially without apyrase, to which 0.02 U/mL apyrase was added 30 min before ADP.

ADP **(Fig. 5A)**. When apyrase is omitted, the platelets become refractory to ADP and are unable to change shape or aggregate **(Fig. 5B)**. This is at least partly due to a leakage of nucleotides, which causes desensitization of one of the two G protein-coupled ADP receptors (P2Y$_1$). It is a transient phenomenon, as addition of apyrase to refractory platelets rapidly (15 min) restores a full ADP response **(Fig. 5C)** *(12)*. Apyrase is also needed to study the P2X$_1$ receptor, a nonselective cation channel activated by ATP *(13)*. To reduce P2X$_1$ receptor desensitization during isolation of platelets, apyrase is added at all steps of the washing procedure at the high concentration of 0.9 U/mL. In platelet suspensions prepared under these conditions, the specific P2X$_1$ agonist α,β-MeATP induces a transient rise in intracellular calcium and shape change *(12)* (*see* Chapter 15, vol. 2).

3.3.2. Rodent Platelets

In many respects, rodent platelets behave in a similar manner to human platelets. However, some differences can be observed in response to several agonists. For example, it is well known that PAF does not activate rat platelets because they lack the PAF receptor. Because rat platelets express both alpha and beta adrenergic receptors, adrenaline is inhibitory, while it amplifies human and mouse platelet responses. Other subtle differences make rodent platelets secrete low amounts of granule contents in response to ADP. Importantly, mouse and rat platelets do not aggregate in response to PAR1-agonist peptides *(14)*.

3.4. Limitations of the Method

Washed platelet suspensions have the distinct advantage that platelet function can be studied in the absence of an anticoagulant. Furthermore, provided that the necessary precautions are taken to avoid thrombin generation and platelet activation during the preparation, the cells resuspended in the final medium containing apyrase retain their discoid shape and functional properties for storage periods of 5–8 h at 37°C. However, compared with gel filtration, the platelet yields from PRP are lower and more time is required to carry out the successive centrifugation and incubation steps. A further limitation of the method described in this chapter is the possibility that subpopulations of platelets may be selected during centrifugation, either when isolating PRP from whole blood or in subsequent steps of the washing procedure.

3.5. Related Preparative Methods

Platelets can also be isolated from human blood by density gradient centrifugation. In the albumin technique described by Walsh et al. *(15)*, citrated PRP is layered onto a continuous albumin gradient at 300 mOsm in calcium-free Tyrode's buffer containing apyrase at pH 6.5. After centrifugation, the platelets are resuspended and the washing procedure is repeated in the absence of apyrase.

In order to avoid preparing PRP by centrifugation, and thus reduce the risk of selecting subgroups of the platelet population, Corash et al. *(16)* have developed a method whereby whole blood is centrifuged through an arabinogalactan (Stractan) gradient. The platelets are thus separated in a single step from the plasma and other cellular blood components and the Stractan is later removed on an iso-osmolar albumin gradient.

Gel filtration of PRP on Sepharose 2B is another alternative method *(17,18)*. Using this technique, the platelets appear in the void volume, while the majority of plasma proteins are retained in the gel and eluted later. The separation is rapid and reproducible with minimal loss of platelets from the initial PRP, an advantage when only small blood volumes are available, but the platelet count in the resulting suspension is often low and the technique is not readily adapted to the preparation of sufficient quantities of platelets for experimental work. In addition, it does not enable the elimination of larger plasma components, e.g., immunoglobulins, factor V, and factor VIII-von Willebrand.

The principal advantages of the centrifugation technique for the isolation of platelets are that washed platelet suspensions may be prepared in large quantities with the required platelet count and in the absence of red blood cells and plasma proteins, including high-molecular-weight constituents such as the multimeric von Willebrand factor. Use of an artificial buffer medium as the suspending fluid further allows adjustment of the pH, osmolarity, and divalent cation concentrations to physiological levels.

4. Conclusion

This chapter describes a method for the isolation of non-activated platelets from human or rodent blood. Platelets that are resuspended in a well-defined medium under physiological conditions (pH, temperature, osmolarity, ions, and proteins) can respond for several hours to platelet agonists, or may be used in different protocols such as radiolabeling, electron microscopy, fluorescent labeling, immunolabeling, secretion experiments, or reinjection. To reproduce this technique over time, it should be kept in mind that all stages of the procedure are important and any modification can result in erroneous results.

5. Notes

1. ACD solution has the advantage that it not only chelates the calcium in blood and thereby prevents coagulation but also lowers the pH of the blood to 6.5. Platelets do not aggregate at this pH *(19)*.

2. To facilitate the dissolution of the different salts, it is better to add the NaCl, KCl, and NaH$_2$PO$_4$ together into 600 mL and the NaHCO$_3$ separately into 200 mL, which must be warmed to 80°C to obtain dissolution. When all salts have dissolved, mix the NaHCO$_3$ solution with the NaCl, KCl, and NaH$_2$PO$_4$ solution and bring the volume to 1 L. The stock solution can be stored for several weeks at 4°C but it must be filtered through a 0.22-µm filter under vacuum.

3. HEPES is used as the pH buffer in the Tyrode's salines. pH buffers such as Tris[tris (hydroxymethyl)aminomethane] should be avoided because, like other amines, they inhibit some platelet responses and potentiate others.

4. Before adding the different stock solutions, 50 mL of distilled water should be poured into the beaker to prevent the precipitation of calcium phosphate or calcium carbonate when adding stock I and stock III. All washing solutions are kept at 37°C throughout the preparation.

5. Diluted apyrase should not be frozen a second time but can be stored for several weeks at 4°C. Some commercially available preparations are not suitable because they contain impurities (e.g., potato lectin, a platelet-agglutinating agent) and 5′-nucleotidase activity, which hydrolyses AMP to adenosine. In the final suspending medium, use a concentration of apyrase capable of converting 0.25 µM ATP to AMP in 120 s at 37°C. Alternatively, choose an apyrase concentration that maintains platelet sensitivity to ADP, but does not have an appreciable inhibitory effect on ADP-induced aggregation (tested in the presence of fibrinogen) *(3)*. If too much apyrase is used, ADP-induced aggregation will be diminished; if too little is used, the platelets will become refractory to ADP (desensitization of platelet ADP receptors). The ratio of the ADPase to the ATPase activity is highly variable, depends on the origin of the potatoes, and can change during storage.

6. Some heparin preparations cause platelet aggregation and make platelets stick to the walls of their container. Batches of heparin should therefore be screened before use to ensure that this does not occur.

7. Transient platelet activation during the preparation may be inhibited by using PGI$_2$ in the centrifugation and resuspension steps *(3)*. Since the half-life of PGI$_2$ is short (a few minutes), it must be added to the washing solution just before centrifugation or platelet resuspension. The PGI$_2$ solution should be stored at 4°C immediately after thawing and should not be frozen again.

8. Institutional guidelines for collection and disposal of human blood should be followed at all times. As many drugs affect platelet responses (particularly aspirin and other nonsteroidal anti-inflammatory drugs, and thienopyridines like ticlopidine or clopidogrel), donors should be asked carefully about the medication they have taken during the previous two weeks. The manipulation of blood samples is also subject to strict hygiene controls and all donors are screened for the absence of viral infections (HCV, HBV, HIV).

9. It is particularly important to avoid generating traces of thrombin during the preparation of washed platelet suspensions *(3)*. Therefore, blood should be drawn with a minimum of vessel trauma and a rapid blood flow, while attention should be paid to eliminating all traces of plasma from the centrifuge tube before resuspending the platelet pellet after centrifugation of PRP. Platelets stimulated by exposure to low concentrations of thrombin may have reduced granule contents or be more sensitive to ADP- or adrenaline-induced aggregation *(2,3)*.

10. In order to stabilize the pH of the platelet suspension at about 7.3, the operator should breathe air (containing elevated CO_2 levels compared to atmospheric air) into the tube before closing it at each step of the washing procedure *(6)*.

11. The washed platelet preparation is kept at 37°C in a closed tube under a 5% CO_2/95% air atmosphere and under these conditions is stable for 5–8 h *(6)*.

12. Human fibrinogen 4% (w/v, Grade L, Kabi, Stockholm, Sweden). The lyophilized powder is dissolved in 0.9% NaCl (4 g in 100 mL) and treated with diisopropylfluorophosphate (DiFP, Sigma-Aldrich-Fluka) *(3)* to inactivate traces of contaminant plasma serine proteases. Aliquots (1 mL at about 10 mg/mL) are stored at –20°C and thawed and warmed to 37°C before use. Note that DiFP is highly toxic and should only be used under appropriate conditions (gloves, mask, fume hood).

Acknowledgments

The authors wish to thank Monique Freund for animal care and J. N. Mulvihill for reviewing the English of the manuscript. This work was supported by INSERM, EFS-Alsace, and ARMESA.

References

1. Ludlam, C. (1981) Assessment of platelet function. In *Thrombosis and Haemostasis* (Bloom, A. L., and Thomas, D. P., eds.), Churchill Livingstone, New York, pp. 775–795.
2. Kinlough-Rathbone, R. L., Packham, M. A., and Mustard, J. F. (1983) Platelet aggregation. In *Methods in Hematology* (Harker, L. A. and T.S., Z., eds.), Vol. 8, Churchill Livingstone, New, York, pp. 64–91.
3. Cazenave, J. P., Hemmendinger, S., Beretz, A., Sutter-Bay, A., and Launay, J. (1983) Platelet aggregation: a tool for clinical investigation and pharmacological study. Methodology. *Ann. Biol. Clin. (Paris)* **41,** 167–179.
4. Mustard, J. F., Perry, D. W., Ardlie, N. G., and Packham, M. A. (1972) Preparation of suspensions of washed platelets from humans. *Br. J. Haematol.* **22,** 193–204.
5. Ardlie, N. G., Perry, D. W., Packham, M. A., and Mustard, J. F. (1971) Influence of apyrase on stability of suspensions of washed rabbit platelets. *Proc. Soc. Exp. Biol. Med.* **136,** 1021–1023.
6. Han, P. and Ardlie, N. G. (1974) The influence of pH, temperature, and calcium on platelet aggregation: maintenance of environmental pH and platelet function for in vitro studies in plasma stored at 37 degrees C. *Br. J. Haematol.* **26,** 373–389.
7. Kinlough-Rathbone, R. L., Mustard, J. F., Packham, M. A., Perry, D. W., Reimers, H. J., and Cazenave, J. P. (1977) Properties of washed human platelets. *Thromb. Haemost.* **37,** 291–308.
8. Molnar, J. and Lorand, L. (1961) Studies on apyrases. *Arch. Biochem. Biophys.* **93,** 353.
9. Ardlie, N. G., Glew, G., and Schwartz, C. J. (1966) Influence of catecholamines on nucleotide-induced platelet aggregation. *Nature* **212,** 415–417.
10. Gachet, C., Stierle, A., Ohlmann, P., Lanza, F., Hanau, D., and Cazenave, J. P. (1991) Normal ADP-induced aggregation and absence of dissociation of the membrane GPIIb-IIIa complex of intact rat platelets pretreated with EDTA. *Thromb. Haemost.* **66,** 246–253.
11. Lanza, F., Beretz, A., Stierle, A., Hanau, D., Kubina, M., and Cazenave, J. P. (1988) Epinephrine potentiates human platelet activation but is not an aggregating agent. *Am. J. Physiol.* **255,** H1276–H1288.

12. Baurand, A., Eckly, A., Bari, N., Leon, C., Hechler, B., Cazenave, J. P., et al. (2000) Desensitization of the platelet aggregation response to ADP: differential down-regulation of the P2Y$_1$ and P2$_{cyc}$ receptors. *Thromb. Haemost.* **84,** 484–491.

13. Rolf, M. G., Brearley, C. A., and Mahaut-Smith, M. P. (2001) Platelet shape change evoked by selective activation of P2X$_1$ purinoceptors with α,β-methylene ATP. *Thromb. Haemost.* **85,** 303–308.

14. Sinakos, Z. and Caen, J. P. (1967) Platelet aggregation in mammalians (human, rat, rabbit, guinea-pig, horse, dog). A comparative study. *Thromb. Diath. Haemorrh.* **17,** 99–111.

15. Walsh, P. N., Mills, D. C., and White, J. G. (1977) Metabolism and function of human platelets washed by albumin density gradient separation. *Br. J. Haematol.* **36,** 287–296.

16. Corash, L., Tan, H., and Gralnick, H. R. (1977) Heterogeneity of human whole blood platelet subpopulations. I. Relationship between buoyant density, cell volume, and ultrastructure. *Blood* **49,** 71–87.

17. Tangen, O., McKinnon, E. L., and Berman, H. J. (1973) On the fine structure and aggregation requirements of gel filtered platelets (GFP). *Scand. J. Haematol.* **10,** 96–105.

18. Lages, B., Scrutton, M. C., and Holmsen, H. (1975) Studies on gel-filtered human platelets: isolation and characterization in a medium containing no added Ca^{2+}, Mg^{2+}, or K$^+$. *J. Lab. Clin. Med.* **85,** 811–825.

19. Aster, R. H., and Jandl, J. H. (1964) Platelet sequestration in man. I. Methods. *J. Clin. Invest.* **43,** 843.

3

Platelet Counting

Paul Harrison, Carol Briggs, and Samuel J. Machin

1. Introduction

The assessment of the platelet count is essential within both routine hematology and research laboratories. Accurate and precise enumeration of platelets is not only critical to assist in diagnosis and treatment of various clinical disorders, but it is also a vital research tool particularly for standardizing counts within whole blood, platelet-rich plasma (PRP), or purified platelet preparations. The normal platelet count is widely quoted as between $150-400 \times 10^9$/L of whole blood.

In this chapter, both the existing and newly proposed international reference methods for platelet counting will be described in detail, as they can be performed in any laboratory with suitable equipment. However, the full range of alternative automated methodologies will also be reviewed so that readers will be able to understand their relative advantages and disadvantages and utilize the most appropriate platelet-counting procedure within their laboratory. As these analyzers are relatively easy to use it is not necessary to describe how to utilize them, but quality control and assurance procedures will be briefly discussed. The four main analytical procedures for platelet counting are (1) manual counting using phase-contrast microscopy, (2) impedance analysis and (3) optical light scatter/fluorescence analysis using various commercially available analyzers, and (4) immunoplatelet counting using flow-cytometric principles. Although manual methods have been largely replaced by automated instrumentation, many research and nonspecialized laboratories interested in a reliable method for accurately counting platelets can still either perform manual counting or utilize small impedance analyzers if access to a larger automated blood counter is not possible.

Early methods for enumerating platelets in blood were usually inaccurate and irreproducible until the mid-20th century. In 1953, Brecher et al. *(1)* developed a manual phase-contrast microscopy method enabling platelets to be easily discriminated from lysed red cells within a counting chamber or hemocytometer. Although the development of the Coulter principle in the 1950s revolutionized blood counting, platelet counts were not added to the automated full blood count until the late 1970s. Within early

From: *Methods in Molecular Biology, vol. 272:*
Platelets and Megakaryocytes, Vol. 1: Functional Assays
Edited by: J. M. Gibbins and M. P. Mahaut-Smith © Humana Press Inc., Totowa, NJ

impedance analyzers platelet counting could be performed only by analysis of PRP or purified platelet preparations and was thus prone to considerable error. Until the wide-spread availability of the full blood count, the majority of platelet counts were still performed manually via phase contrast microscopy. The manual phase count is still recognised as the gold standard or international reference method *(1,2)*. Thus until very recently, the calibration of platelet counts on automated blood cell counters and qual-ity control material was still routinely performed via the manual method by the major-ity of instrument manufacturers. The method is not only time-consuming, subjective, and tedious, but it also results in high levels of imprecision with typical interobserver coefficients of variation (CVs) in the range of 10 to 25% *(3)*. At low platelet numbers, because fewer cells are counted, observed CVs also increase proportionally. Although relatively imprecise, the method still offers a cheap, simple, and viable means to enumerate platelets in the nonspecialized laboratory.

The introduction of automated full blood counters using impedance technology resulted in a dramatic improvement in precision with typical CVs of less than 3% *(4)*, particularly as much higher numbers of platelets are counted *(5)*. Impedance platelet counting methods still have significant limitations, however, despite their widespread use. One of the major problems is that cell size analysis cannot discriminate platelets from other similarly sized particles, such as small or fragmented red cells, immune complexes, and so on *(6)*. These may be erroneously included in the platelet count, and in severely thrombocytopenic samples the number of interfering particles may even exceed the number of true platelets. Large or giant platelets may be excluded from the count on the basis of their size, as they cannot be resolved from red blood cells. There may also be significant variations in the results obtained on different analyzers within the same sample due to differences in the method analysis, linearity over the entire measuring range and the number of events actually counted. More recently multiple light-scatter parameters and/or fluorescence, rather than impedance sizing alone, have been introduced for platelet counting within automated hematology analyzers. This has improved the ability of automated analyzers to discriminate platelets. Despite these newer methods there are still occasional cases in which absolute accuracy of the platelet count remains a challenge. Thus, there has been renewed interest in the development of an improved reference procedure to enable optimization of automated platelet counting. This method utilizes specific monoclonal antibodies to platelet cell surface antigens (e.g., anti-CD41, 42, or 61) conjugated to a suitable fluorophore. By performing flow-cytometric analysis of the ratio of fluorescent platelet events to nonfluorescent red cell events, a highly accurate and precise technique is now available for counting platelets in whole blood *(3)*. This relatively new approach permits the possible implementation of a new international reference method to calibrate cell counters, assign values to cal-ibrators, and obtain a direct count on a wide variety of pathological samples. This should, it is hoped, lead to an improved accuracy of platelet counting in thrombocy-topenia and facilitate further studies into proving whether current platelet transfusion thresholds can be safely lowered without the risk of bleeding. The method can also be adapted so that platelets can be quantified within purified preparations via the addition of precise numbers of fluorescent beads *(3)*.

Table 1
Examples of Major Hematological Analyzers Currently Available

Manufacturer	Instrument	Principle of platelet count
Abbott Diagnostics	CELL-DYN 4000	Impedance, optical, and immunological
ABX Diagnostics	Pentra-120	Impedance
Bayer Corporation	ADVIA 120	Optical
Beckman Coulter	LH-750	Impedance
	GEN-S	Impedance
Sysmex Corporation	SE-9500	Impedance
	XE-2100	Impedance and Optical

1.1. Manual Counting

Despite the widespread use of automated technology, manual counting of platelets is still widely performed in less-resourced laboratories and within research laboratories with no access to specialized instrumentation. It is also common practice to use manual counting methods in the routine laboratory if the platelet count is low or there are atypical platelets present in the sample. The current international reference method for platelet counting is still performed by the standard manual method using phase-contrast microscopy and was established by the International Committee for Standardisation in Haematology (ICSH) *(2,7)*. Within whole blood, platelet counts are usually performed on EDTA anticoagulated blood obtained by standard clean venipuncture. To discriminate platelets from red cells, manual counting is usually performed by visual examination of diluted and lysed whole blood using a Neubauer counting chamber that contains a precise volume of fluid. Purified platelet preparations can also be counted with this method.

1.2. Automated Platelet Counting

There are now several methods using commercial analyzers for counting platelets, including aperture impedance, optical scattering, and fluorescence. **Table 1** lists the currently available large hematology analyzers that incorporate platelet counting. Normal platelets give a classical log-normal volume distribution curve, which is particularly useful as the basis for determining a valid platelet count **(Fig. 1)**. Other derived platelet parameters are highly dependent on the individual technology and are influenced by the anticoagulant and delay time from sampling to analysis (e.g., EDTA-induced swelling). Within impedance analyzers, the mean platelet volume (MPV) and platelet distribution width (PDW) are derived from the platelet distribution curve. Although these derived platelet parameters must be interpreted carefully, there is an established inverse relationship between MPV and the platelet count that contributes to the maintenance of hemostatic function. There is also evidence that MPV is an important risk factor for myocardial infarction. If MPV is to be reliably measured then the potential influence of anticoagulant on the MPV must be controlled for either by using an alternative anticoagulant or standardizing the time delay between sampling and analysis.

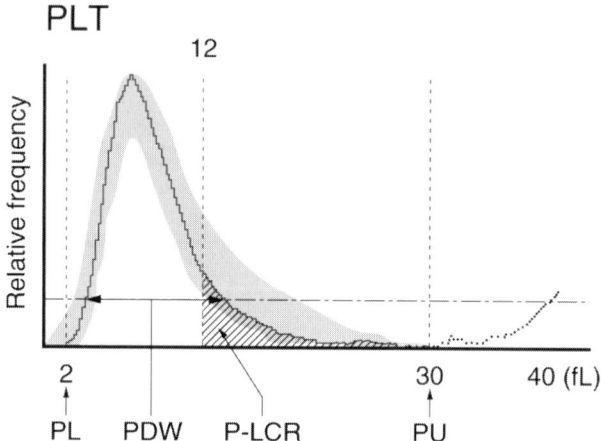

PL   : Lower discrimination for platelet size distribution
PDW : Platelet distribution width
P-LCR : Platelets-large cell ratio
PU   : Upper discrimination for platelet size distribution

Fig. 1. Typical platelet size distribution. (Courtesy of Sysmex Corporation.)

Whichever automated method is used for platelet counting, it must be demonstrated that it is precise, shows minimum fluctuation in repeated results on the same sample, and gives linear results over the entire analytical range. At high counts there is a growing probability of coincidence—two or more cells passing through the sensing zone at the same time—as well as possible sample carryover if a high count precedes a low count. With thrombocytopenic samples it is important that added counts due to spurious signals caused by electronic noise are not included within the reported result. It is also desirable that there be minimal method variation between different analyzers; results obtained with different systems on the same sample should be comparable. For information on quality control *see* **Notes 12** and **13**.

1.2.1. Impedance Platelet Counting

Wallace Coulter first described the resistance detection method, usually referred to as the "Coulter principle" or impedance method *(8)* (**Fig. 2**). In this method biological cells are regarded as completely nonconductive resistivity particles. When a blood cell passes through an aperture (sensing zone) suspended in electrolyte solution, the change in electric impedance is detected. Each individual cell gives an impedance signal that is proportional to the volume of the cell detected, and so this method can be used to size and count individual cells. This method was originally used for the counting of red cells and white cells; the first Coulter platelet counter required the use of platelet-rich plasma to avoid counting red cells as platelets. Many research laboratories still utilize such small analyzers to count platelets in PRP or in purified preparations (**Table 2** shows

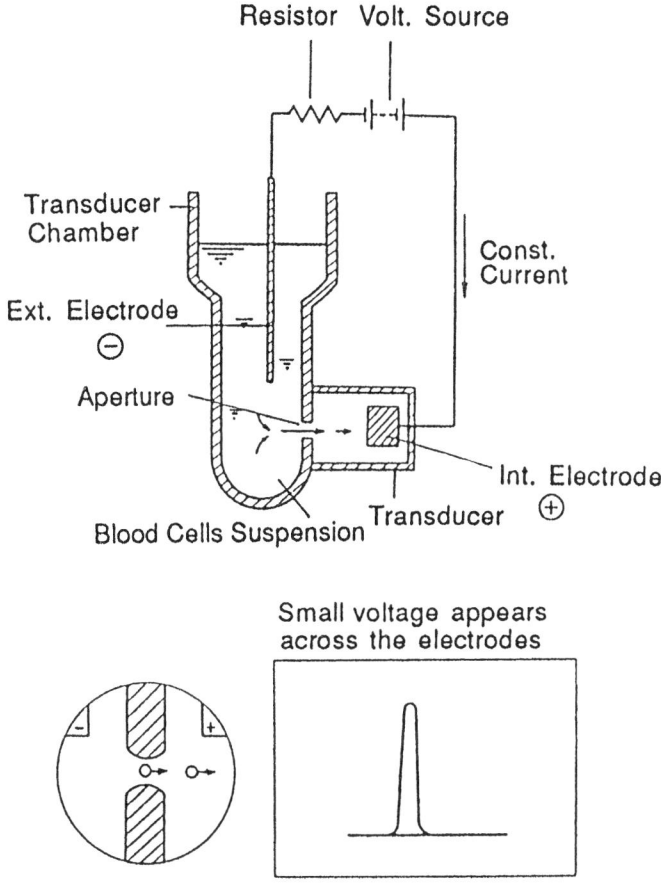

Fig. 2. Electrical impedance method or Coulter principle. (Courtesy of Sysmex Corporation.)

examples of commercially available compact impedance analyzers that are often used within smaller hematology or research laboratories). It was not until the 1970s that improvements in technology, including coincidence correction and hydrodynamic focusing, allowed the discrimination of platelets from red cells to enable an accurate platelet count to be produced from a whole blood sample. Ideally, if cells go through the sensing zone one by one, the total number detected are counted. However, simultaneous occupancy of the sensing zone by more than one particle occurs. This phenomenon is called "coincidence" and the resulting count error is known as the coincidence error. The magnitude of coincidence error increases with the concentration of cells suspended. For major hematology analyzers, the coincidence correction formula can be established

Table 2
Examples of Compact Impedance Analyzers Currently Available

Manufacturer	Instrument	Principle of platelet count
Abbott Diagnostics	CELL-DYN 1200	Impedance
ABX Diagnostics	Pentra 60	Impedance
	Micros 60	Impedance
Bayer Corporation	Advia 60 & 70	Impedance
Beckman Coulter	A^{C}T	Impedance
Sysmex Corporation	KX21	Impedance

by measuring the results from several samples of different concentrations. The correction formula may be integrated into the analyzer's computer and the coincidence corrected result reported. In order to minimize coincidence physically, the hydrodynamic focusing method has been developed for some analyzers. If two cells pass through the sensing zone together, the count may be corrected by the coincidence correction but a large single pulse will be generated, and it is not possible to determine if this arises from one large cell or two small cells.

If a cell passes through the sensing zone close to the wall, where high current density exists, an M-shaped pulse is generated; while the count result may be valid because of the coincidence correction, there is no way to correct the measurement of the cell volume. Hydrodynamic focusing resolves these problems. In hydrodynamic focusing a steady flow of diluent is drawn through the aperture and the cell suspension is injected into this moving body of liquid in a fine stream close to the aperture entrance **(Fig. 3)**. The likelihood of two cells passing through the aperture together is dramatically decreased and no cell goes near the wall or the entrance angle of the sensing zone where high current density exists. Hydrodynamic focusing produces a clear discrimination between red cells and platelets.

Within the currently available Beckman Coulter analyzers (e.g., GEN-S and LH 750), particles between 2 and 20 femtoliter (fL) are counted as platelets *(9)*. Pulses are obtained from three red cell/platelet orifices to obtain 64-channel size-distribution histograms for each orifice. These histograms are smoothed and a high point and two low points are identified in the distribution. A log-normal curve is fitted to these points. The curves have a range of 0–70 fL and the platelet count and parameters are derived from this curve.

Within the Sysmex counting systems (e.g., SE-9500 and XE-2100) platelets are also counted by the orifice-impedance method *(9)*. A platelet size distribution plot is produced using three thresholds. One is fixed at the 12 fL level and the other two are allowed to hunt the upper and lower ends of the platelet population between certain limits **(Fig. 1)**. The lower platelet size threshold may move between 2 and 6 fL, the higher between 12 and 30 fL. The purpose of these thresholds is to endeavor to distinguish platelets from small red cells or red cell fragments at the upper end of the platelet population and debris at the lower end. Analyzers using the standard imped-

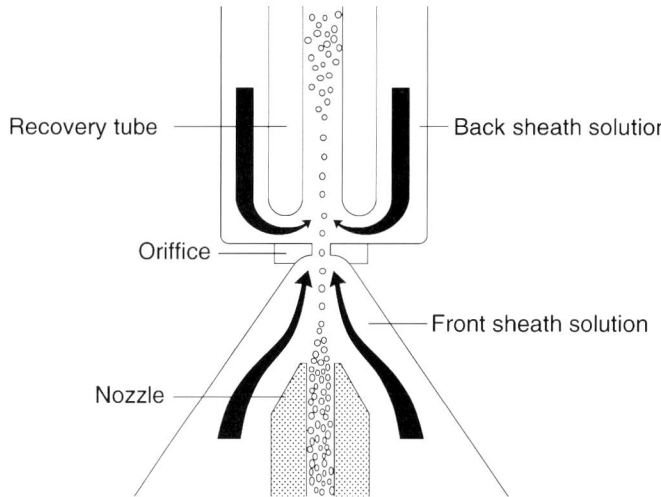

Fig. 3. Schematic diagram of sheath flow and the principle of hydrodynamic focusing. Platelets and erythrocytes are analysed by a hydrodynamic focusing system that eliminates potential errors of coincidence, recirculation, and stress changes associated with traditional methods of analysis. This results in more accurate RBC and platelet counts and cell sizing even when cell counts are low or high. (Courtesy of Sysmex Corporation.)

ance measurements are able (for most samples) to provide an accurate platelet count down to 20×10^9/L. Below this level, impedance analyzers become less accurate due to decreasing statistical confidence, fewer events analyzed, and the increasing influence of background and plasma nonplatelet particulate matter. A major disadvantage of the electrical impedance method for counting platelets is the difficulty in distinguishing large platelets from extremely microcytic or fragmented red cells even using hydrodynamic focusing methods. False increases will occur when erythrocyte or white cell fragments, microcytic red cells, immune complexes, bacteria, or cell debris are included in the reported platelet count (6). False underestimates in the count will occur when there are large platelets present or platelet clumping, as seen with pseudothrombocytopenia by ethylene diamine tetraacetic acid (EDTA)-dependent agglutinins or with platelet satellism (6).

1.2.2. Optical Platelet Counting

More recently, optical light scatter methods have been introduced. In one-dimensional platelet analysis platelets are counted and sized by a flow-cytometry system, in which the cells in a suitable diluent pass through a narrow beam of light (i.e., helium-neon laser) illumination and the light scatter by each cell is measured at a single angle (2° to 3°). This allows assessment of the number of electrical pulses generated proportional to the number of cells and cell volume. In these automated systems (H*3, Bayer, or the CELL-DYN

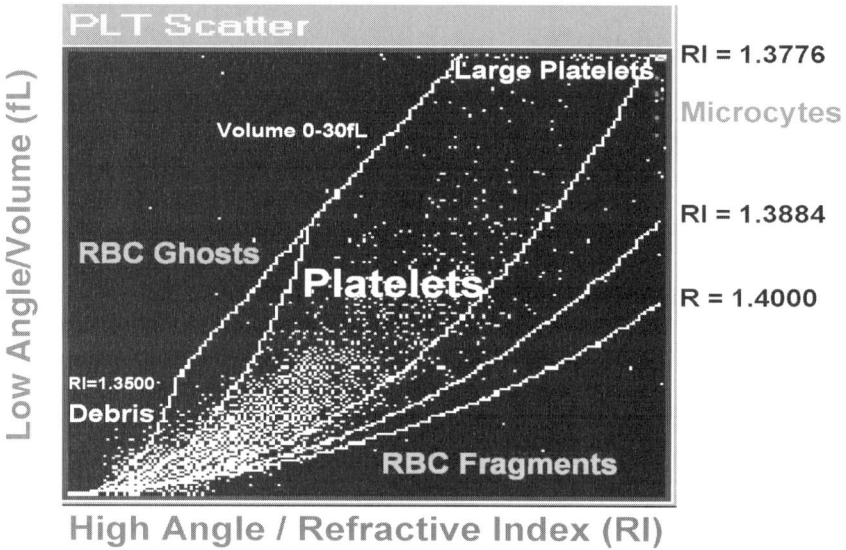

Fig. 4. Identification of Platelets by the Bayer ADVIA 120 hematology analyzer. The vertical axis indicates low angle light scatter or cell volume. The horizontal axis indicates high angle light scatter or refractive index. (Courtesy of Bayer Corporation.)

3500, Abbott), a series of algorithms or a smoothing or fitting routine on the platelet volume histogram is used to establish validity of each platelet count.

To improve discrimination of platelets accurately from nonplatelet particles, two-dimensional laser light scatter was developed. The ADVIA 120 analyzer (Bayer Corporation) uses two-dimensional platelet analysis; volume and refractive index of effectively sphered individual platelets are simultaneously determined on a cell-by-cell basis by measuring two angles of laser light scatter at 2–3° and at 5–15° *(10)*. The two scatter measurements are converted to volume (platelet size) and refractive index (platelet density) values using the Mie theory of light scattering for homogenous spheres *(11)*. The platelet scatter cytogram map resolves volumes between 1 and 30 fL and refractive index values between 1.35 and 1.44. Large platelets, red-cell fragments, red-cell ghosts, microcytes, and cellular debris are distinguished. Platelets are identified within the map on the platelet scatter cytogram based on their volume and refractive index (1.35–1.40) **(Fig. 4)**. Red-cell fragments and microcytes with the same volume range have a greater refractive index than platelets and fall below and to the right of the grid; red cell ghosts with a refractive index less than platelets fall above and to the left of the grid **(Fig. 4)**. Large platelets with volumes between 30 and 60 fL are identified in the large platelet area of the red-cell map. The reported two-dimensional platelet count is the sum of platelets and large platelets identified in the platelet and red-cell scatter cytograms. Recent published data suggests that the two-dimensional platelet count improves the accuracy of the platelet count in thrombocytopenic samples *(3,10)*.

Optical Platelets

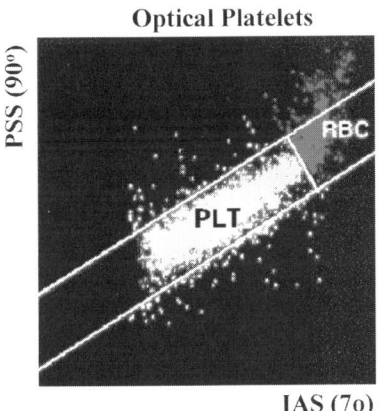

IAS (7o)

Impedance Platelets

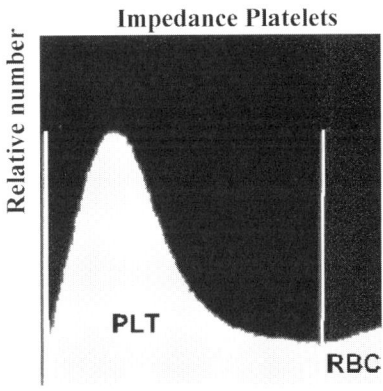

Fig. 5. An example of a scattergram produced by the Abbott Cell Dyn-4000 showing the optical platelet count and impedance platelet size distribution. (Courtesy of Abbott Diagnostics.)

The CELL-DYN 4000 instrument also routinely reports an optical platelet count (as well as an impedance count) based on two light scatter parameters, intermediate light scatter (7°) and a wide-angle scatter (90°). An algorithm is used to identify platelets using these two parameters to exclude, as far as possible, nonplatelet particles while including all platelets. This is a two-dimensional analysis in which platelets must fall within a region that defines the correlation between the two light scatter parameters (a sloping window) and between a lower threshold and an upper discriminator (**Fig. 5**). The three discriminator lines are set dynamically; the lower threshold is fixed. A simultaneous determination of the impedance platelet count is performed; discrepancies between the two counts generate an alert flag suggesting the presence of sample interferences. The combination of two-dimensional optical analysis and flow impedance counting on the CELL-DYN 4000 has made a significant contribution to improving the accuracy and precision of platelet counting (*6*).

1.2.3. Optical Fluorescence Platelet Counting

An optical fluorescent platelet count has been introduced on the Sysmex XE 2100 analyzer, in addition to the traditional impedance count (*12*). The optical fluorescent platelet count is measured in the reticulocyte channel. A polymethine dye is used to stain the RNA/DNA of reticulated cells and the platelet membrane and granules. This technology allows the simultaneous counting of the red-cell reticulocytes, erythrocytes, and fluorescent platelets (**Fig. 6**). Within the flow cell, each single cell is passed through the light beam of a semiconductor diode laser; the fluorescence intensity of each cell is analyzed, which allows the separation of the platelets from the red cells and reticulocytes. The fluorescent staining of the platelets not only allows the exclusion of nonplatelet particles from the count but also allows the inclusion of large or giant platelets.

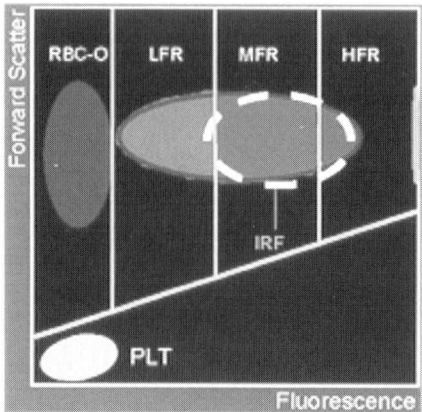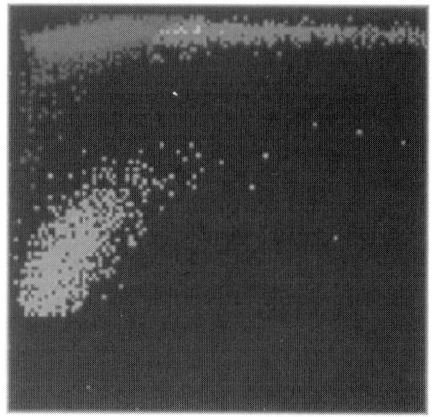

Fig. 6. An example of a scattergram produced by the Sysmex XE-2100 hematology analyzer in both cartoon (left) and dot plot (right) formats. The vertical axis indicates forward scattered light or cell volume and the horizontal axis indicates fluorescence intensity. The scattergram is divided into PLT area, mature RBC area (RBC-O), and the various immature reticulocyte fractions (LFR, MFR, and HFR). (Courtesy of Sysmex Corporation.) See color insert following p. 44.

The optical fluorescent count is more reliable at levels below 100×10^9/L and may allow more appropriate clinical decisions to be made, particularly with regard to platelet transfusions *(12)*.

1.2.4. Immunological Platelet Counting

With the widespread availability of flow cytometers within hematology and research laboratories, a number of different groups began to investigate the applicability of this technology to accurately enumerate various cells within whole blood including platelets. The principle of this methodology involves simply labeling EDTA-anticoagulated blood with a suitable antiplatelet monoclonal antibody (e.g., conjugated to FITC). As most flow cytometers cannot measure a fixed volume of sample, counting procedures involve indirect derivation of cell number using the ratio of fluorescent platelets to either added bead preparations or inherent number of RBCs within the sample. Recently a number of flow-cytometric counting procedures were reviewed by the ICSH (International Council for Standardisation in Haematology) expert panel on cytometry *(3,13–15)*. The ICSH panel identified the variables and problems associated with this methodology which enabled the ISLH (International Society of Laboratory Haematology) task force panel to develop, evolve, and test a new candidate reference method within a multilaboratory study *(16,17)*. The preferred method simply derives the platelet count from the ratio of fluorescent platelets to RBCs within the sample. The main advantage of the RBC ratio is that, providing the blood sample is well mixed and that coincident events

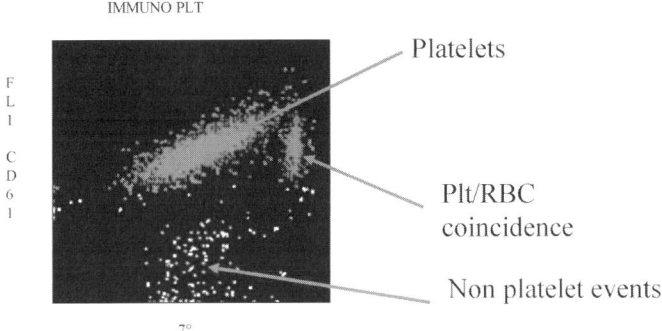

IMMUNO PLT

F
L
I

C
D
6
1

7°

Platelets

Plt/RBC
coincidence

Non platelet events

Fig. 7. An example of an ImmunoPLT™ scattergram of light scatter vs fluorescence produced by the Abbott Cell Dyn-4000. The fluorescent platelets are clearly resolved from nonplatelet events and Plt/RBC coincidence events. (Courtesy of Abbott Diagnostics.)

(RBC/RBC and RBC/platelet) are eliminated by optimal dilution, the count obtained is not only accurate and precise but independent of potential pipetting artifacts. The method is also superior to derived counts from bead ratios *(3)* as these methods are dependent on a stable bead preparation (with an accurate bead count) in combination with very accurate/precise pipetting. However, bead-derived platelet counts may be useful for simply counting platelets within purified preparations as the RBC have been removed (*see* **Note 11**).

1.2.5. Automated Immunological Counting

With the more recent convergence of flow cytometry and analyzer technology it became feasible not only to perform optical counting by light scatter and fluorescence (*see* **Subheadings 3.2.** and **3.3.**) but also to simultaneously measure cells identified with fluorescent monoclonal antibodies. Currently the only available instrument that can measure antibody-labeled platelets is the Abbott CELL-DYN 4000. Unlike the flow cytometric method, the ImmunoPLT® method is a fully automated procedure and labels platelets within whole blood by using anti-CD61 antibodies contained within a lyophilized pellet within special evacuated tubes (Becton Dickinson, San Jose, CA). During analysis the CELL DYN 4000 simply aspirates 40 µL of blood into the antibody-containing tube and performs a standard incubation. Final counting is perfomed within a fixed volume and includes PLT/RBC coincidence events but hence is not based on a cell ratio **(Fig. 7)**. The method has been shown to provide an accurate platelet count, especially within thrombocytopenic samples *(18,19)*. As expected, it has also been recently shown to agree closely with immunocounting by flow cytometry *(19)*. However, a fully automated immunological technique has obvious advantages and will be very useful in clinical situations in which accurate platelet counts are required.

2. Materials

2.1. Manual Counting

1. Phase-contrast microscope with ×40 objective and ×6 or ×10 eyepieces.
2. Hemocytometer: Improved Neubauer counting chamber (according to the British Standard for Haemocytometer and Particle Counting Chambers—BS 748: 1982) (*see* **Note 6**).
3. Thick cover slip (different from ordinary coverslips).
4. Clean glassware.
5. Mechanical mixer.
6. 0.22-μm filter.
7. Diluent—1% (1 g/100 mL) ammonium oxalate solution (filtered) in sterile distilled water—stored at 4°C. Centrifuge at 1500*g* for 15 min each day to remove debris.
8. Petri dish with a moisture chamber.
9. Capillary tubes or Pasteur pipets.

2.2. Immunological Platelet Counting

1. Flow cytometer: For platelet and red-cell enumeration a fluorescent flow cytometer with hydrodynamic focusing and the capability of measuring both forward light scatter and fluorescence is used. The instrument should have sufficient sensitivity to both scattered and fluorescein fluorescent light to reliably count fluorescein isothiocyanate (FITC)-labeled spherical particles of 2 μm diameter.
2. Impedance counter: For the whole blood red blood cell count a semiautomated, single-channel aperture impedance particle counter is used.
3. Diluent: phosphate-buffered saline (PBS), 10 mM, pH 7.2–7.4 with 0.1% bovine serum albumin (BSA). Dissolve 1.15 g dibasic, anhydrous sodium phosphate (Na_2HPO_4, CAS 7558-79-4, molecular mass 142.0) in approx 750 mL of deionized or distilled water. Add 210 mg monobasic, anhydrous potassium phosphate (KH_2PO_4, CAS 7778-77-0, molecular mass 136.1), 8.0 g sodium chloride (NaCl, CAS 7647-14-5, molecular mass 58.44), 200 mg potassium chloride (KCl, CAS 7447-40-7, molecular mass 74.55), and 1.0 g bovine serum albumin, fraction V. Dilute to 1000 mL with deionized or distilled water. Store at 4 to 8°C. Filter the diluent through a low-binding, low-release membrane filter, 0.20–0.25 μm mean pore diameter, before use. (Good results have been obtained with, e.g., Millex-GV Millipore filters.)
4. Monoclonal antibodies: directly conjugated, FITC-labeled antibodies against two distinct epitopes on the GpIIb/IIIa complex of platelets are used, e.g., antibodies anti-CD 41 (clone P2, Beckman Coulter, High Wycombe, UK) and anti-CD 61 (clone RUU-PL 7F12, Becton Dickinson, Oxford, UK) (*see* **Note 7**).
5. Positive displacement pipets.

3. Methods

3.1. Manual Counting

1. Obtain EDTA anticoagulated blood, check for blood clots (if present, reject sample), and mix well.
2. Dilute mixed blood 1:20 with 1% filtered ammonium oxalate solution and mix for 10 min (*1,2,7*). Typically, 100 μL of blood is added to 1.9 mL of ammonium oxalate within a

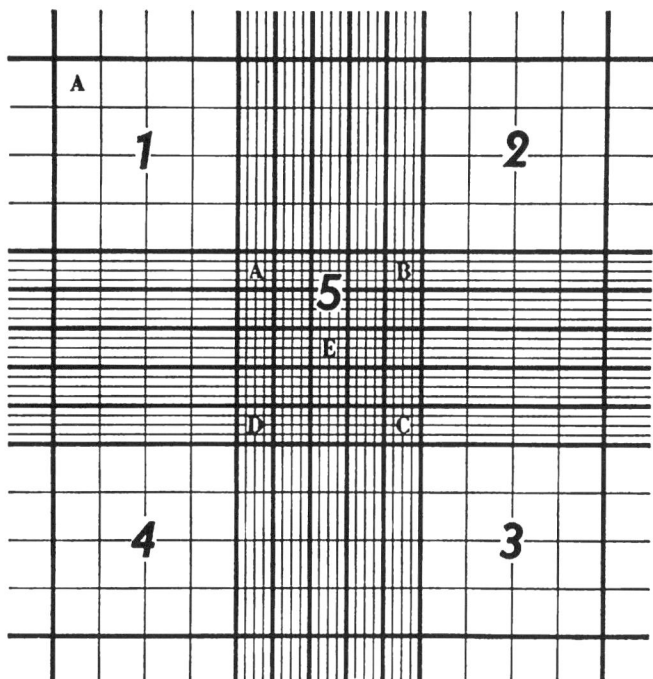

Fig. 8. Improved Neubauer counting chamber. The solid black lines are triple lines. Platelets and erythrocytes are counted in the central square (5) within the 25 smaller squares (e.g., 5A, 5B, 5C, 5D, 5E, until the count is >200). (Reprinted with permission from the publisher from *The Successor to Thomas Hale Ham's Syllabus of Laboratory Examinations in Clinical Diagnosis*, edited by Lot B. Page and Perry J. Culver, Cambridge, MA, Harvard University Press, Copyright 1950, 1960 by the President and Fellows of Harvard College, p. 28.)

glass container. Mix for 15 min on a mechanical mixer. The ammonium oxalate lyses the red cells but leaves the platelets and white cells intact (*see* **Note 4**).

3. Ensure that the counting chamber and cover slip are clean (*see* **Note 3**). Apply special thick cover slip firmly onto counting chamber. Newtonian rings should be visible if the cover slip is correctly in place.
4. Fill counting chambers with diluted lysed blood using a capillary tube or Pasteur pipet.
5. Place the counting chamber into the moist Petri dish. Ensure that it is flat and leave for at least 20 min to allow the platelets to settle. Use phase-contrast microscope to count the platelets, which appear as small but highly refractile particles. Ensure that platelets and not cell debris are counted (*see* **Note 2**). Check for platelet clumping at low power (*see* **Note 5**). If platelets are uniformly spread, then proceed with counting. The improved Neubauer hemocytometer consists of rulings etched on metallized glass within two counting chambers with a depth of 0.1 mm. Each ruled area is 9 mm^2 with a central area of 1 mm^2

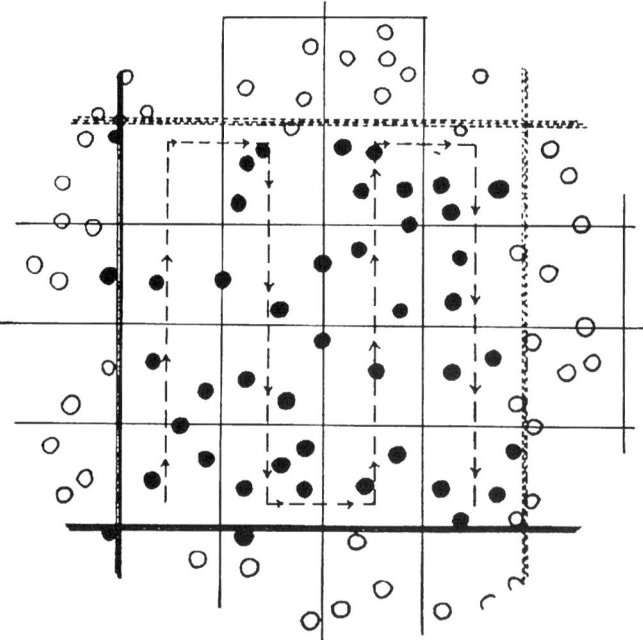

Fig. 9. A typical counting sequence for cells in square 5A within Fig. 8. (Reprinted with permission from the publisher from *The Successor to Thomas Hale Ham's Syllabus of Laboratory Examinations in Clinical Diagnosis*, edited by Lot B. Page and Perry J. Culver, Cambridge, MA: Harvard University Press, Copyright 1950, 1960 by the President and Fellows of Harvard College, p. 29.)

(square 5 in **Fig. 8**), which is divided into 25 squares and then further divided into 16 smaller squares (hence 400 smallest squares, each 0.05 × 0.05 mm). The 25 squares are surrounded by triple lines for easy identification by microscopy (*see* **Figs. 8,9**). This central area is used for either red-cell or platelet counting via phase-contrast microscopy. White cells can be counted in the four-corner 1-mm^2 squares (1–4 in **Fig. 8**).

6. Count the platelets according to a specific sequence within the central 1-mm^2 area or 0.1 μL total volume—*see* **Fig. 9**. Platelets touching the lines on two sides of the square are counted as in the square but those touching the other two sides are not counted, as they are outside the square. This avoids duplicate counting of the same cell.

7. The total number of platelets to be counted should be greater than 200 to lower the CV down to <10% (*see* **Note 1**).

8. Calculation of the platelet count is performed with the following equation:

$$\frac{\text{Number of platelets counted }(N)}{\text{Volume counted }(\mu L)} \times \text{Dilution factor (20)} \times 10^6$$

The number of platelets in one liter of blood therefore = $N \times 10 \times 20 \times 10^6$

3.2. Immunological Platelet Counting

1. Pipet 5 µL of the well-mixed (at least 8 complete, gentle inversions of the specimen tube) blood specimen into 100 µL of the filtered PBS-BSA diluent.
2. Add 5 µL of the CD41 and 5 µL of the CD61 staining solution; mix by gentle inversion and incubate for 15 min in the dark, at ambient (room; 18–22°C) temperature (*see* **Note 9**).
3. After 15 min, mix well by gentle inversions and prepare a final 1:1000 dilution for counting by adding 4.85 mL of the PBS-BSA diluent (*see* **Note 10**). Mix well by gentle inversions to ensure proper and equal distribution of red cells and platelets.
4. With the flow cytometer, count a minimum of 50,000 events with a minimum of 1000 platelet events. Analyze by plotting log FL1 versus log forward scatter (FS) (*see* **Fig. 10**) (*see* **Notes 7** and **8**). Events that are positive for red-cell scatter signal, as well as for platelet fluorescence, are considered to be red-cell/platelet coincidence events and are added to both the red-cell and the platelet events.
5. Both quadrant and bit-map analysis are acceptable, but bit-map analysis is recommended (**Fig. 10**).
6. Following the ICSH reference method for enumeration of erythrocytes (and leukocytes), determine the red blood cell concentration of the original blood specimen with a semiautomated single-channel aperture-impedance particle counter.
7. From the flow cytometry data determine the red cell:platelet ratio to at least three decimal places. (In a series of 357 apparently healthy, racially mixed, male and female volunteers, median age 26 years, a ratio of 21.572 ± 5.134 was found.)
8. Divide the red-cell count determined in the original specimen by this RBC/Plt ratio to arrive at the platelet count.

$$\text{Example: red cell count } 5.44 \times 10^{12}/\text{L; RBC/Plt ratio} = 20.4896$$
$$\text{Platelet count} = 5.44 \times 10^{12} : 20.4896 = 265.5 \times 10^{9}/\text{L}$$

4. Notes

1. The subjectivity and the number of cells being counted limits the accuracy of manual counting. At low platelet numbers, because fewer cells are being counted, observed CVs increase proportionally. The total number of platelets counted should exceed 200. The degree of imprecision of the manual count is exemplified by reported interobserver coefficients of variation in the range of 10 to 25% (*3*).
2. Other disadvantages of manual counting are the possible errors in the manual dilution of the blood and that red-cell debris may be mistaken for platelets.
3. Cleanliness is crucial for the success of manual counting. Ensure that the counting chamber and coverslip are clean.
4. Ammonium oxalate solution must be filtered and centrifuged at 1500*g* for 15 min to remove debris.
5. Platelets should be evenly dispersed and not clumped together. Occasional clumps of two to three cells are often seen. The presence of larger aggregates will invalidate the count.
6. For phase-contrast microscopy a special thin counting chamber for platelets enhances the phase-contrast effect.
7. Laboratories must verify that a specific clone/batch of antibodies results in adequate fluorescent staining of the platelets when performing the flow cytometry method.

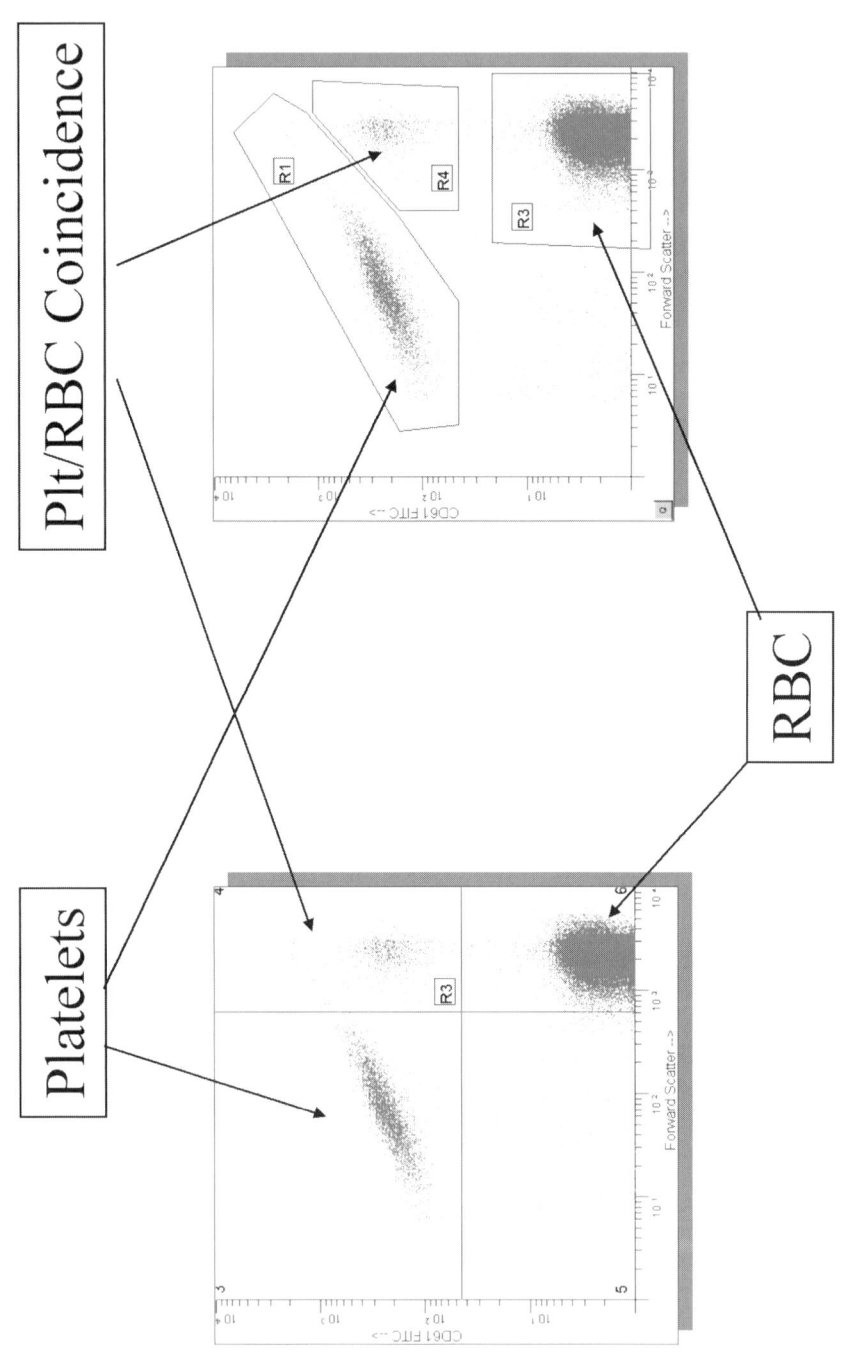

Plt/RBC Coincidence

Platelets

RBC

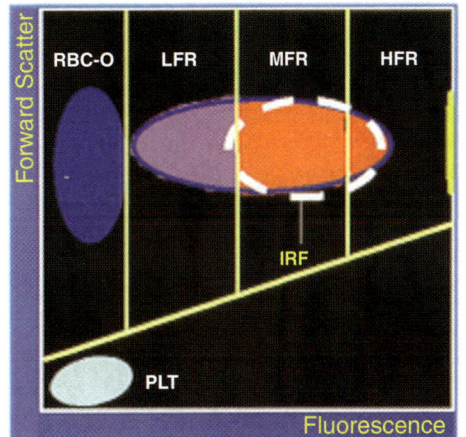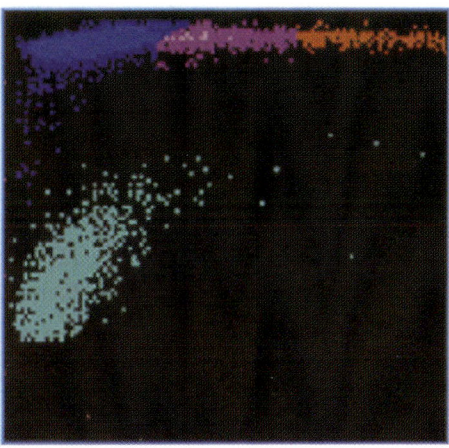

Color Plate 1, Fig. 6 (*see* discussion in Chapter 3, p. 38.) An example of a scattergram produced by the Sysmex XE-2100 hematology analyzer in both cartoon (left) and dot plot (right) formats. The vertical axis indicated forward scattered light or cell volume and the horizontal axis indicates fluorescence intensity. The scattergram is divided into the PLT area, mature RBC area (RBC-O), and the various immature reticulocyte fractions (LFR, MFR, and HFR). (Courtesy of Sysmex Corporation.)

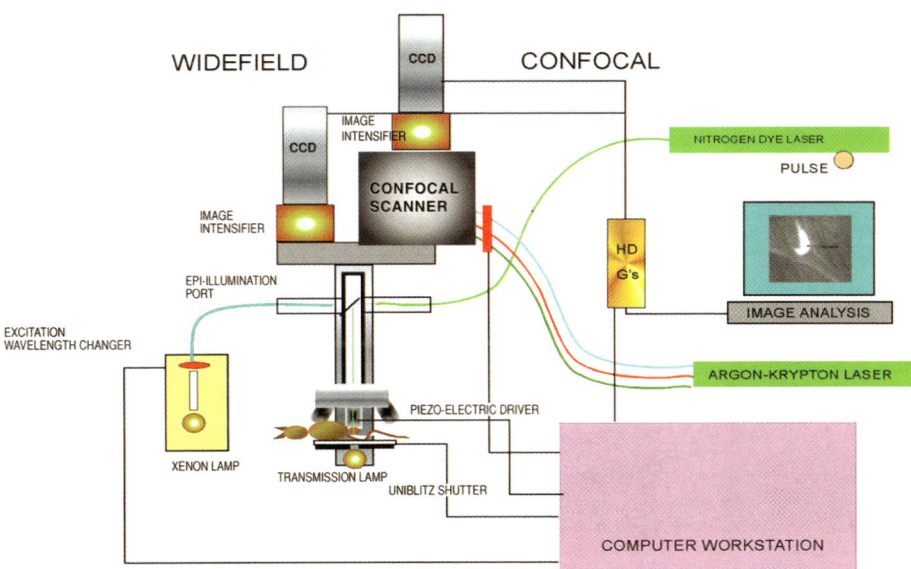

Color Plate 2, Fig. 2 (*see* discussion in Chapter 16, p. 190.) Schematic representation of intravital setup for evaluation of real-time thrombus formation. Microvessel data can be obtained by intravital microscopy using a fluorescence microscope fitted with a water-immersion objective and long-distance condenser. The microscope's dual ports allow for both confocal and wide-field imaging systems. Images of the intravascular interactions are captured using a CCD camera and an image intensifier onto a computer workstation. (Reproduced from *ref. 12* with permission.)

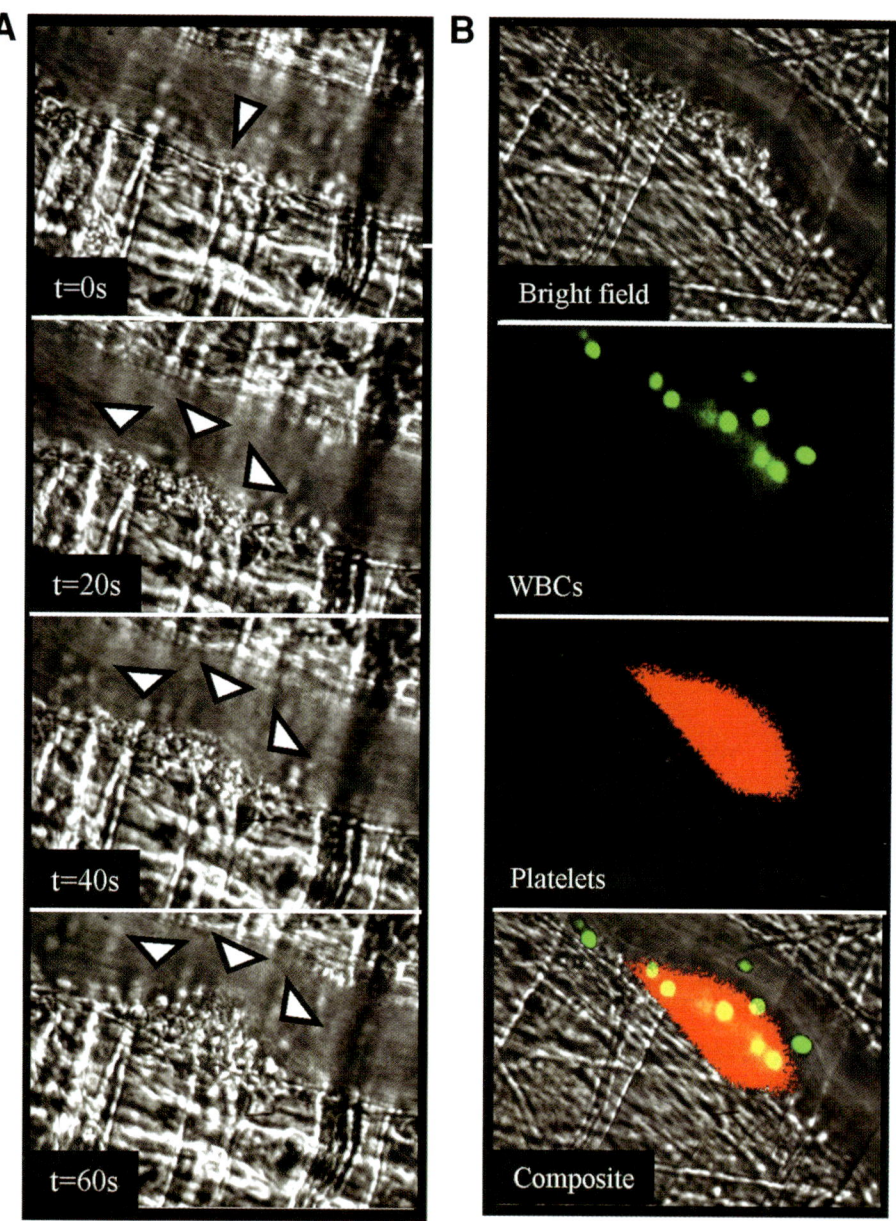

Color Plate 3, Fig. 3 (*see* full caption and discussion in Chapter 16, p. 195.) Time course of thrombus formation in vivo and fluorescent labeling of venous thrombus components. Initiation and propagation of thrombus formation after laser ablation is here shown in four time points in bright field (**A**). Surgical preparation of mouse, laser ablation, and acquisition of data are detailed in text.

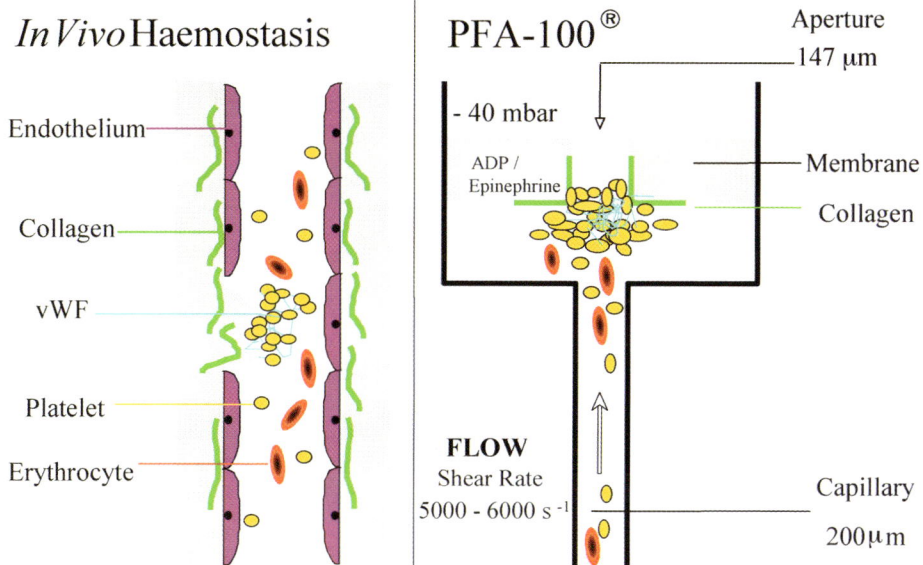

Color Plate 4, Fig. 2 (*see* discussion in Chapter 18, p. 217.) Cross-section of cartridge (right-hand side) showing the principle of the PFA-100 test, which mimics the high-shear-dependent platelet adhesion and aggregation (left-hand side) (courtesy of Dade-Behring).

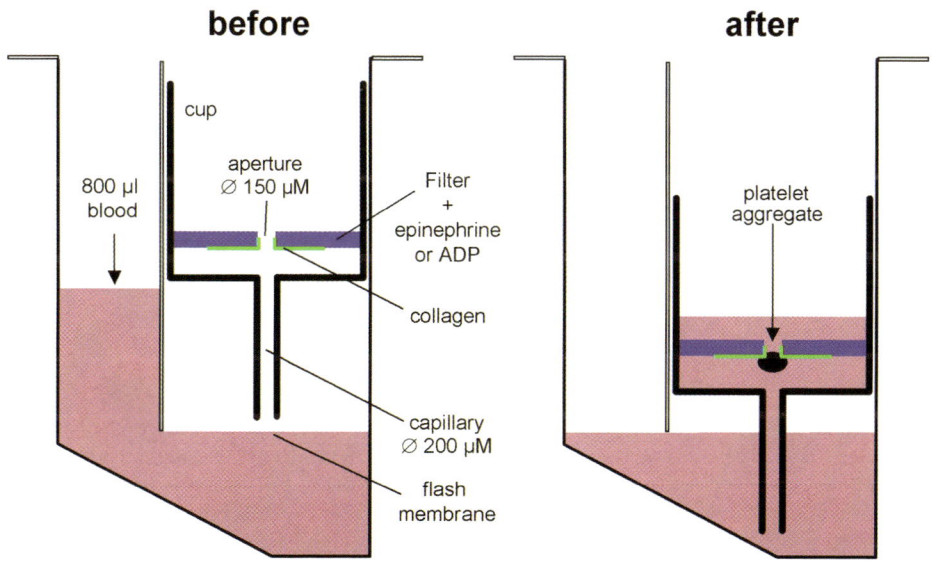

Color Plate 5, Fig. 3 (*see* discussion in Chapter 18, p. 217.) Cross-section of a cartridge before and after performing the PFA-100 test (courtesy of Dade-Behring).

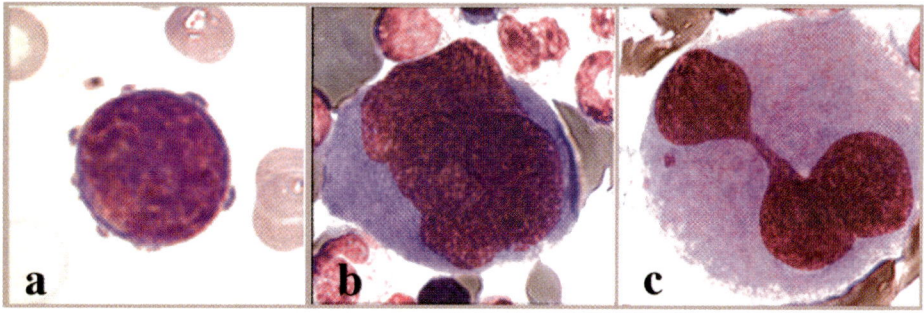

Color Plate 6, Fig. 1 (*see* discussion in Chapter 25, p. 331.) Light microscopic appearance of MKs from a normal bone marrow smear, stained by the Romanovski technique. The 3 sequential maturation stages are represented: **(A)** Immature MK or megakaryoblast: the relatively large size of this otherwise poorly differentiated hemoblast (high nucleus:cytoplasm ratio, thin chromatin, basophilic cytoplasm) allows it to be assigned to the MK lineage. **(B)** MK of an intermediate maturation: large size, convoluted large polyploid nucleus, surrounded by a uniformly basophilic cytoplasm; some azurophilic granules appear toward the cell center. **(C)** Mature MK: Large cell with a polylobulated nucleus, and a uniformly granular and azurophilic cytoplasm.

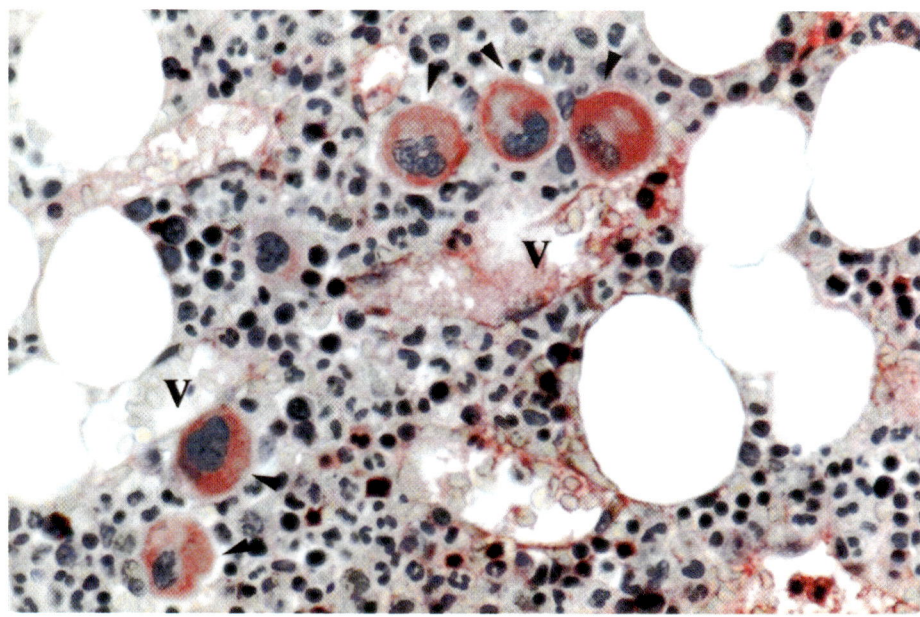

Color Plate 7, Fig. 2 (*see* discussion in Chapter 25, p. 332.) Human normal bone marrow biopsy immunostained for fibrinogen by the APAAP technique. MKs are frequently grouped and located along a vascular sinusoid (v). Fibrinogen displays peripheral staining in mature MK (arrowheads). The staining intensity is weak in the small immature MK while it is maximal in the large mature MK. The cell periphery is intensely stained, and the juxta nuclear region appears to be weakly labeled. This staining pattern is typical of an alpha-granule protein endocytosed from the extracellular medium.

8. When setting up the flow cytometer, ensure that the forward scatter discriminator is set to eliminate noise but does not interfere with the lower portion of the platelet cloud. Set FL1 PMT so that fluorescent platelets are clearly discrimated from noise/debris on the log scale (*see* **Fig. 10**). Typical flow cytometer settings are published in Harrison et al. (*17*).

9. Consistent flow cytometry results have been obtained when the blood and the CD41 and CD61 staining solutions are pipetted as separate beads in the bottom of the reaction tube, the PBS-BSA diluent is added, and the solution is mixed well by at least eight complete inversions.

10. At 1:1000 final dilution the coincidence error should be negligible on the flow cytometer. Coincidence correction can be applied according to the equations in Harrison et al. (*17*). This should not be necessary at this final dilution factor.

11. If measuring platelets within a purified preparation flow cytometry using the platelet/RBC ratio cannot be used as the RBCs are absent. Use calibration beads instead (e.g., Trucount, Becton Dickinson, Oxford, UK) according to Harrison et al. (*3*).

12. Modern automated analyzers are very precise but care needs to be taken to ensure that they are producing accurate platelet counts. Most modern instruments tend to be precalibrated by the manufacturer but often perform adjustments according to the individual blood sample characteristics. Despite improved calibration, each instrument requires regular maintenance and cleaning (according to the manufacturer's specifications) to ensure optimum performance. Each laboratory also should establish an in-house reference range for each measured cell type, including the platelet count. Quality control procedures should be performed regularly (e.g., daily) to check for accuracy. Each analyzer manufacturer produces quality-control material that can be purchased to monitor performance of the instrument. The control can usually be used on those manufacturers' instruments only with their specific reagents. The control consists of treated stabilized human erythrocytes in an isotonic bacteriostatic medium with the addition of a stabilized platelet-sized component and white blood cells or fixed erythrocytes to simulate leukocytes and red blood cells. The controls are usually available with low, normal, or high levels of WBCs, RBCs, and platelets. Each control has assigned values and expected ranges. Expected ranges include variations between lots and between individual instruments, and represent 95% confidence limits for well-maintained instrument systems.

13. If analyzing clinical samples, each laboratory should participate in a national quality assurance scheme (e.g., UK NEQAS). These schemes usually involve regular analysis of stabilized blood preparations (with a range of counts) that are treated as normal patient samples. Results are returned to the quality-control service, which then provides regular reports on the individual center's performance compared with that of other laboratories using the same test method or analyzer. Performance is usually assessed individually within instrument groups against the consensus target value.

Fig. 10. (*see opposite page*) Flow-cytometry scattergrams (left) and bit-map analysis (right) of log fluorescence (FL1) vs log forward scatter. The fluorescent platelets are clearly resolved from noise/debris, RBCs, and Plt/RBC coincidence events.

References

1. Brecher, G., Schneiderman, M. and Cronkite, E. P. (1953) The reproducibility of the platelet count. *Am. J. Clin. Pathol.* **23,** 15–21.
2. England, J. M., Rowan, R. M., Bins, M., Bull, B. S., Groner, W., Jones, A. R., et al. (1998) Recommended methods for the visual determination of white cell and platelet counts. *WHO LAB* **88,** 1.
3. Harrison, P., Horton, A., Grant, D., Briggs, C. and Machin, S. J. (2000) Immunoplatelet counting: A proposed new reference procedure. *Br. J. Haematol.* **108,** 228–235.
4. Bentley, S. A., Johnson, A., and Bishop, C. A. (1993) A parallel evaluation of four automated haematology analyzers. *Am. J. Clin. Pathol.* **100,** 626–632.
5. Bull, B. S., Schneiderman, M. A., and Brecher, G. (1965) Platelet counts with the Coulter counter. *Am. J. Clin. Pathol.* **44,** 678–688.
6. Ault, K. A. (1996) Platelet counting. Is there room for improvement? *Laboratory Haematol.* **2,** 139–143.
7. Rowan, R. M. (1991) Platelet counting and assessment of platelet function. In *Practical Laboratory Haematology* (Koepke, J. A., ed.), Churchill Livingstone, New York, p. 157.
8. Coulter, W. H. (1953) Means for counting particles suspended in a fluid. US Patent 2,656,508.
9. Patterson, K. (1997) Platelet parameters generated by automated blood counters. *CME Bull. Haematol.* **1,** 13–16.
10. Kunicka, J. E., Fischer, G., Murphy, J., and Zelmanovic, D. (2000) Improving platelet counting using two-dimensional laser light scatter. *Am. J. Clin. Pathol.* **114,** 283–289.
11. Tycko, D. H., Metz, M. H., and Epstein, E. A. (1985) Flow-cytometric light scattering measurement of red blood cell volume and haemoglobin concentration. *Appl. Optics* **24,** 1355–1365.
12. Briggs, C., Harrison, P., Grant, D., Staves, J., and Machin, S. J. (2000) New quantitative parameters on a recently introduced automated blood cell counter—the XE 2100. *Clin. Lab. Haematol.* **17,** 163–172.
13. Davis, B. and Bigelow, N. C. (1999) Indirect immunoplatelet couting by flow cytometry as a reference method for platelet count calibration. *Lab. Haematol.* **5,** 15–21.
14. Tanaka, C., Isii, T., and Fujimoto, K. (1996) Flow cytometric platelet enumeration utilising monoclonal antibody CD42a. *Clin. Lab. Haematol.* **118,** 265–269.
15. Groner, W., Mayer, K., and Chapman, E. (1994) An indirect platelet count using platelet specific monoclonal antibody and flow cytometry can produce reliable platelet counts for assessing thrombocytopenia *(abstract)*. *Blood* **84(Suppl. 1),** 687a.
16. International Council for Standardization in Haematology (ICSH) Expert Panel on Cytometry and International Society of Laboratory Haematolgy (ISLH). Task Force on Platelet Counting (2000). Platelet Counting by the PLT/RBC ratio—a reference method. *Am. J. Clin. Pathol.* **115(3),** 460–464.
17. Harrison, P., Ault, K. A., Chapman, S. E., Davis, B., Fujimoto, K., Houwen, B., et al. (2000) An inter-laboratory study of a candidate reference method for platelet counting. *Am. J. Clin. Pathol.* **115(3),** 448–459.
18. Ault, K. A., Mitchell, J., Knowles, C., and Van Hove, L. (1997) Implementation of the immunological platelet count on a haematology analyzer—the Abbott CELL-DYN 4000. *Lab. Haematol.* **3,** 125–128.
19. Kunz, D., Kunz, W. S., Scott, C. S., and Gressner, A. M. (2001) Automated CD61 Immunoplatelet analysis of thrombocytopenic samples. *Br. J. Haematol.* **112,** 584–592.

4

Electron Microscopy Methods for Studying Platelet Structure and Function

James G. White

1. Introduction

Platelets are very small—the smallest of cellular elements in circulating blood. They lack a nucleus and their cytoplasm is relatively clear. As a result it was impossible to visualize platelets in the crude instruments used by early microscopists. In fact, platelets were not identified until many years after red blood cells and leukocytes were well known *(1,2)*. It took the development of the compound and achromatic microscopes *(3)* to see platelets, and even then they were considered fragments of erythrocytes or white blood cells *(4,5)*. Difficulties in anticoagulating blood and preparing samples for study in microscopes complicated the problem and delayed for decades the realization that platelets were involved in blood clotting and thrombosis *(6)*. That platelets were critical cellular elements for hemostasis in vivo took even longer *(7)*. It was not until the electron microscope became available that insights into relationships among platelet structure, function, and pathology began to evolve *(8,9)*. Even then, the problems of fixing platelets to preserve their fine structure and relate physical changes following activation to their role in hemostatic physiology took considerable time *(10)*.

Fortuitously, methods for isolating viable platelets, procedures for carrying out studies of their physiology and biochemistry, and techniques for preserving fine details of ultrastructural anatomy were developed at about the same time that members of the blood research community began to appreciate the greater importance of platelets in hemostasis and vascular pathology. Glutaraldehyde was one of several dialdehyde fixatives introduced in the early 1960s *(11)*. Fixation of blood cells in various combinations of glutaraldehyde and osmium tetroxide separately or together was soon found to be superior, at least in most situations, to preservation in osmic acid alone. Initially, dual fixation with glutaraldehyde and osmic acid was carried out in the same manner as when osmium had been used alone *(12)*. Platelets were separated from whole blood collected in EDTA anticoagulant by centrifugation in a refrigerated centrifuge at 4°C.

From: *Methods in Molecular Biology, vol. 272:*
Platelets and Megakaryocytes, Vol. 1: Functional Assays
Edited by: J. M. Gibbins and M. P. Mahaut-Smith © Humana Press Inc., Totowa, NJ

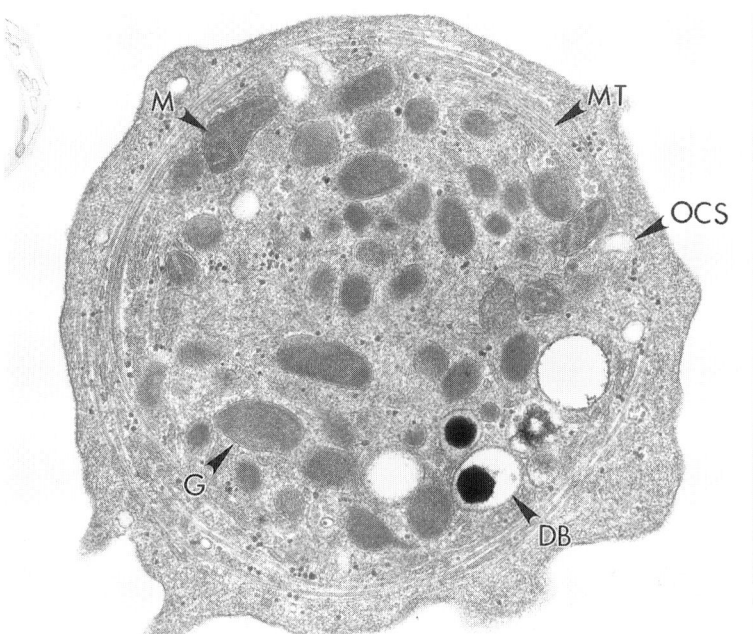

Fig. 1. Equatorial section of normal human platelet. The disk form is supported by a circumferential coil of microtubules (MT) lying just under the cell membrane. Organelles, including numerous alpha granules (G), a few dense bodies (DB), and occasional mitochondria (M) are randomly dispersed in the cytoplasm. (Original magnification ×36,000.)

The isolated cells were kept chilled and sedimented in the cold a second time to obtain pellets. The supernatant plasma was discarded and chilled glutaraldehyde was layered over the pellet. After 15–30 min the pellet was broken up into small pieces and fixed for an additional 60 min at a low temperature. Following this, the aldehyde fixative was discarded and the cell fragments were washed in cold buffer or distilled water several times, then combined with chilled osmic acid for about 1–2 h. The fixed sample was again washed and dehydrated in a graded series of acetone. After exposure to pure acetone, the fixed samples were infiltrated with liquid plastic, usually methacrylate or vestopal-W. After polymerization, sections were cut from plastic blocks with glass knives on hand-driven microtomes. The sections were usually stained with a lead salt to enhance contrast and evaluated in the electron microscope.

Photographs of platelets prepared in this manner revealed morphological details that had not been apparent when osmic acid was used as the only fixative (**Fig. 1**) *(13,14)*. In particular, initial exposure to glutaraldehyde prior to incubation with osmic acid preserved a new platelet organelle that had not been recognized previously *(15)*. The structure was smaller than the more numerous α granules, and appeared to consist of an electron-dense core surrounded by a clear space separating the opaque substance from its enclosing membrane. Some initial studies suggested that glutaraldehyde acted

Table 1
Anticoagulant

1. 0.1 *M* citric acid, 10.508 g, to 500 mL with distilled H_2O.
2. 0.1 *M* sodium citrate. $2H_2O$, 14.706 g, to 500 mL with distilled H_2O.

To make the reagent:
a. 35 mL 0.1 *M* citric acid.
b. 465 mL 0.1 *M* sodium citrate.
c. 12.25 g dextrose (0.1 *M*).
d. Add 5+ drops 10 *N* NaOH (0.1 *M*) to pH 6.5.
e. Refrigerate.

as a Schiff base to stabilize the structure and as a mordant to attract osmic acid. Based on these observations, the term "osmiophilic dense body" was proposed as the eponym for the new organelle. Subsequent studies, however, demonstrated that this hypothesis for preservation of dense bodies was incorrect because the organelles were inherently electron-opaque. Yet the discovery had an important influence on the near-universal adoption of dual fixation in glutaraldehyde and osmic acid to preserve platelet fine structure.

Even though the improved ultrastructural preservation achieved with dual fixation represented a significant advance, many morphological features remained obscure or were completely missed because of inherent errors in the fixation procedure. Most of these difficulties were recognized and resolved in subsequent years, and form the basis of our current approach to platelet fixation.

The methods described in this chapter for preserving platelet structure and carrying out special procedures have been in use in our laboratory for decades. They are not foolproof, but are very reliable. Others trying to use them have occasionally had difficulty and called for assistance or visited our laboratory. When they have learned the methods in detail and follow them precisely, they obtain the same results as we do. In the interest of space limitations, we have not described many other methods we have found useful. Cytochemical and immunocytochemical techniques have helped to advance our knowledge of platelet structural physiology. For particular applications, the reader should consult the literature.

2. Materials

1. Anticoagulant: citrate-citric acid dextrose, pH 6.5 (*see* **Table 1**) (for further information regarding the choice of anticoagulant, *see* **Note 1**).
2. A "butterfly" infusion set with 30 cm (12 in) of loose plastic tubing between the hub and a 19-gauge needle, and 35-mL or 50-mL plastic syringes (*see* **Notes 2** and **3**).
3. Centrifuge.
4. A water bath to allow blood and platelet preparation to be maintained at a temperature between 23 and 37°C. (For information regarding the importance of temperature during blood collection, and platelet preparation and fixation, *see* **Note 4**.)

Table 2
Stock Solutions for White's Saline

A. NaCl	14.0 g
KCl	0.75 g
$MgSO_4$	0.55 g
$Ca(NO_3)_2•4H_2O$	1.5 g
Add distilled H_2O to 100 mL.	
Refrigerate.	
B. $NaHCO_3$	1.1 g
$Na_2HPO_4•7H_2O$	0.22 g
KH_2PO_4 anhydrous	0.052 g
Phenol red	0.01 g
Add distilled H_2O to 100 mL.	
When dissolved at room temperature bubble CO_2 in for about 15 s, if	
necessary. Mix well, and adjust pH to 7.4.	
Refrigerate.	

Table 3
Fixatives

1. 0.1% glutaraldehyde in White's saline:
   8.9 mL distilled H_2O
   0.5 mL White's A
   0.5 mL White's B
   0.1 mL 10% glutaraldehyde
2. 3% glutaraldehyde in White's saline:
   6 mL distilled H_2O
   0.5 mL White's A
   0.5 mL White's B
   3 mL 10% glutaraldehyde
3. 1% (w/v) OsO_4: Prepare and keep in a dark brown glass-stoppered bottle.
   2.5 mL 4% (w/v) OsO_4 aqueous
   2.0 mL stock buffer (Zetterquist's)
   0.68 mL stock salt solution
   2.0 mL 0.1 N HCl
   2.82 mL distilled H_2O
   Keeps 1 wk in refrigerator.

5. A supply of 95% O_2, 5% CO_2 gas to prevent a spontaneous rise in the pH of C-PRP, which affects platelet morphology (for further details *see* **Note 5**).
6. Glutaraldehyde.
7. Osmic acid.
8. Many different solutions are used to buffer glutaraldehyde and osmic acid. We favor the use of White's saline (*see* **Table 2,3** and **Note 6**) containing NaCl, KCl, $MgSO_4$, $Ca(NO_3)_2•4H_2O$, $NaHCO_3$, $Na_2HPO_4•7H_2O$, KH_2PO_4, and phenol red.

Table 4
Zetterquist's Veronal Buffer

1. Stock buffer	
Sodium barbital	14.7 g
Sodium acetate•3H$_2$O	9.7 g
Dilute to 500 mL with distilled H$_2$O.	
2. Stock salt solution	
NaCl	20 g
KCl	1 g
CaCl$_2$	0.5 g
Dilute to 250 mL with distilled H$_2$O.	

9. Zetterquist's Veronal acetate buffer (*see* **Table 4**) containing sodium barbitol, CH$_3$CO$_2$Na, NaCl, KCl, CaCl$_2$.
10. Epon 812.
11. Diamond knife on an ultramicrotome.
12. Formvar-coated carbon-stabilized grids.
13. 12-mm round cover slips attached to stubs for standard SEM or on 2 × 4 mm glass chips for low-voltage, high-resolution scanning electron microscope (LVHR-SEM), precoated in polylysine.
14. Liquid freon and liquid nitrogen.
15. Balzer's freeze-fracture unit (for freeze-fracture technique only).
16. Tannic acid.
17. 0.1 *M* cacodylate buffer, pH 7.2.
18. Tris-HCl.
19. Diaminobenzidine.
20. Hydrogen peroxide.
21. Dimethylsulfoxide.
22. Potassium ferrocyanide.

3. Methods

3.1. Standard Fixation

The simple procedure established in our laboratory many years ago is still routinely used to fix platelets for study in the electron microscope. Ordinarily the number of platelets present in 1 mL of C-PRP is sufficient to make a good preparation. The pellet derived from smaller volumes is often too small and hard to follow during subsequent steps of fixation, dehydration, and embedding. If the patient is thrombocytopenic, larger volumes of C-PRP will be required and longer periods of centrifugation at higher sedimentation rates will help.

1. Samples of platelets are combined with an equal volume of 0.1% glutaraldehyde in White's saline, pH 7.3.
2. After 15 min at 37°C, during which the sample can be mixed gently, the platelets are sedimented to pellets by centrifugation at room temperature and 800*g*.

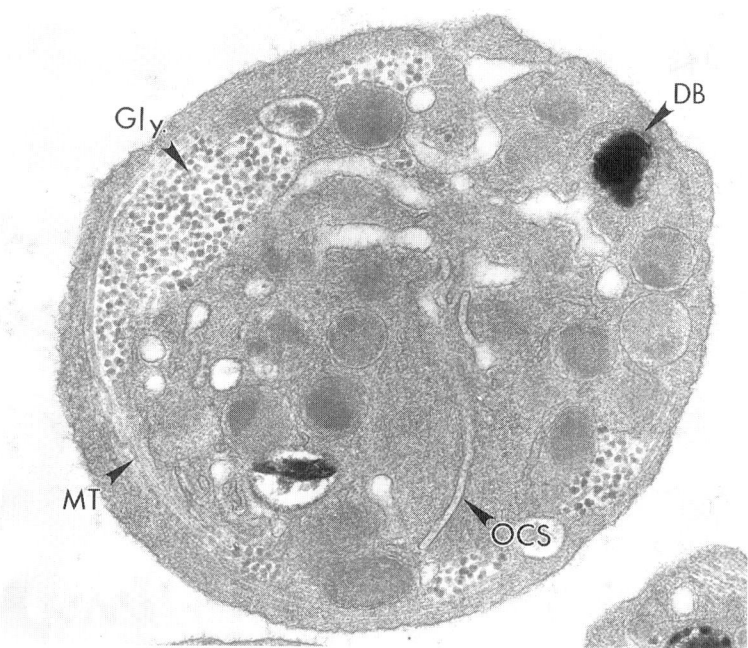

Fig. 2. Equatorial section of discoid platelet from PRP collected in citrate anticoagulant and then combined with EDTA. Discoid shape is preserved by citrate, but EDTA
does cause physical changes in membranes of the open canalicular system (OCS).
Microtubule (MT) coils are located under the cell surface. Glycogen is present in
masses (Gly) or single particles. Granules, mitochondria, and dense bodies (DB) are
randomly dispersed. (Original magnification ×45,000.)

3. The supernatant is discarded and replaced with 3% glutaraldehyde in White's saline.
4. Fixation is continued either at room temperature or 4°C for 40–60 min. The supernatant is
   then discarded and the cells washed once with buffer and then combined with 1% (w/v)
   osmic acid in White's saline (**Table 3**) or Zetterquist's Veranol acetate buffer (*see* **Table 4**).
5. After exposure to osmic acid fixation at 4°C for 1 h, the cells are dehydrated in a graded
   series of alcohol and embedded in Epon 812. The contrast of thin sections cut with a
   diamond knife on an ultramicrotome is usually enhanced with uranyl acetate and lead
   citrate (**Figs. 1–4**) (*see also* Chapter 25, vol. 1).
6. For further details on conditions for fixation, *see* **Note 7**.
   For further details regarding the choice of concentration of glutaraldehyde during fixation,
   see **Note 8**.
   For further details regarding osmic acid fixation, *see* **Notes 9** and **10** and **Tables 3** and **4**.

3.2. Whole Mount Procedure

The formed organelles in the cytoplasm of human and animal platelets have been
characterized in many previous studies *(22–25)*. They include alpha granules, mito-

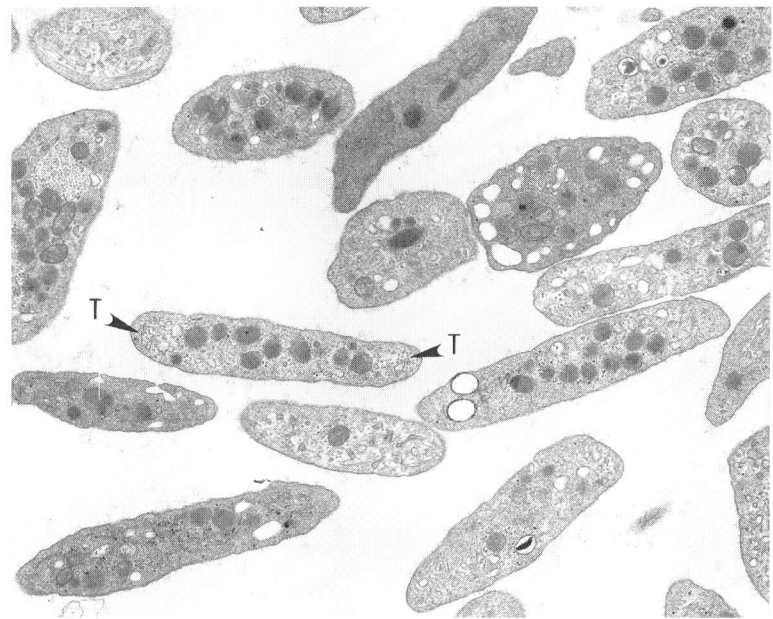

Fig. 3. Transverse section of discoid human platelets. Microtubule coils (T) appearing as a cluster of small circles at each pole of the cell support the disklike form. (Original magnification ×17,000.)

chondria, lysosomes, and dense bodies **(Fig. 4)**. Other membrane-enclosed structures, such as glysosomes, are also present, but do not constitute a significant population. Most of the organelles are easily visualized in thin sections of glutaraldehyde-osmic acid fixed, plastic embedded platelets **(Figs. 1–3)**. Dense bodies are present in thin sections, but are more easily identified as a single population in unfixed, unstained whole-mount preparations *(26)*.

1. Small drops of PRP are placed on Formvar-coated, carbon-stabilized grids, rinsed within 10–15 s with drops of distilled water, dried from the edge with pieces of filter paper, and waved in the air to remove residual moisture.
2. The grids are inserted into the electron microscope without fixation or staining.
3. Dense bodies are present in almost every normal platelet **(Fig. 5)**, but absent from platelets of patients with the Hermansky–Pudlak syndrome **(Fig. 6)**.

3.3. Scanning Electron Microscopy

Scanning electron microscopy (SEM) and low-voltage–high-resolution SEM (LVHR-SEM) have been useful for following alterations on the exterior surface of activated platelets **(Fig. 7; *27*)**.

1. Samples of PRP or washed suspensions, before or after activation, are fixed in suspension with an equal volume of 0.1% glutaraldehyde in White's saline for 15 min.

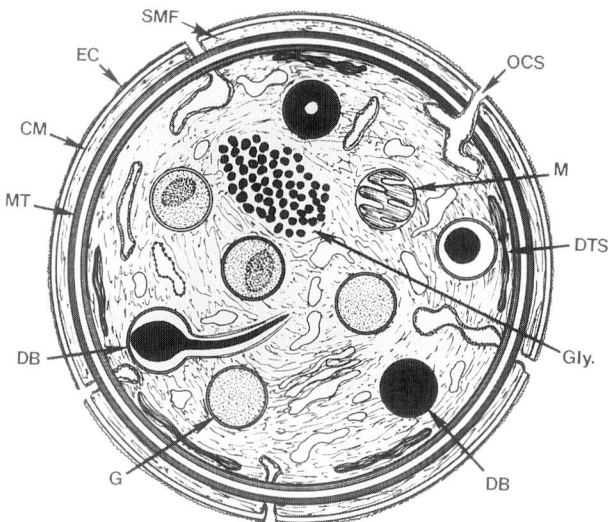

Fig. 4. The diagram summarizes ultrastructural features observed in thin sections of discoid platelets cut in the equatorial plane. Components of the *peripheral zone* include the exterior coat (EC), trilaminar unit membrane (CM), and submembrane area containing specialized filaments (SMF), which form the wall of the platelet and line channels of the surface-connected open canalicular system (OCS). The matrix of the platelet interior is the *sol-gel zone* containing actin microfilaments, structural filaments, the circumferential band of microtubules (MT), and glycogen (Gly). Normal elements embedded in the sol-gel zone include mitochondria (M), alpha granules (G), and dense bodies (DB). Collectively, they constitute the *organelle zone*. The *membrane systems* include the surface-connected open canalicular system (OCS) and the dense tubular system (DTS), which serve as the platelet sacroplasmic reticulum.

2. After the initial step the samples are centrifuged to pellets, the supernatant discarded and replaced with 3% glutaraldehyde in White's saline. After a short interval (5–10 min) the pellet is resuspended in the fixative.
3. Small drops are placed on 12-mm round cover slips attached to stubs for standard SEM or on 2 × 4 mm glass chips for LVHR-SEM.
4. The samples are allowed to settle and stick on the glass fragments, which are precoated with polylysine.
5. The glass is then rinsed with distilled water, dehydrated in a graded series of alcohols, or critical-point-dried. For study at high resolution the samples are examined for example in the Hitachi 450 SEM.

3.4. Freeze-Fracture Technique

A method for splitting lipid bilayers allowing the study of the inner side of the outside layer and the outside of the inner layer of membranes seemed very attractive when first introduced. It has provided some useful information about the platelet open

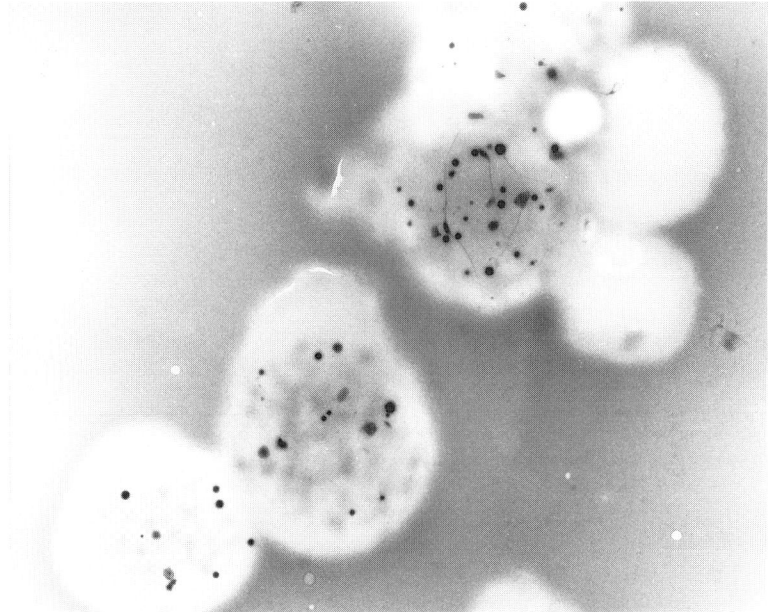

Fig. 5. Whole-mount technique. This simple procedure permits recognition of inherently electron-dense bodies containing serotonin and adenine nucleotides. Note that some dense bodies have whiplike extensions. (Original magnification ×6000.)

canalicular system, dense tubular system, and their association in membrane complexes (**Fig. 8**; *28*). References to the method applied to platelet structural physiology, however, have virtually disappeared from the recent literature.

1. Preparation of platelets for freeze-fracture begins after the second step of fixation in 3% glutaraldehyde for 1–2 h (*see* **Subheading 3.1., step 3**). At that time, the fixative is discarded and replaced with 20% glycerol in White's saline for 10 min.
2. The pellet is then cut into small pieces, transferred to special holders, and dropped immediately into receptacles containing liquid freon suspended in liquid nitrogen.
3. After the initial step of freezing, the samples are placed in liquid nitrogen until ready for fracturing. Holders with the frozen platelet samples are transferred quickly to the stage of a Balzer's freeze-fracture unit cooled with liquid nitrogen and exposed immediately to high vacuum.
4. The frozen platelets are fractured at −120°C, allowed to etch at that temperature for 30 s, and then freed from tissue by soaking the samples in 30% chlorine bleach. The replicas are washed in distilled water, mounted on uncoated 200- or 300-mesh grids, and examined in the electron microscope.

3.5. Tannic Acid Procedure

Study of the platelet open canalicular system and the secretory process has been greatly facilitated by staining platelets with tannic acid during fixation (**Fig. 9**; *29,30*).

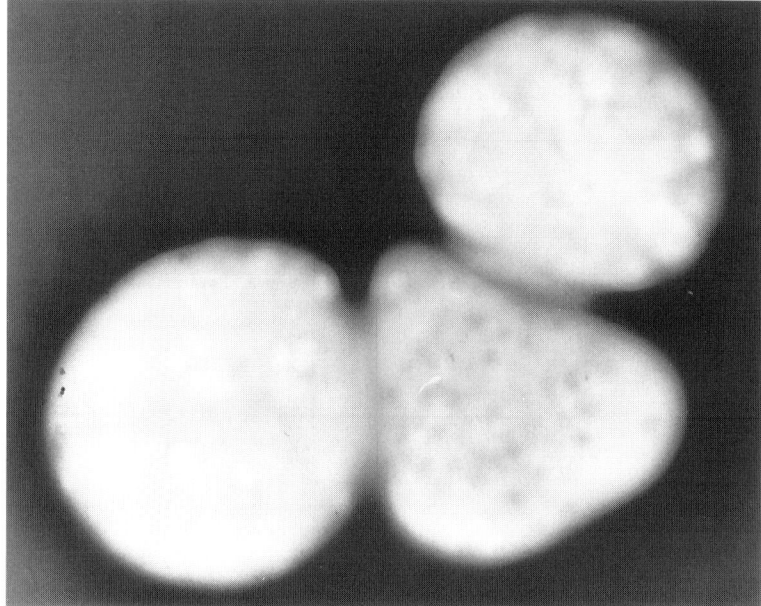

Fig. 6. Whole-mount preparation of platelets from a patient with storage pool deficiency. These platelets lack dense bodies and their content of serotonin and nucleotides.
(Original magnification ×12,000.)

1. After completion of the initial fixation steps, pellets are washed three times and stored
   overnight in 0.1 *M* cacodylate buffer, pH 7.2.
2. The buffer is decanted the following day and replaced with 2% (w/v) tannic acid in 0.1 *M*
   cacodylate buffer, pH 7.2, for 4 h at room temperature.
3. The supernatant is decanted, the pellets washed in cacodylate buffer, and the samples post
   fixed in 2% (w/v) osmic acid alone or combined with 1.5% (w/v) potassium ferrocyanide
   for 2 h at 4°C.
4. The samples are then dehydrated in a series of alcohols and embedded in Epon for
   preparation of thin sections.

3.6. Platelet Peroxidase

The platelet dense tubular system is an important anatomical and physiological component. Its localization in the cell and interaction with the dense tubular system have
been greatly facilitated by the histochemical procedure for staining platelet peroxidase
(Fig. 10; *31*).

1. Samples of platelet-rich plasma or washed platelet suspensions are fixed initially at 37°C
   with an equal volume of 0.1% glutaraldehyde in 0.1 *M* cacodylate buffer at room
   temperature.
2. The fixed samples are washed three times in 0.05 *M* Tris-HCl buffer at either pH 6.0 or
   pH 9.0, then incubated in a modification of the media described by Graham and

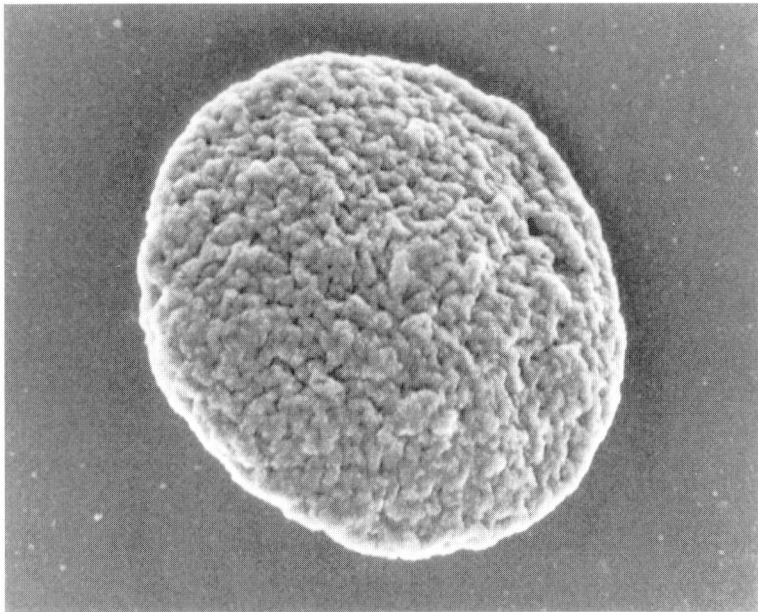

Fig. 7. Discoid platelet viewed in the low-voltage, high-resolution scanning electron microscope (LVHR-SEM). The surface is rugose, resembling the surface of the brain. Red blood cells viewed in the same sample have smooth, unruffled surfaces. (Original magnification ×30,000.)

Karnovsky for demonstration of endogenous peroxidase and adapted by others for localizing catalase (see below). Our contribution consisted of adding 1% glutaraldehyde to the incubation system in order to improve penetration of substrate into the platelets. The final media contained the following reagents:

diaminobenzidine	25 mg
3% hydrogen peroxide	0.1 mL
dimethylsulfoxide	0.1 mL
0.05 M Tris-HCl buffer	10 mL
glutaraldehyde	1%

3. Samples of platelets fixed in this manner described are incubated in the solution for 60 min at room temperature.
4. Reacted platelets are then washed twice in 0.05 M Tris-HCl buffer, pH 6.0 or pH 9.0, and fixed for 1.5 h in 2% (w/v) osmic acid in 0.1 M cacodylate buffer.
5. The fixed samples were dehydrated and embedded in the routine manner. Controls to determine the specificity of the enzyme reaction included the following:
   a. Fixing platelets in 0.1% glutaraldehyde in White's saline and then in 3% glutaraldehyde in White's saline before washing and exposure to complete media.
   b. Incubating platelets fixed in glutaraldehyde-paraformaldehyde in media without hydrogen peroxide (H_2O_2), without diaminobenzidine (DAB), with excess H_2O_2 (3%), or with reduced amounts of H_2O_2 (0.003%).

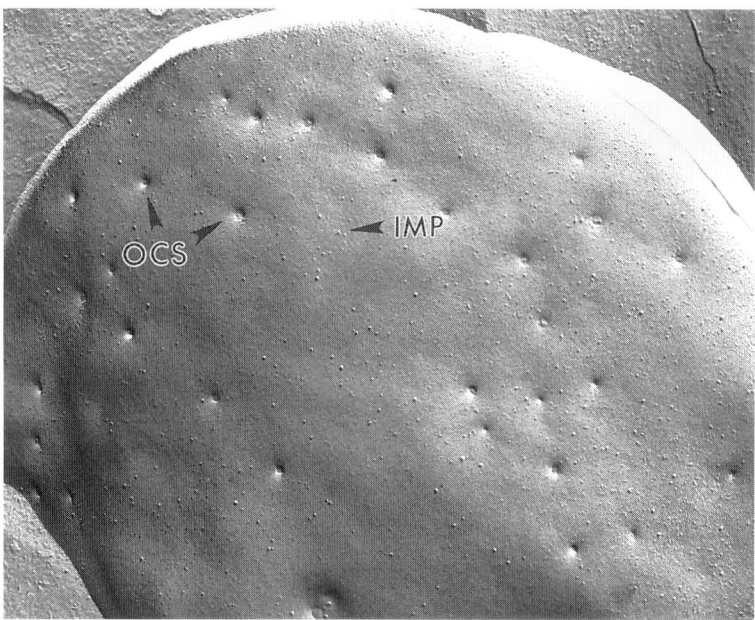

Fig. 8. Replica of a freeze-fractured platelet. It represents the outside of the inner layer of the surface membrane. Intramembranous particles (IMP) and pores of the surface-connected open canalicular system (OCS) cover the surface. (Original magnification ×48,000.)

    c. Incubating glutaraldehyde-paraformaldehyde fixed platelets in complete media containing 0.02 *M* potassium cyanide for 1–2 h.

4. Notes

1. EDTA is a useful anticoagulant. It keeps blood in a fluid state by chelating the calcium necessary for the coagulation process. Unfortunately, it also affects platelet membranes (**Fig. 2**). Platelets lose the discoid form characteristic of their appearance in circulating blood and become irregularly convoluted, resembling spiny spheres. As a result, the morphology of circulating platelets is not well preserved in samples prepared for electron microscopy from blood collected in EDTA anticoagulant. This problem was resolved quite simply by employing one of several different citrate anticoagulant solutions (**Table 1**). Our choice has been citrate-citric acid dextrose, pH 6.5. Other formulae for citrate anticoagulants are probably just as effective, but this variation has worked well for us.

2. Blood for our studies is usually collected from an anticubital vein distended by application of a tourniquet to the upper arm. A "butterfly" infusion set with 30 cm (12 in) of loose plastic tubing between the hub and a 19-gauge needle is routinely employed in adults and children. Venous blood is drawn into 35-mL plastic syringes and then mixed immediately in a ratio of 9 parts blood to 1 part anticoagulant. In some cases the first few milliliters of blood are drawn into a 5- or 10-mL plastic syringe and discarded before collecting the blood to be used for study in the larger-volume plastic syringes. Occasionally 50-mL syringes are used,

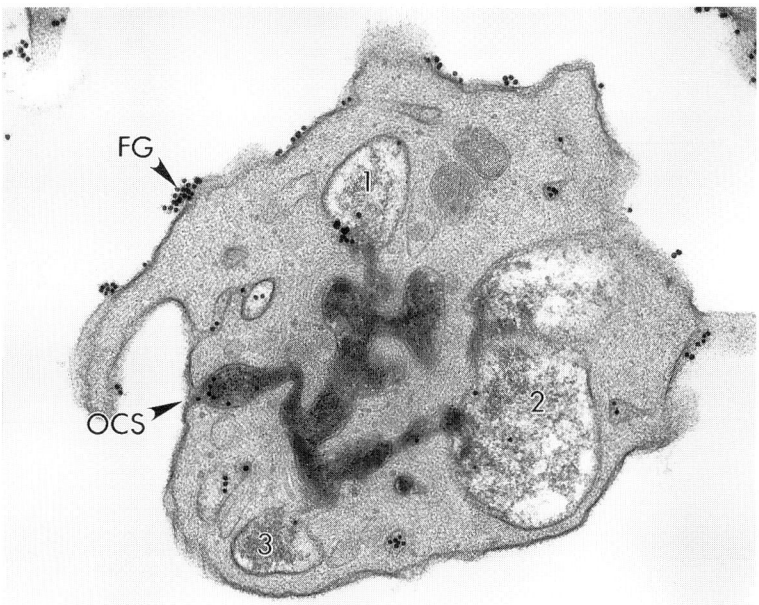

Fig. 9. Thin section of a human platelet activated by thrombin during exposure to fibrinogen-coated gold particles (FG) and stained with tannic acid during fixation. Alpha granules (1,2,3) are swollen and connected to channels of the open canalicular system (OCS) filled with fibrinogen and fibrin stained by tannic acid. The procedure demonstrates that the OCS is the secretory pathway for products (fibrinogen) stored in alpha granules and a two-way street allowing fibrinogen-coated gold particles to reach the interior of the discharging organelles. (Original magnification ×45,000.)

but in general, 35-mL syringes are preferred because they are less unwieldy and blood can be mixed with anticoagulant sooner. We have not found it necessary to insert large-gauge needles to collect venous blood by free flow, as suggested by other workers.

3. On occasion heparin anticoagulant is used in place of citrate, but for electron microscopy we prefer the citrate-citric acid-dextrose. In some cases EDTA or EGTA is desirable to maximally reduce levels of calcium in plasma without disturbing platelet disk form. This can be achieved by adding EDTA or EGTA to citrate-rich plasma **(Fig. 2)**. Discoid form in the presence of the chelating agents will be preserved under these conditions for about 30 min **(Fig. 3)**.

4. The importance of temperature for preserving the morphology of discoid platelets was demonstrated several years ago *(16,17)*. Samples of citrate-platelet-rich plasma (C-PRP) rapidly lose their discoid form on chilling. After a few minutes in an ice bath at 2–4°C all platelets are irregular in form with multiple pseudopods. The shape change was shown to be associated with disappearance of the circumferential bundle of microtubules, which acts as a cytoskeletal system to support the lentiform appearance of unstimulated platelets. Rewarming the chilled platelets restores their discoid form, and the recovery is associated with reassembly of the annular band of tubules. However, the cells are somewhat deformed

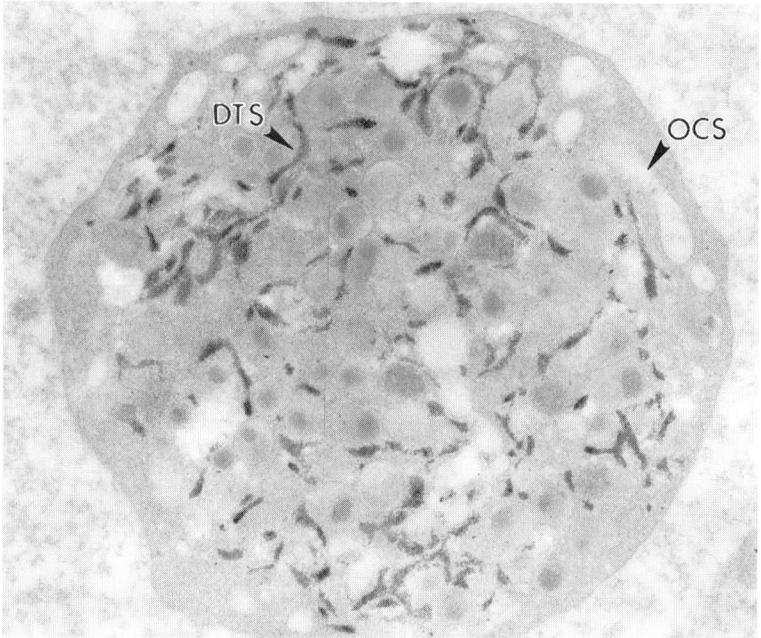

Fig. 10. Platelet from a sample stained for endogenous peroxidase. The reaction product is localized to channels of the dense tubular system (DTS). Channels of the open canalicular system (OCS) are devoid of reaction product. (Original magnification ×37,000.)

   by the cycle of chilling and rewarming. Therefore, to avoid the effects of cold, platelets should be collected and separated from whole blood at room temperature and maintained at 23°C (or 37°C). Initial fixation in glutaraldehyde should be carried out in this same temperature range (**Subheading 3.1., step 1**).

5. Blood collected in the citrate anticoagulant described will have a pH of about 7.2–7.3. The pH will be maintained during separation of C-PRP if the procedure is carried out soon enough after blood collection. Within an hour after obtaining blood the pH of the C-PRP will rise spontaneously, and the alkaline conditions will favor discocyte-to-echinocyte transformation, just as in the case of erythrocytes. The pH rise can be avoided by exposing the air above the C-PRP to a stream of 95% O_2, 5% CO_2 gas and then sealing the tube with a cork *(18)*. However, maintenance under these conditions for prolonged periods will cause a fall in pH. The initial fall from pH 7.3 to 6.5 will tend to make platelets more discoid. However, at pHs below 6.0, platelets undergo disk-to-sphere transformation in the same manner as erythrocytes. Therefore, it is best to avoid wide swings in pH if optimal morphology is a major goal.

6. Many different solutions are used to buffer glutaraldehyde and osmic acid. Some are used to facilitate cytochemical procedures carried out after initial fixation. Others are employed because the ionic composition tends to favor retention of specific chemical constituents or structures in cells. It is for that reason that White's saline (**Table 2**) is used to buffer glutaraldehyde in most of our routine studies of platelet ultrastructural morphology. Many

Table 5
Osmium Ferrocyanide

1% (w/v) OsO$_4$ potassium ferrocyanide	2% (w/v) OsO$_4$ 1.5% (w/v) potassium ferrocyanide
0.75 mL distilled water 15 mg potassium ferrocyanide Shake to dissolve. Add 0.25 mL 4% (w/v) aqueous OsO$_4$.	0.5 mL distilled water 15 mg potassium ferrocyanide 0.5 mL 4% (w/v) aqueous OsO$_4$

years ago we found that a high concentration of calcium in the buffer preserved platelet-dense bodies while phosphate ions tended to extract them during fixation. For this reason we were able to demonstrate that thin sections of normal platelets contained one to two dense bodies per cell, rather than the 1 dense body per 1300 platelet thin sections reported earlier. Many workers worry about the osmolarity contributed by glutaraldehyde to the buffer solution and reduce the concentrations of salts to adjust for it. This has been found to be unnecessary. Though glutaraldehyde does contribute significantly, it appears that the buffer strength and osmolarity in relation to that of plasma need to be the only major concerns. Thus, for other cells we often use Hanks' balanced salt solution, Ringer's lactate, or other isotonic buffers as the vehicle for the fixative.

7. When osmic acid was the only fixative in common use, it was standard practice to sediment platelets to a pellet before combining with osmium. This set of conditions continued to be employed after dual fixation was introduced. However, studies carried out many years ago demonstrated that close cell contact caused by centrifugation activated platelets and resulted in shape change *(19)*. Therefore, in most cases, it is advisable to fix platelets in suspension. To accomplish this we simply mix the platelet sample with an equal volume of fixative solution, stir gently, and allow it to stand at 37°C or room temperature for 15 min before centrifugation to a pellet. A similar procedure is used for platelet aggregates prepared on a platelet aggregometer. Under these conditions glutaraldehyde appears to penetrate quite rapidly and to terminate both physical and biochemical reactions.

8. Early investigators demonstrated that excellent preparations of discoid platelets could be obtained for electron microscopy by collecting native blood directly into fixative solution containing 6% glutaraldehyde. We have found it easier to combine samples of C-PRP with an equal volume of 0.1% glutaraldehyde in White's saline (**Table 3**) for a few minutes, centrifuge the sample to a pellet, discard the supernatant, and replace it with 3% glutaraldehyde in White's saline. The low final concentration of glutaraldehyde (0.05%) stabilizes the discoid shape and fine structure of platelets without precipitating plasma proteins *(20)*.

9. This facet is particularly important when platelets are being prepared for study in the scanning electron microscope. Other workers feel that 0.05% glutaraldehyde is too low a concentration to achieve fixation, but it has worked very well for us and is strongly recommended. The second step involving 3% glutaraldehyde may seem too high and 1 or 2% could work as well. We continue to use 3% because it has proven effective.

10. In general we have preferred to use Zetterquist's veranol acetate buffer for osmic acid fixation (**Tables 3, 4**). However, White's saline also works well and recently we have used osmic acid in distilled water combined with 1% potassium ferrocyanide *(21)*. Osmium-ferrocyanide is very useful, particularly if the sample has been in glutaraldehyde for a long time (**Table 5**). It provides a nearly selective stain for glycogen and preserves the

lipid bilayer structure of membrane better than other fixatives. Unfortunately, it influences the stability of dense bodies negatively, and many are extracted during dehydration and embedding. Clearly, one has to make a choice, depending on what aspects of platelet structure are of most interest.

References

1. Lee, P. Y. H. (1988) in pursuit of platelets—the third element of blood. *Pharos Alpha Omega Honor Med. Hon. Soc.* **51,** 8–13.
2. Robb-Smith, A. H. T. (1967) Why the platelets were discovered. *Br. J. Haematol.* **13,** 618–637.
3. Clay, R. S. and Court, T. H. (1932) *The History of the Microscope.* Charles Griffin & Co., London, p. 20.
4. Donné, A. (1842) De l'origine des globules du sang, de leur mode de formation et de leur fin. *CR Seances Acad. Sci.* **14,** 366–368.
5. Howell, W. H. (1884) The new morphological element of the blood. *Science* **3,** 46–49.
6. Bizzozero, J. (1882) Uber einen formestandtheil de saugethierblutes und die bedeutung derselben fur die thrombose und blutgerinnung uberhaupt. *Centralbl. Med. Wissensch.* **20,** 17–20.
7. Bizzozero, J. (1983) D'un nouvel element morphologique de sang et de son importance dans la thrombose et dans la coagulation. *Arch. Ital. Biol.* **2,** 345–362; (1982) **3,** 94–121.
8. Wolpers, C. and Ruska, H. (1939) Strukturuntersuchungen zur blutgerinnung. *Klinische Wochenschrift* **23,** 1077–1081; 1111–1117.
9. David-Ferreira, J. F. (1964) The blood platelet: electron microscopic studies. *Int. Rev. Cytol.* **55,** 89–103.
10. Rebuck, J. W., Riddle, J. M., Johnson, S. A., Monto, R. W., and Sturrock, R. M. (1959) Contributions of electron microscopy to the study of blood platelets. *Proceeding of the Third Conference on Platelets.* Detroit, MI, pp. 2–22.
11. Sabatini, D. D., Bensch, K. G., and Barnett, R. S. (1962) Preservation of ultrastructure and enzymatic activity by aldehyde fixation. *Anatom. Rec.* **142,** 274–283.
12. White, J. G. and Krivit, W. (1965) Fine structural localization of adenosine triphosphosphatase in human platelets and other blood cells. *Blood* **26,** 554–568.
13. White, J. G. (1971) Platelet morphology. In *The Circulating Platelet* (Johnson, S. A., ed.), Academic Press, New York, pp. 45–121.
14. White, J. G. (1971) The ultrastructural cytochemistry and physiology of blood platelets. In *The Platelet* (Mostafi, F. K. and Brinkhous, K. M., eds.), Williams and Wilkins, Baltimore, MD, pp. 83–115.
15. Wood, J. G. (1965) Electron microscopic localization of 5-hydroxytryptamine (5-HT). *Texas Reports on Biology and Medicine* **23,** 828–837.
16. Behnke, O. (1996) Incomplete microtubules observed in mammalian blood platelets during microtubule polymerization. *J. Cell Biol.* **34,** 697–701.
17. White, J. G. and Krivit, W. (1967) An ultrastructural basis for the shape changes induced by chilling. *Blood* **30,** 625–635.
18. Tang, S. S. and Frojmovic, M. M. (1977) The effects of pCO2 and pH on drug-induced platelet sphering and aggregation for human and rabbit platelet-rich plasma. *Thromb. Res.* **10,** 135–145.
19. O'Brien, J. R. and Woodhouse, M. A. (1968) Platelets: their size, shape and stickiness in citro: degranulation and propinquity. *Exper. Biol. Med.* Karger, Basel **3,** 90–102.

20. White, J. G. (1968) Fine structural alterations induced in platelets by adenosine diphosphate. *Blood* **31,** 604–622.
21. Karnovsky, M. J. (1971) Use of ferrocyanide reduced osmium terroxide in electron microscopy. American Society of Cell Bioliogy, Annual Meeting, New Orleans.
22. White, J. G. (1971) Platelet Morphology. In *The Circulating Platelet* (Johnson, S. E., ed.), Academic Press, New York, 45–121.
23. White, J. G. (1971) The ultrastructural cytochemistry and physiology of blood platelets. In *The Platelet* (Mostafi, F. K. and Brinkhous, K. M., eds.), Williams and Wilkins, Baltimore, MD, 873–915.
24. Breton-Gorius, J. and Guichard, J. (1975) Two different types of granules in mega-karyocytes and platelets as revealed by the diaminobenzidine reaction. *J. Micros. Biol.* **23,** 197–202.
25. Bentfield, M. E. and Bainton, D. F. (1975) Cytochemical localization of lysosomal enzymes in rat megakaryocytes and platelets. *J. Clin. Invest.* **56,** 1635–1639.
26. White, J. G. (1969) The dense bodies of human platelets: inherent electron opacity of serotonin storage organelles. *Blood* **33,** 598–606.
27. White, J. G. and Escolar, G. (1993) Current concepts of platelet membrane response to surface activation. *Platelets* **4,** 176–189.
28. White, J. G. and Conard, W. J. (1973) The fine structure of freeze-fractured blood platelets. *Am. J. Pathol.* **70,** 45–56.
29. White, J. G. and Clawson, C. C. (1980) Biostructure of blood platelets. *Ultrastruct. Pathol.* **1,** 533.
30. White, J. G. and Clawson, C. C. (1980) The surface-connected canalicular system of blood platelets-A fenestrated membrane system. *Am. J. Pathol.* **101,** 353.
31. Breton-Gorius, J. and Guichard, J. (1972) Ultrastructural localization of peroxidase activity in human platelets and megakaryocytes. *Am. J. Pathol.* **66,** 277–286.

5

Platelet Aggregation

Turbidimetric Measurements

Gavin E. Jarvis

1. Introduction

Of all the functional responses of platelets, aggregation is probably the mostly widely investigated. This is for two main reasons. First, the pathophysiological processes of most interest to medical scientists studying platelets are hemostasis and arterial thrombosis: the formation of hemostatic plugs and occlusive thrombi. As both of these events directly involve the clumping of platelets, aggregation presents itself to us as a functional response of singular clinical relevance. This is reflected in the fact that antiplatelet and antithrombotic drugs are characterized essentially as antiaggregatory agents. Whether this emphasis on aggregation is justified is a subject for another occasion; however, the central role of aggregometry in the academic study of platelet function and the pharmaceutical development of novel therapeutic agents is undeniable.

Second, the development of the technique of turbidimetric aggregometry has greatly facilitated the investigation of platelet aggregation. Turbidimetric (or optical) aggregometers can be found in many clinical hematology laboratories and probably every platelet laboratory throughout the world. It is this technique that is the subject of this chapter. This combination of pathophysiological significance and methodological ease has contributed to making turbidimetric aggregometry the *sine qua non* of platelet research.

1.1. Basic Principles

Turbidimetric aggregometry in its modern form was initially described in the 1960s *(1,2)*. The basic principle of the technique is simple. Light is passed through a stirred turbid suspension of platelets. The presence of the platelets in suspension causes the light to be scattered such that a reduced proportion of the light passes directly through the platelet suspension unobstructed. The amount of transmitted light is recorded and provides a measure of the optical density of the platelet suspension. On addition of a

From: *Methods in Molecular Biology, vol. 272:*
Platelets and Megakaryocytes, Vol. 1: Functional Assays
Edited by: J. M. Gibbins and M. P. Mahaut-Smith © Humana Press Inc., Totowa, NJ

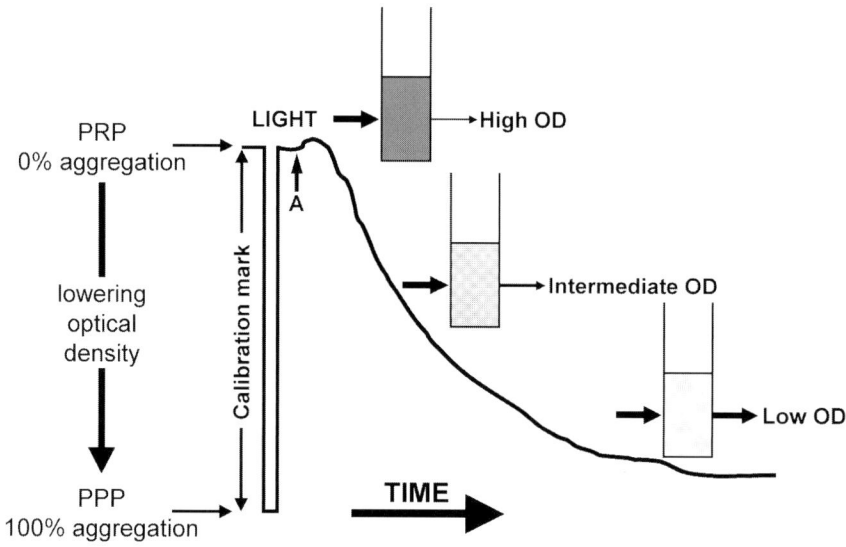

Fig. 1. Diagram of a typical turbidimetric aggregometry trace. The unstimulated suspension of platelet-rich plasma (PRP) has a relatively high optical density (OD), which represents 0% aggregation. Following addition of the agonist (A) the platelets aggregate, allowing more light to pass through the suspension of platelets and resulting in a reduction in the optical density. Autologous platelet-poor plasma (PPP) provides the measured optical density equivalent to 100% aggregation as indicated by the calibration mark. The transient increase in optical density that is typically observed following addition of the agonist is commonly attributed to the phenomenon of platelet shape change.

proaggregatory stimulus, the platelets form clumps, as a result of which the amount of light that is scattered is reduced until it passes mostly unobstructed through the platelet suspension (**Fig. 1**). Hence, as the platelets aggregate, the optical density of the suspension is reduced. It is immediately apparent that this technique is dependent on using a preparation of platelets through which light will pass, such as platelet-rich plasma or a washed or gel-filtered platelet preparation (*see* Chapter 2 on platelet preparation). Thus, this technique cannot be used for measuring platelet aggregation in whole blood, as the presence of the erythrocytes obscures the transmission of the light through the platelet medium.

1.2. Optical Density and Aggregation

In earlier studies, platelet aggregation was measured in terms of absolute optical density (2); however, more typically, output from turbidimetric aggregometers is expressed in percentage terms. This is achieved by calibrating the aggregometer in such a way that the optical density of the unstimulated basal platelet suspension (e.g., platelet-rich plasma) represents 0% aggregation, while the optical density of the medium in which the platelets are suspended without any platelets present (e.g., platelet-poor plasma) represents 100% aggregation (*see* **Fig. 1**). The simplicity of this process and the familiarity of the percentage scale can seduce the investigator into believing that the quantitative output of the aggregometer is a straightforward indicator of the extent of actual platelet aggregation. However, it is important to realize that turbidimetric aggregometry measures the optical density of platelet suspensions; therefore, so-called 50% aggregation is really a 50% reduction in optical density, relative to the platelet-rich plasma (0%) and the platelet-poor plasma (100%). An appreciation of the relationship between optical density and actual aggregate formation is therefore desirable for subsequent interpretation of data. Unfortunately, despite the apparent simplicity of the technique, this relationship is far from straightforward *(3)*.

1.3. Factors That Influence the Optical Density of Platelet Suspensions

A full account of this relationship is beyond the scope of this text; however, it is worth noting that the optical density of a suspension of platelets will be determined by the concentration, shape, size, and internal architecture of the platelets, and the composition and stirring rate of the suspending medium *(4,5)*. The extent of the absolute and relative changes in optical density of a suspension of platelets following the addition of an activatory stimulus will potentially depend on all these factors, and even on the make and model of the instrument employed *(6)*. Not only aggregation, but also the change of shape of a resting platelet from a biconvex disk to a sphere, and subsequent pseudopod formation, will result in changes in optical density *(7–9)*, as will the release of platelet contents present in the cytoplasm *(10,11,11a)*.

Numerous studies have been conducted to investigate how the sizes and numbers of platelet aggregates are related to measured optical density *(3,5,12)*. An important and consistent conclusion is that the turbidimetric aggregometer is very insensitive to the formation of microaggregates, such that the presence of aggregates comprising 2–8 platelets is typically undetectable by changes in optical density *(3,5,8)*. In fact, it has been claimed that turbidimetric aggregometry is insensitive to the formation of any aggregates that cannot be detected with the naked eye *(13)*. Methods that detect aggregation by measuring the reduction in the single-platelet count (*see* Chapter 6) are much more sensitive to the formation of microaggregates and clearly indicate that substantial microaggregate formation can occur before any indication of aggregation is manifest using a turbidimetric aggregometer *(14)*.

The complexity of the relationship between platelet responses and turbidity is most apparent in relation to small increases and decreases in optical density. Small changes can result as a consequence of shape change, release of platelet granules, and aggregation *(12)*. Although the small increase in optical density frequently observed immediately following platelet activation is typically attributed to platelet shape change *(15,16)*, it has also been shown that the formation of small platelet aggregates can result, paradoxically, in an increase in turbidity *(12,13,17)*. Despite this, the substantial reduction in optical density (from 0% to 100%) measured by the aggregometer is most obviously associated with the formation of large and increasingly dense platelet aggregates *(3)*.

1.4. Mechanisms of Aggregation

The molecular basis for aggregation is the conversion of the platelet surface $\alpha_{IIb}\beta_3$ integrin (also known as GPIIbIIIa) from a conformational state with low affinity for fibrinogen to one with high affinity for fibrinogen. Since fibrinogen is a bipolar molecule, it can bind simultaneously to two integrin complexes, as a result of which it cross-links activated platelets, causing them to aggregate *(18,19)*. The term "aggregation" is most commonly used to refer to this process of $\alpha_{IIb}\beta_3$-mediated platelet clump formation.

However, other molecular mechanisms exist that can cause platelets to adhere to each other. For example, addition of ristocetin to platelet-rich plasma causes clumping as a result of a von Willebrand factor (vWF)-mediated cross-linking of platelets *(20,21)*. Unlike $\alpha_{IIb}\beta_3$-mediated aggregation, this process is not dependent on metabolically active intracellular processes but is a result of the binding of vWF to GPIb on the platelet surface, which causes passive cross-linking of platelets. Ristocetin has its effect by altering the conformation of the vWF such that it will bind GPIb. The response to ristocetin is frequently referred to as agglutination, in order to indicate that the process is metabolically passive, and to distinguish it from the metabolically active process of $\alpha_{IIb}\beta_3$-mediated aggregation. However, it is important to note that there are no definitive characteristic features of the trace recordings of ristocetin-induced agglutination that enable the phenomenon to be distinguished from metabolically active aggregation using a turbidimetric aggregometer.

Platelet clumping can also arise as a result of thrombin-induced conversion of fibrinogen to fibrin and the subsequent trapping of the platelets in the fibrin mesh *(11a)*. Clearly, this phenomenon is also not dependent on a metabolically active platelet response and has been observed not only with platelets but also with inert latex particles *(22)*.

Therefore, it is important to stress that turbidimetric aggregometers measure changes in optical density, whatever the underlying phenomena and molecular mechanisms responsible.

1.5. Indices of Platelet Aggregation

The output from a turbidimetric aggregometer comes in the form of a real-time trace recording, which can be captured either by a simple paper chart recorder or by computer software systems that are usually designed for specific platelet aggregometers. These recordings encapsulate information not only about the extent of the response at any given moment, but also about the kinetics of both aggregation and disaggregation. The distillation of this information into one or two numerical indices inevitably discards much potentially useful information that is generated by the aggregometer.

Numerical indices that are frequently used to report aggregation responses include the rate and extent of the response, and the delay from application of the activating stimulus to the onset of the response. The final extent of aggregation is clearly dependent on the period of time for which the assay is allowed to proceed, unless a clear plateau is reached. Perhaps the most commonly reported measure, though, is the maximum extent of aggregation. However, in cases in which there is an obviously biphasic response to a stimulus, the choice of this index can result in values that are substantially time-dependent and therefore potentially misleading. In addition, measurements of maximum extent will not distinguish between situations in which there is significant disaggregation and those in which there is no reversibility at all. Furthermore, when there is no reversibility in the response, the maximum extent of aggregation will be as dependent on the assay time as the final extent of aggregation.

The initial rate of aggregation is typically reported as a function of the maximum initial slope of the trace recording (rather than a first-order rate constant) and may be considered to more accurately reflect the magnitude of the initial stimulus to the platelet, since the extent of aggregation is frequently an all-or-nothing response and can be dependent on secondary activatory phenomena, such as the generation of thromboxane A_2 and the release of ADP *(23)*. In addition, the initial rate of aggregation is not dependent on the period of time for which the assay is allowed to proceed, provided that the initial rapid rate of aggregation has obviously slowed down.

The choice of aggregation index can have a significant bearing on the conclusions drawn about the pharmacology and physiology of the platelet. For example, it has been shown that the initial rate of ADP-induced platelet aggregation is heavily dependent on the degree of activation of the $P2Y_1$ receptor, whereas the final extent of the ADP-induced aggregation response is a function of the activation of the $P2Y_{12}$ (formerly known as P_{27}) receptor *(24)*. A failure to appreciate the significance of different measurement indices could easily lead an investigator into drawing erroneous conclusions about the physiological significance of platelet stimuli and their receptors.

1.6. Reproducibility of Aggregation Data

In general terms, turbidimetric aggregometry is a robust and reproducible technique, which makes it a valuable tool in both clinical and basic science laboratories. However, like all scientific methods, there are many significant sources of variability that the investigator must appreciate in order to interpret the raw data in a reasonable and intelligent manner *(25,26)*. First, it is well established that differences between donors can be reflected in the responsiveness of their platelets to a range of agonists. Differences in age, sex, lifestyle choices such as smoking and alcohol consumption, exercise and fitness, health status, and concurrent medication can all influence results *(27–31)*. Even the time of day at which blood is drawn from patients or volunteers can have a significant impact on subsequent aggregation results. In patient studies, it must also be recognized that certain conditions may influence platelet responsiveness.

Since aggregation concentration-response relationships are typically quite steep (particularly for the extent of aggregation), unless the provoking concentration of an agonist is carefully selected and adequately controlled, differences in responsiveness may be inadvertently ascribed to a particular treatment regime (either ex vivo or in vitro) when in fact they could simply be due to small and essentially random variations in platelet sensitivity or agonist concentrations. Problems with interpretation of data are less likely when the relevant responses range from "almost complete" to "almost no" aggregation. However, when the differences concerned are in the order of 10, 20, or even 30%, then a great deal more caution ought to be exercised, and any conclusions supported by appropriate statistical analyses.

2. Materials

Many of the materials and reagents required to perform turbidimetric aggregometry are supplied specifically for that purpose and can be purchased from specialist companies.

Clearly, the most important piece of equipment is the aggregometer itself; these are available from a variety of sources. The choice of instrument will depend on many factors, including the proposed use of the machine, the circumstances of that use, and of course the cost.

In addition to the aggregometer, a paper chart recorder or computerized data capture system is usually required, although some aggregometers are manufactured with built in paper and computerized output systems.

In addition to the aggregometer and chart recorder, the basic materials required for aggregometry are as follows:

Cuvets—These are usually made of siliconized glass, although polystyrene ones can be used. They are frequently supplied for use with specific makes and models of aggregometers.
Stir bars—These are also usually supplied for use with specific cuvets and aggregometers.
Gel-loading tips—Although any number of means can be found for adding agents to stirred samples of platelets, disposable gel-loading tips are both convenient and easy to use.

3. Methods

Platelet preparations for use in turbidimetric aggregometry must be able to transmit light. Hence, platelets need to be in platelet-rich plasma (PRP) or a washed or gel-filtered platelet preparation. Details of how to prepare platelets can be found in Chapters 1 and 2, vol. 1. Briefly, anticoagulated human blood can be centrifuged for 15–20 min at approx $200–250g$ and the platelet-rich supernatant removed. In addition, it is necessary to prepare a sample of the suspending medium without any platelets present to serve as a 100% aggregation standard. When PRP is used to measure platelet aggregation, then platelet-poor plasma (PPP) can easily be prepared from autologous blood for this purpose (*see* **Note 1**).

Once the platelets are prepared, it is possible to proceed immediately to the assay; however, it is frequently recommended to allow the platelets to rest for approx 30 min in the case of PRP; for washed platelets, an adequate period of time (1–2 h) has to elapse to allow responsiveness to return when prostacyclin has been used during the washing procedure. Fresh platelet preparations can be used for aggregation studies for several hours, often for as long as 6 to 8 h. However, this period of time will vary depending on various factors, including the species and preparation of platelets used. It is also recognized that the responsiveness of platelets can change over time *(32–34)*; therefore, it is both essential to use appropriate control measurements to identify any significant time-dependent changes, and desirable to complete any investigative work as quickly as possible once the platelets are prepared.

3.1. Choosing a Platelet Preparation

The decision to use platelet-rich plasma or washed platelets in aggregometry studies will be determined by a variety of factors, including the choice of agonist, subsequent investigations, availability of blood samples, and so forth. However, it is undoubtedly the case that different preparations of platelets can produce different results, and other factors, such as the choice of anticoagulant (*see* Chapters 1 and 2, vol. 1) or the detailed methodology of washed platelet preparation, can also have a significant impact on results. A few considerations are discussed further below.

The principle mechanism by which platelet aggregation is mediated is through the binding of fibrinogen to activated $\alpha_{IIb}\beta_3$ integrins. When aggregation is measured in PRP, there is adequate fibrinogen in the medium to easily support aggregation. However, in washed platelet preparations, the levels of fibrinogen are much lower and may not be able to sustain aggregation, despite activation of the platelets. This is rarely a problem when the platelet agonist in use is potent (e.g., thrombin or collagen) since this will induce release of fibrinogen from platelet alpha granules; nevertheless, even in these cases, addition of exogenous fibrinogen can significantly increase the rate of aggregation of the platelets. However, when the agonist is not sufficiently potent (e.g., ADP, 5-HT, epinephrine) no detectable aggregation may occur in the absence of added fibrinogen. Hence, the desirability of adding exogenous fibrinogen to the platelets must be considered *(35)*. A concentration of 0.2–2.0 mg/mL fibrinogen is usually adequate to support ADP-induced platelet aggregation in washed platelets *(36,37)*.

ADP will consistently induce aggregation of human platelets in PRP. However, the nature of the response can vary depending on the choice of anticoagulant. Citrate, the most commonly used anticoagulant, acts by reducing the calcium concentration sufficiently to prevent thrombin generation, but not so much as to prevent the function of the $\alpha_{IIb}\beta_3$ integrin. In citrated PRP, ADP will induce both aggregation and the generation of thromboxane A_2 (TxA_2), which further activates the platelets. However, this response to ADP is contingent on the abnormally low levels of calcium, and under circumstances in which physiological calcium levels are present (e.g., when an anticoagulant such as heparin or hirudin is employed), ADP does not cause TxA_2 generation *(23)*.

In washed platelets, the aggregation response to ADP is exquisitely dependent on the precise details of the protocol for platelet preparation *(35)*. For example, washed platelets prepared according to the method of Watson et al. *(38)* do not aggregate at all in response to ADP, those prepared according to the methods of Gear *(37)* and Cazenave et al. *(39)* manifest a consistent and reversible response to ADP *(40)*, whereas those prepared using the method of Humphries et al. *(36)* respond in a reproducible and sustained manner. It is not the purpose of this text to explore the possible reasons for these differences, nor to imply that any one preparation is better than another; rather, the intention is simply to impress on the minds of platelet researchers that the choice of experimental conditions is not a trivial matter, but requires appropriate care and consideration.

3.2. Aggregometry Protocols

Turbidimetric platelet aggregometry is technically very straightforward. Although the precise details of how to perform the assay vary depending on the aggregometer being used, the basic principles are in all cases the same (*see* **Note 8**). The following steps outline the basic procedure for conducting the assay.

1. Accurately pipet a fixed volume of the platelet suspension into a cuvet. The volume required will vary depending on the aggregometer and the circumstances of the experiment, but typically will be from 250–1000 µL.

2. Add a stir bar to the cuvet. The stir speed of the aggregometer can often be set manually, although not in all cases. A stir speed of 1000 rpm is frequently used (*see* **Note 2**).

3. Ensure that the aggregometer is warmed up and at the required temperature. Most aggregometers measure aggregation at 37°C.

4. Incubate the platelets for several minutes at the final temperature at which the assay is to be run. This is usually 37°C and many aggregometers have incubation wells specifically for this purpose (*see* **Note 3**).

5. At this stage it will be necessary to calibrate the aggregometer. Calibration procedures vary depending on the equipment. Some aggregometers produce a trace output with a superimposed time and calibration grid, whereas others produce a single calibration deflection for subsequent reference. However, the principles of calibration are the same in all cases. A cuvet containing the suspending medium (usually either platelet-poor plasma or water) is used as a fixed standard for optical density representing a theoretical 100% aggregation. In some cases the PPP is left in a single recording well for the duration of the experiment. In other cases the PPP has to be set individually prior to each individual aggregation measurement (*see* **Notes 4**, **5**).

6. Calibration of the 0% aggregation reference point is usually achieved using the assay sample itself. Even small differences in platelet count can influence the optical density of a platelet suspension, so it is important to recalibrate the 0% aggregation point for each individual measurement. With some aggregometers, it is impossible to run the aggregation assay without doing this—in other cases it can be (accidentally) omitted.

7. Once the calibration procedure is complete, there should be an observable flat and slightly noisy trace. It is a good idea to leave the trace to run for 30–60 s to ensure that there is no spontaneous aggregation (*see* **Note 6**).

8. Addition of aggregating stimuli is usually in the form of soluble agonists in small volumes. Agonist dilutions are typically 1:50 or 1:100. If larger volumes are used, then this can produce a dilution artifact in the trace. Smaller volumes can of course be used; however, difficulties in quantitative accuracy are more likely to be encountered with addition volumes of 1 μL or less (*see* **Note 7**).

9. Aggregation will proceed as indicated by the trace recording following addition of the agonist. The period of time for which the assay is run will depend on the precise experimental circumstances and is at the discretion of the investigator. However, 6 min is a period that is frequently used for clinical aggregometry assays, and most aggregation will be complete by this time.

10. When the assay is complete, the trace recording can be stopped. Calculation of the rate and extent of aggregation is carried out manually or electronically, depending on the equipment used. Manual calculation of results is straightforward and simply involves relating the agonist-induced deflection in the trace to the calibration markings of the trace. Calculation of the rate of aggregation also depends on the speed of the chart recording device, which should be noted.

4. Notes

1. Where the supply of blood is limited, PPP can be prepared from the unwanted red cells that are sedimented out following the initial centrifugation step of the isolation of platelet-rich plasma.

2. Platelet aggregation will not take place unless the sample is stirred. If a stir bar is not added to the cuvet or if the stirring mechanism on the aggregometer is disabled, then the aggregation response will not occur. It is possible to identify a cuvet to which the stir bar

has not been added since there will not be the usual "noisy" appearance to the trace. In addition, the trace will often drift up and down in the absence of stirring.

3. As a technique, measurement of optical density is not greatly influenced by temperature. However, platelet function is probably best measured at a physiologically relevant temperature whenever possible. Although it has been reported that cooling platelets can induce premature activation *(2)*, other investigators have successfully maintained functional preparations of washed platelets for up to 6 h by keeping them at temperatures of approx 4°C *(36)*. Keeping platelets at room temperature prior to use is usually acceptable, although it has also been suggested that this can activate platelets *(41,42)* and therefore, some investigators prefer to keep them at 37°C. Obviously, when this is the case, pre-incubation of the platelets prior to running the assay is less important.

4. Some aggregometers have covers with which to occlude light from the cuvets when the aggregation is measured. In these models it is important to shut these covers, as external sources of light can interfere with measurement of aggregation and movement across the aggregometer can produce artifactual deflections in the trace recordings.

5. Since the sample of PPP used is the same throughout the course of an experiment, and will therefore influence each recording, it is essential that it is prepared fastidiously. If, for example, not all the platelets are centrifuged from the plasma, or if the platelet pellet is disturbed, resulting in some platelets remaining in the PPP, then the 100% aggregation reference point will be calibrated incorrectly. In this case, the percentage aggregation measured will be artifactually high and aggregation values of greater than 100% may be obtained. In addition, it is essential to use platelet-poor plasma as the 100% reference when using platelet-rich plasma as the assay sample. Although if water is used instead, reproducible results will be obtained, aggregation values obtained will be lower than would be observed using PPP, since the optical density of PPP is greater than that of water.

6. *Spontaneous aggregation* is the name given to the phenomenon of platelets aggregating prior to addition of any activating stimulus. Since platelets do not aggregate efficiently until they are stirred, such a problem may arise because of the presence in the platelet preparation of an agonist, manifest only when the sample is added to the stirring assay well. Spontaneous aggregation can also occur as a result of preactivation of platelets, which can occur during blood sampling and platelet preparation. Different preparations of platelets are more predisposed to spontaneous aggregation than others; for example, heparinized platelets are more prone to this problem than citrated platelets.

7. Once in the aggregometer assay well, the platelet suspension is completely hidden from view. It is, of course, essential to ensure that the agonist is added completely and directly into the platelet suspension. Disposable gel-loading tips are ideal for extending to the bottom of most aggregometer cuvets.

8. Although use of a proprietary aggregometer is the most common way of performing turbidimetric aggregometry, it is possible to use microplate methodologies that also exploit the change in optical density of aggregating platelets. Such methods have the advantage of allowing the acquisition of large quantities of data simultaneously and rapidly *(43)*.

References

1. Born, G. V. R. (1962) Aggregation of blood platelets by adenosine diphosphate and its reversal. *Nature* **194,** 927–929.
2. Born, G. V. R. and Cross, M. J. (1963) The aggregation of blood platelets. *J. Physiol.* **168,** 178–195.

3. Born, G. V. and Hume, M. (1967) Effects of the numbers and sizes of platelet aggregates on the optical density of plasma. *Nature* **215,** 1027–1029.

4. Latimer, P., Born, G. V., and Michal, F. (1977) Application of light-scattering theory to the optical effects associated with the morphology of blood platelets. *Arch. Biochem. Biophys.* **180,** 151–159.

5. Thompson, N. T., Scrutton, M. C., and Wallis, R. B. (1986) Particle volume changes associated with light transmittance changes in the platelet aggregometer: dependence upon aggregating agent and effectiveness of stimulus. *Thromb. Res.* **41,** 615–626.

6. Latimer, P. (1983) Blood platelet aggregometer: predicted effects of aggregation, photometer geometry, and multiple scattering. *Applied Optics* **22,** 1136–1143.

7. Michal, F. and Born, G. V. (1971) Effect of the rapid shape change of platelets on the transmission and scattering of light through plasma. *Nat. New Biol.* **231,** 220–222.

8. Frojmovic, M. M. and Panjwani, R. (1975) Blood cell structure-function studies: light transmission and attenuation coefficients of suspensions of blood cells and model particles at rest and with stirring. *J. Lab. Clin. Med.* **86,** 326–343.

9. Patscheke, H., Dubler, D., Deranleau, D., and Luscher, E. F. (1984) Optical shape change analysis in stirred and unstirred human platelet suspensions. A comparison of aggregometric and stopped-flow turbidimetric measurements. *Thromb. Res.* **33,** 341–353.

10. Hugues, J. (1971) What does the optical platelet aggregation test actually measure? Introductory remarks. *Acta Med. Scand. Suppl.* **525,** 39–40.

11. Milton, J. G. and Frojmovic, M. M. (1983) Turbidometric evaluations of platelet activation: relative contributions of measured shape change, volume, and early aggregation. *J. Pharmacol. Methods* **9,** 101–115.

11a. Jarvis, G. E., Atkinson, B. T., Frampton, J., and Watson, S. P. (2003) Thrombin-induced conversion of fibrinogen to fibrin results in rapid platelet trapping which is not dependent on platelet activation or GPIb. *Br. J. Pharmacol.* **138,** 574–583.

12. Kitek, A. and Breddin, K. (1980) Optical density variations and microscopic observations in the evaluation of platelet shape change and microaggregate formation. *Thromb. Haemost.* **44,** 154–158.

13. Malinski, J. A. and Nelsestuen, G. L. (1986) Relationship of turbidity to the stages of platelet aggregation. *Biochim. Biophys. Acta* **882,** 177–182.

14. Frojmovic, M. M., Milton, J. G., and Duchastel, A. (1983) Microscopic measurements of platelet aggregation reveal a low ADP-dependent process distinct from turbidometrically measured aggregation. *J. Lab. Clin. Med.* **101,** 964–976.

15. Born, G. V. (1970) Observations on the change in shape of blood platelets brought about by adenosine diphosphate. *J. Physiol.* **209,** 487–511.

16. McLean, J. R. and Veloso, H. (1967) Change of shape without aggregation caused by ADP in rabbit platelets at low pH. *Life Sci.* **6,** 1983–1986.

17. Maurer-Spurej, E. and Devine, D. V. (2001) Platelet aggregation is not initiated by platelet shape change. *Lab. Invest.* **81,** 1517–1525.

18. Leung, L. and Nachman, R. (1986) Molecular mechanisms of platelet aggregation. *Annu. Rev. Med.* **37,** 179–186.

19. Zucker, M. B. and Nachmias, V. T. (1985) Platelet activation. *Arteriosclerosis* **5,** 2–18.

20. Howard, M. A. and Firkin, B. G. (1971) Ristocetin—a new tool in the investigation of platelet aggregation. *Thromb. Diath. Haemorrh.* **26,** 362–369.

21. Cooper, H. A., Mason, R. G., and Brinkhous, K. M. (1976) The platelet: membrane and surface reactions. *Annu. Rev. Physiol.* **38,** 501–535.

22. Chao, F. C., Tullis, J. L., Conneely, G. S., and Lawler, J. W. (1976) Aggregation of platelets and inert particles induced by thrombin. *Thromb. Haemost.* **35,** 717–736.

23. Mustard, J. F., Perry, D. W., Kinlough-Rathbone, R. L., and Packham, M. A. (1975) Factors responsible for ADP-induced release reaction of human platelets. *Am. J. Physiol.* **228,** 1757–1765.

24. Jarvis, G. E., Humphries, R. G., Robertson, M. J., and Leff, P. (2000) ADP can induce aggregation of human platelets via both $P2Y_1$ and P_{2T} receptors. *Br. J. Pharmacol.* **129,** 275–282.

25. Harrison, M. J., Emmons, P. R., and Mitchell, J. R. (1967) The variability of human platelet aggregation. *J. Atheroscler. Res.* **7,** 197–205.

26. Tiffany, M. L. (1983) Technical considerations for platelet aggregation and related problems. *Crit. Rev. Clin. Lab. Sci.* **19,** 27–69.

27. Taylor, R. R., Sturm, M., Vandongen, R., Strophair, J., and Beilin, L. J. (1987) Whole blood platelet aggregation is not affected by cigarette smoking but is sex-related. *Clin. Exp. Pharmacol. Physiol.* **14,** 665–671.

28. Fusegawa, Y., Goto, S., Handa, S., Kawada, T., and Ando, Y. (1999) Platelet spontaneous aggregation in platelet-rich plasma is increased in habitual smokers. *Thromb. Res.* **93,** 271–278.

29. Torres Duarte, A. P., Dong, Q. S., Young, J., Abi-Younes, S., and Myers, A. K. (1995) Inhibition of platelet aggregation in whole blood by alcohol. *Thromb. Res.* **78,** 107–115.

30. Piret, A., Niset, G., Depiesse, E., Wyns, W., Boeynaems, J. M., Poortmans, J., et al. (1990) Increased platelet aggregability and prostacyclin biosynthesis induced by intense physical exercise. *Thromb. Res.* **57,** 685–695.

31. Davis, R. B., Boyd, D. G., McKinney, M. E., and Jones, C. C. (1990) Effects of exercise and exercise conditioning on blood platelet function. *Med. Sci. Sports Exerc.* **22,** 49–53.

32. Rossi, E. C. and Louis, G. (1975) A time-dependent increase in the responsiveness of platelet-rich plasma to epinephrine. *J. Lab. Clin. Med.* **85,** 300–306.

33. Taylor, R. R., Strophair, J., Sturm, M., Vandongen, R., and Beilin, L. J. (1988) Time dependence of whole blood aggregation in response to platelet activating factor (PAF). *Thromb. Haemost.* **59,** 162–163.

34. Coller, B. S., Franza, B. R., Jr., and Gralnick, H. R. (1976) The pH dependence of quantitative ristocetin-induced platelet aggregation: theoretical and practical implications—a new device for maintenance of platelet-rich plasma pH. *Blood* **47,** 841–854.

35. Kinlough-Rathbone, R. L., Mustard, J. F., Packham, M. A., Perry, D. W., Reimers, H. J., and Cazenave, J. P. (1977) Properties of washed human platelets. *Thromb. Haemost.* **37,** 291–308.

36. Humphries, R. G., Tomlinson, W., Ingall, A. H., Cage, P. A., and Leff, P. (1994) FPL 66096: a novel, highly potent and selective antagonist at human platelet P2T-purinoceptors. *Br. J. Pharmacol.* **113,** 1057–1063.

37. Gear, A. R. (1982) Rapid reactions of platelets studied by a quenched-flow approach: aggregation kinetics. *J. Lab. Clin. Med.* **100,** 866–886.

38. Watson, S. P., Poole, A., and Asselin, J. (1995) Ethylene glycol bis(beta-aminoethyl ether)-N,N,N′,N′-tetraacetic acid (EGTA) and the tyrphostin ST271 inhibit phospholipase C in human platelets by preventing Ca^{2+} entry. *Mol. Pharmacol.* **47,** 823–830.

39. Cazenave, J. P., Hemmendinger, S., Beretz, A., Sutter-Bay, A., and Launay, J. (1983) Platelet aggregation: a tool for clinical investigation and pharmacological study. Methodology. *Ann. Biol. Clin. (Paris)* **41,** 167–179.

40. Gachet, C. (2001) ADP receptors of platelets and their inhibition. *Thromb. Haemost.* **86,** 222–232.

41. Maurer-Spurej, E., Pfeiler, G., Maurer, N., Lindner, H., Glatter, O., and Devine, D. V. (2001) Room temperature activates human blood platelets. *Lab. Invest.* **81,** 581–592.

42. Gear, A. R. (1981) Preaggregation reactions of platelets. *Blood* **58,** 477–490.

43. Salmon, D. M. (1996) Optimisation of platelet aggregometry utilising micotitreplate technology and integrated software. *Thromb. Res.* **84,** 213–216.

6

Platelet Aggregation in Whole Blood

Impedance and Particle Counting Methods

Gavin E. Jarvis

1. Introduction

Platelet aggregation and its measurement using the turbidimetric method were discussed in the previous chapter. Many of the same considerations relating to aggregometry that were raised there are equally valid in the context of this chapter and it is recommended that readers acquaint themselves with Chapter 5, vol. 1 prior to commencing this one.

1.1. Whole Blood Aggregometry

Turbidimetric aggregometry is probably the most commonly used technique for the measurement of platelet aggregation. However, it has certain drawbacks, perhaps the most obvious of which is that it needs to be carried out using a preparation of platelets capable of transmitting light, such as platelet-rich plasma (PRP) or washed platelets. It is not possible to use conventional turbidimetric methods for measuring platelet aggregation in whole blood, which may be considered more physiologically relevant than plasma or media such as modified Tyrode's solutions. Indeed, the functional responses of platelets to certain stimuli and drugs may be dependent on interactions with leukocytes and erythrocytes *(1)*, and therefore may not be identified in PRP or washed platelets. For example, it has been shown that endotoxin can induce activation of equine platelets in a manner that is dependent on the presence of leukocytes *(2)* and the effectiveness of dipyridamole as an antiplatelet agent is dependent on the presence of erythrocytes *(3)*.

The preparation of PRP or washed platelets requires significant manipulation of a whole blood sample, and can potentially introduce artifactual alterations in the platelets' functional properties. For example, the initial centrifugation step in preparing PRP may result in the loss of a proportion of larger platelets, resulting in a nonrepresentative population of platelets in the final preparation. Subsequent washing procedures can induce activation of platelets and influence their functional properties. Furthermore, such

From: *Methods in Molecular Biology, vol. 272:*
Platelets and Megakaryocytes, Vol. 1: Functional Assays
Edited by: J. M. Gibbins and M. P. Mahaut-Smith © Humana Press Inc., Totowa, NJ

procedures are time-consuming and demand that substantial quantities of blood be taken for the required purpose.

For these and other considerations *(4)*, the ability to measure platelet aggregation in whole blood can offer significant advantages under particular circumstances. In this chapter, two further techniques for investigating platelet aggregation will be described, both of which are applicable to whole blood measurements. These are impedance aggregometry and particle counting aggregometry *(5)*. As with turbidimetric aggregometry, the principles on which these techniques are based are relatively straightforward and an appreciation of them will help investigators to interpret data correctly and identify and control for any confounding influences in their experiments.

1.2. Impedance Aggregometry

Impedance aggregometry was initially described in 1980 by Cardinal and Flower *(6)*. Although this method can be used to measure aggregation in any preparation of platelets, it was developed specifically for use with whole blood and will be discussed with this application primarily in mind.

The method involves the insertion of a pair of palladium electrodes into a cuvet containing a stirred sample of whole blood, which is diluted 50:50 with a physiological buffer (e.g., phosphate-buffered saline). A current is passed across the electrodes through the blood, giving the electrodes a net charge. The platelets, which have a surface negative charge, rapidly form a monolayer on the positive electrode. Since the gap between the electrodes is the part of the electrical circuit where the resistance is greatest, when the platelets are activated and aggregate around the monolayer of platelets on the electrodes they increase the resistance within the circuit as a whole. The aggregometer measures the effect of the aggregating platelets on the total electrical resistance within the circuit (*see* **Fig. 1**).

When a direct current is used, the platelets preferentially accumulate around one electrode *(6)*. For this reason, an alternating current is used, so that the charge on each electrode rapidly and continuously changes. It is also for this reason that this method is known as impedance aggregometry, since impedance is the name given to the total electrical resistance within a circuit of specifically alternating rather than direct current. Therefore, as the platelets aggregate, the impedance of the circuit gradually increases. The changing impedance is recorded as a deflection of a trace using a conventional chart recorder or a computerized data capture system.

Many factors can affect the impedance of the circuit and can therefore influence the measurement made by the aggregometer:

1. As the distance between the electrodes increases, so will the impedance of the circuit. Although electrodes are made specifically for impedance aggregometry, it is essential that they be handled with great care to prevent any damage, which may result in a change in the consistency with which the impedance is measured.
2. Electrical currents flow more easily with higher temperature. As a result, this method is much more sensitive to changes in temperature than turbidimetric aggregometry and thermostatic control must therefore be accurate and reliable.

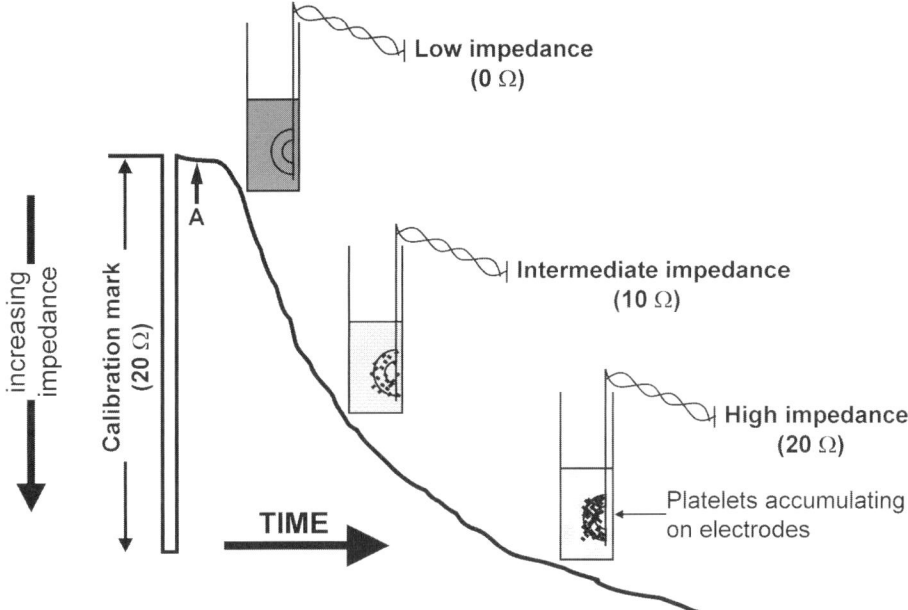

Fig. 1. Diagram of a typical impedance aggregometry trace. Once the platelets are activated, they begin to aggregate and accumulate around the electrodes. This causes an increase in the impedance of the current passed across the electrodes. The extent of aggregation can be quantified in ohms (Ω) by comparing the deflection of the trace with the calibration mark that represents 20 Ω. The rate of aggregation can be determined if the speed of the chart recorder is known.

3. Foreign bodies (e.g., small clots) present in the blood sample can affect the impedance measurement by becoming lodged between the electrodes. If this happens intermittently, this can result in a jumpy trace and interfere with platelet function.
4. Stirring is essential for efficient aggregation of platelets in suspension. However, impedance aggregometry is particularly dependent on smooth and consistent stirring in order to produce reproducible traces.
5. The cellular and electrolyte composition of the sample will also affect the results obtained with an impedance aggregometer. For example, differences in the hematocrit can result in variable impedance output *(7)*, and significant addition artifacts can also be produced by agonists that have different electrolytic properties to the sample as a whole.

Calibration of the impedance aggregometer is achieved by increasing the impedance across the circuit by a known amount and measuring the deflection that this produces on the recording device. This increase is usually fixed at 20 ohms (Ω). The relative size of the deflection induced by the 20 Ω change can be modified to maximize the size of deflection on the chart recorder caused by any subsequent platelet aggregation. With impedance aggregometry, the extent and rate of aggregation are therefore measured in ohms and ohms per unit time, respectively. There is no equivalent of the 100% aggregation represented by platelet-poor plasma with turbidimetric measurements. Supramaximal stimuli frequently result in aggregation values in the order of 20 to 30 Ω.

Impedance aggregometry is considered to be an insensitive technique for detecting platelet aggregates. Formation of aggregates in the sample will have no effect on the measured impedance unless those aggregates become attached to the electrodes. Small and transient aggregates are less likely to remain intact if they do become attached to the electrode because they would then have to withstand the additional shear forces that being held stationary in a stirred sample would inevitably generate. Furthermore, small numbers of attached platelets are unlikely to have a significant impact on the measured impedance in the circuit. Even responses of a few ohms are usually the result of the accumulation of small but visible quantities of platelets on the electrodes. However, as more platelets aggregate, the response becomes greater and maximal responses usually produce substantial aggregates on the electrodes. Therefore, impedance aggregometry is particularly insensitive to low levels of platelet activation and is not a useful technique for measuring the formation of microaggregates. By contrast, however, it is able to distinguish between variations in substantial stimuli that result in the production of different-sized platelet macroaggregates. This level of sensitivity in aggregate detection is in sharp contrast to the following method to be described, particle counting aggregometry.

Although impedance aggregometry is insensitive to the formation of microaggregates, the preservation of a physiological milieu can nevertheless result in the platelets in whole blood being more biologically sensitive to particular agonists. Aggregation responses may therefore still be detected at low concentrations of agonists, although it must be remembered that any aggregation detected by this method is inevitably substantial macroaggregate formation.

1.3. Particle Counting Aggregometry

Particle counting aggregometry is based on the principle that as platelets aggregate, the number of single particles present in the sample is reduced. Methods that exploit this phenomenon have been used by many investigators and have the advantage that specialized aggregometry equipment is not required, although for this same reason, many diverse protocols have been used. Fortunately, a full account of these is unnecessary. The specific method that will be described in this chapter is based on the one that has been developed in the laboratory of Professor Stan Heptinstall (University of Nottingham, UK) *(8–10)*.

In order to use this method, a means of counting cells in suspension is required. In theory, it is possible to use hemocytometers to count the platelets; however, the method is expedited by the use of automatic particle counters such as Coulter counters. Coulter counters work by drawing a fixed volume of a sample through a small aperture. As each particle passes through the aperture this causes a change in the electrical conductance of the aperture as a whole. This change is measured as a distinct voltage for each particle. The rapid voltage pulses caused by a stream of cells or particles enable a count, and therefore a final concentration of the sample, to be determined. In addition, each voltage pulse is proportional to the volume of fluid displaced by the particle. As a result, Coulter counters are able to provide detailed information about the size of the particles in the sample, and limits can be set on the sizes of particles to be counted. (This is done to prevent the counting of either very small or very large pieces of irrelevant debris.) Coulter counters do not distinguish between the shapes, colors, or densities of particles. Therefore, if two identical particles are inadvertently drawn through the aperture at the same time, the displaced volume will be double that which one alone would have caused. As a result, the counter will detect only one particle of double the volume rather than two of actual volume. Coulter counters report the size of particles in terms of volume or diameter. It is the displaced volume that affects the conductance, and the diameter readings that are produced are derived using simple calculations based on the assumption that the particle is a sphere.* Needless to say, this is not necessarily the case.

As platelets aggregate in response to an activating stimulus, they stick together to form ever-increasing sizes of aggregates until no single platelets remain. Performing a count on such a sample will clearly result in a very low value no different from that obtained using a buffer containing no cells. Thus, as the degree of aggregation in a sample increases, the platelet count falls. An aggregate that is visible to the naked eye is likely to contain many platelets, but a Coulter counter would not detect it at all with typical limit settings. However, a Coulter counter could detect microaggregates that contain two (or even three or four) platelets (although it will count this as one particle). Therefore, if all the platelets in a sample formed aggregates of two platelets per aggregate, which were measured by the Coulter counter, then the platelet count would be expected to fall by 50%. Such a degree of aggregation would almost certainly go undetected by a conventional turbidimetric aggregometer and an impedance aggregometer. Therefore, particle counting aggregometry is recognized as being much more sensitive to low levels of activation and to microaggregate formation than these other methods. However, it is also evident that the maximal aggregation detectable by this method is reached when all the platelets have been incorporated into aggregates of a relatively small size. Therefore, although particle counting aggregometry is very sensitive to variations in low levels of activation, it is completely insensitive to variations in high levels of activation, which are better detected by turbidimetric and impedance methods.

Low levels of activation of platelets frequently result in transient aggregation responses. The final platelet count then depends on the time at which the sample is taken after addition of the agonist. It is therefore essential to specify this time and, importantly, to stabilize the platelet aggregates in order to obtain comparable results between samples. In order to achieve this, the blood sample and the platelet aggre-

---

*For a sphere: $Volume = \dfrac{\pi \times Diameter^3}{6}$; $Diameter = \sqrt[3]{\dfrac{6 \times Volume}{\pi}}$

gates contained in it can be fixed. Methods of fixation vary considerably, and can be developed for particular circumstances. However, efficient methods can provide samples in which the platelet count remains stable for many hours and days, even if the cells settle out, are stored at variable temperatures, or even subjected to the rigors of the postal service (personal observation).

2. Materials
2.1. Impedance Aggregometry

1. Whole blood impedance aggregometer. As with turbidimetric aggregometry, the most important piece of equipment is the aggregometer itself, which, along with the specific materials and reagents required, is manufactured and supplied by specialist companies.
2. Chart recorder and/or computerized data capture system. Some models of impedance aggregometers generate a numerical readout of the extent of aggregation in ohms after a fixed time. However, it is recommended to still have a real-time trace in order to monitor the ongoing aggregation.
3. Impedance electrode assemblies. These are manufactured specifically for use with particular makes and models of aggregometers.
4. Polystyrene cuvets. These are designed to accommodate the electrode assembly.
5. Teflon-coated disposable magnetic stir bars. These are also designed to fit smoothly in the cuvets.
6. Magnet to remove the stir bars from the cuvets.
7. Phosphate-buffered saline (*see* **Note 1**).
8. Gel-loading tips. Although any number of means can be found for adding agents to stirred samples of platelets, disposable gel-loading tips are both convenient and easy to use.
9. Wash bottle containing distilled water, and waste beaker.
10. Clinical-waste disposal bin.
11. Soft disposable paper tissues.

2.2. Particle Counting Aggregometry

1. Particle counter. Any cell counting equipment can usually be adapted for particle counting aggregometry.
2. Fixative solution. The fixative should be freshly prepared in phosphate-buffered saline to give a pH of 7.4. It should contain 4.5 mM Na$_2$EDTA and 0.15% (w/v) formaldehyde. The fixative and sample are mixed in a ratio of 2:1, which results in a threefold dilution of the platelet count but also a rapid dispersion of the sample. Final concentrations in the fixed sample should be 3 mM Na$_2$EDTA and 0.1% (w/v) formaldehyde (*see* **Note 11**).
3. Stirrer and heating block. Since aggregation proceeds efficiently only when a sample is stirred, some means of stirring must be used. A heating block to maintain a stable temperature of 37°C is also required. Conventional aggregometers can serve these purposes very well, although they may be considered expensive if only put to this use. If an aggregometer is used, then it is a simple matter to obtain suitable cuvets and stir bars for the assay.
4. Polystyrene cuvets.
5. Magnetic stir bars.

3. Methods

3.1. Impedance Aggregometry

1. Turn the aggregometer on and allow it sufficient time to warm to the required temperature (usually 37°C).
2. Accurately pipet 0.5 mL of whole blood into a cuvet (*see* **Notes 2** and **3**).
3. Add 0.5 mL of phosphate-buffered saline to dilute the blood (*see* **Note 1**).
4. Add a magnetic stir bar to the cuvet (*see* **Note 4**).
5. Incubate the platelets for approx 5 min at 37°C. Aggregometers usually have incubation wells specifically for this purpose (*see* **Note 5**).
6. While the cuvet is incubating, ensure that the electrode assembly is clean and leave it in warmed buffer prior to use.
7. Transfer the incubated cuvet containing 1 mL of diluted whole blood to the aggregation well and ensure that the sample is stirring. The stir speed of the aggregometer can often be set manually, although not in all cases. A stir speed of 1000 rpm is frequently used (*see* **Note 4**).
8. Remove the electrodes from the buffer and dry them gently with soft paper tissues. Insert the clean, dry electrode assembly into the cuvet, ensuring that the electrodes are fully inserted into the blood. Connect the electrode assembly to the aggregometer and start the recording device.
9. Calibration of the aggregometer takes place at this stage. In principle, all calibration procedures are the same, although the details can vary depending on the make and model of the aggregometer (*see* **Note 6**). Initially, it is necessary to adjust the zero-aggregation baseline. This can be accomplished with zero controls on both the aggregometer and the chart recorder. However, once the settings on the chart recorder are adjusted they should remain unchanged throughout an experiment, and any necessary readjustment of the baseline position from one sample to the next (which ought to be minimal) should be done using the aggregometer zero control.
10. A fixed increase in the impedance of the circuit is then applied using a calibration button. This should be accompanied by a deflection in the trace recording, the size of which is equivalent to an increase of 20 Ω. While the calibration button is depressed, the size of the deflection can be altered by a gain knob on the aggregometer. This should be adjusted in order to maximize the size of any subsequent aggregation recording but without allowing the aggregation trace to extend out of the range of the recorder. Once this procedure is complete, the gain and zero controls should not be adjusted at all until the next aggregation sample. However, if all the aliquots are replicates from the same blood sample, any subsequent adjustment of the zero and gain controls should be minimal (*see* **Note 6**).
11. Following calibration, there should be an observable flat and slightly noisy trace. It is a good idea to leave the trace to run for at least 60 s to ensure that there is no spontaneous aggregation, and that there are no other indications of an abnormal trace recording (*see* **Note 7**).
12. Accurately add the agonist directly into the blood using a pipet and gel-loading tips. Avoid touching the electrode assembly at any point (*see* **Note 8**).
13. If further aggregation assays are to be performed, then the next cuvet can be incubated (**step 5**) while the current one is aggregating.
14. Allow the assay to run for as long as required. Six minutes is a period of time that is commonly used. When the assay is complete, remove the electrode assembly and carefully dispose of the cuvet and its contents in a clinical-waste bin.

15. Clean the electrode immediately as gently and as thoroughly as possible using distilled water from the wash bottle and the disposable tissues. Be careful not to bend, scratch, or damage the electrodes. If substantial aggregation has occurred, the accumulated mass of platelets is easily visible between and around the electrodes. It is essential to remove all traces of blood and the platelet aggregate before using the electrode again. If the electrode is to be used immediately, leave it in clean warm saline. However, when the experiment is complete, the electrodes must be stored clean and dry. Always ensure that the final wash of the electrodes is with distilled water (*see* **Note 9**).

16. Aggregation data can be expressed as the extent of aggregation in ohms after a given period of time (usually 6 min), or as the rate of aggregation in ohms per minute. Both these variables are easy to calculate from trace recordings by comparing the size of the aggregation deflection with the 20-Ω calibration mark (*see* **Fig. 1**).

3.2. Particle Counting Aggregometry

1. Ensure that the heating block is warmed up to the required temperature.
2. Accurately pipet 0.5 mL of whole blood into a polystyrene cuvet (*see* **Notes 2** and **3**).
3. Add a magnetic stir bar to the cuvet.
4. Incubate the cuvet while stirring for 2 min at 37°C.
5. Remove 15 µL of the sample and add to 30 µL of fixative for an initial platelet count.
6. Add the agonist and then remove 15-µL aliquots of the sample at specified intervals and add them to 30 µL of fixative (*see* **Notes 10** and **11**).
7. Determine the platelet count of the fixed platelet samples using the particle counter.
8. Percentage aggregation can easily be calculated by relating the baseline count to the count at each time point. A platelet count of zero equals 100% aggregation.

4. Notes

1. Phosphate-buffered saline and normal saline are commonly used to dilute whole blood for impedance aggregometry. However, other balanced electrolyte solutions such as Tyrode's can be used. The same diluting solution should be used for all experiments where comparable results are required. Water should not be used, as this will cause lysis of erythrocytes. Since the blood sample has to be incubated to 37°C, it is best to add diluting buffer that is already at this or room temperature. Do not use buffer that is chilled.

2. Good quality whole blood samples are essential for accurate reproducible results, and therefore the blood must be handled as gently as possible. When using a conventional pipetting technique, blood remains on the inside of the pipet tip and the final depression of the pipet can cause bubble formation in the blood. A more accurate way of pipetting that does not generate bubbles is known as reverse pipetting. The pipet is set as normal at 0.5 mL; however, a larger volume than this is drawn up by initially depressing the pipet plunger beyond the usual stop point. When dispensing the blood, though, the pipet should be depressed only as far as the first stop. It is important to ensure that all the blood has been ejected from the tip, including any external drops; this can be achieved by having the end of the tip inserted into the sample itself as it is dispensed.

3. Aggregation of platelets (particularly when measured using impedance aggregometry) is sensitive to variations in the hematocrit and cellular content of the sample. Therefore, it is essential that all the samples be as similar as possible. If a blood sample is allowed to stand for any period of time after being drawn, the red cells will settle and subsequent aliquots of blood will have variable cell content. For this reason it is important to pipet out all the aliquots into the cuvets that will be necessary for the entire experiment. If this is not

done, then blood samples would need to be mixed to resuspend cells; however, platelets can become significantly desensitized as a result of this procedure. Undiluted aliquots of blood can be left in the cuvets at room temperature for several hours (as long as eight hours, in the experience of the author) and still respond normally in the impedance aggregometer. However, it is still advisable to complete the investigations in as short a time frame as possible in order to minimize time-dependent variations in response. Particle counting aggregometry is more sensitive to the formation of microaggregates with time, often resulting in a progressive decline in the baseline platelet count with time *(9)*.

4. Unlike with turbidimetric aggregometry, if a stir bar is not added to the cuvet, this cannot easily be confirmed by examining the cuvet. However, once impedance measurements are started, samples in which there is no stir bar (or in which the stirring mechanism has been disabled) have a very distinctive appearance. While the normal impedance trace should be noisy and flat, these traces are very smooth and un-noisy and often drift gradually. Once this problem is identified it can easily be rectified by dropping a stir bar into the cuvet, at which point the characteristic flat noisy trace should immediately appear.

5. Impedance aggregometry is very sensitive to changes in temperature. If the sample has not been fully incubated to 37°C then the baseline will drift as the temperature increases and the impedance is reduced. (If cold buffer is added to the blood, this problem can be substantial.) It can be prevented by allowing adequate incubation time. A similar problem will arise if the aggregometer is used immediately after it has been switched on without any allowance for the required time to warm up.

6. Some models of aggregometers have a one-step automatic calibration procedure, although in principle the same process is carried out. With these models, the aggregometer waits for one minute to determine whether the baseline is stable before indicating that the agonist can be added to the cuvet.

7. Abnormal traces can arise as a result of many causes:
   a. *Unstable baselines:* A baseline trace that drifts in the opposite direction to aggregation, is usually a result of not allowing the sample to warm up to 37°C (*see* **Note 5**). This problem can easily be overcome by incubating the cuvet for a few extra minutes. A baseline that drifts in the same direction as aggregation may indicate premature spontaneous aggregation; this is often caused by a damaged or dirty electrode. A dirty electrode can also give rise to excessively noisy and irregular traces as debris falls on and off the electrode (*see* **Note 9**).
   b. *A thin drifting trace* is frequently seen when the blood sample remains unstirred (*see* **Note 4**). If PRP is used instead of whole blood, then this will also generate a less noisy baseline than normal.
   c. *Jumping traces:* A change in impedance can be brought about by any foreign object in the sample that interferes with the electrode. Occasionally, small pieces of paper or card are found in cuvets, and if not removed these can become trapped in the electrodes and cause sudden changes in the trace. The best way to prevent this problem is to check that the cuvets are clean, although it is sometimes possible to remove the foreign object from the electrode. Small blood clots can have a similar effect and usually arise from a poorly taken blood sample.

8. Addition of agents is best achieved by using small volumes. Addition ratios of 1:50 and 1:100 are frequently used. Large volumes can induce artifacts as a result of diluting the sample or if the electrolytic properties of the agonist and its vehicle are significantly different from those of the blood. Using a physiological buffer as a vehicle will minimize this problem, although this may not always be possible.

9. *Care of the electrode:* It is essential that, after each individual assay, the electrodes be cleaned immediately and all traces of blood removed. Blood must never be allowed to dry out on the electrode. Residual parts of a platelet aggregate can accumulate where the electrode wires join the assembly mounting and, if not removed, these can influence subsequent results and even provoke spontaneous aggregation or irregular traces (*see* **Note 7**). Never use detergent to clean the electrodes. Distilled water and physiological buffers are perfectly adequate for cleaning. The electrode must be checked prior to each measurement to ensure that it is completely clean and dry.

   The electrode assembly is the most delicate part of the apparatus. It is also where the aggregation takes place. Care of the electrode is therefore essential in order to achieve good quality reproducible results. Most problems with impedance aggregometry arise as a result of failure to use or care for the electrodes properly. When stored and not in use, the electrodes must be kept in a clean and dry condition. They must always be finally washed in distilled water and then dried, after which they can be left in a clean unused cuvet, which will protect them. They must never be stored in saline or water.

10. By taking small aliquots from a sample of 0.5 mL, a time course of aggregation can be determined. However, it is also possible to use particle counting in association with turbidimetric or impedance aggregometry, by fixing the entire sample at the end of the aggregation measurement to obtain a final platelet count reading. This allows direct comparisons to be made between the final extent of aggregation in identical samples determined using two methods.

11. *Fixative solution:* The final concentrations of the active ingredients should be: Na_2EDTA, 3 mM; formaldehyde, 0.1% w/v. The ratio of volumes of fixative to sample can vary. As originally described, this ratio is 2:1. Dilution is not necessarily a problem, as many platelet and particle counters are designed to count highly diluted samples. However, if the counter processes the sample directly, then excessive dilution can be prevented if necessary by mixing the sample with a smaller volume of more concentrated fixative (e.g., 1 in 10). It is more important to ensure efficient and rapid mixing of the fixative in this case.

References

1. De La Cruz, J. P., Paez, M. V., Carmona, J. A., and De La Cuesta, F. S. (1999) Antiplatelet effect of the anaesthetic drug propofol: influence of red blood cells and leucocytes. *Br. J. Pharmacol.* **128,** 1538–1544.
2. Jarvis, G. E. and Evans, R. J. (1994) Endotoxin-induced platelet aggregation in heparinised equine whole blood in vitro. *Res. Vet. Sci.* **57,** 317–324.
3. Heptinstall, S., Fox, S., Crawford, J., and Hawkins, M. (1986) Inhibition of platelet aggregation in whole blood by dipyridamole and aspirin. *Thromb. Res.* **42,** 215–223.
4. Riess, H., Braun, G., Brehm, G., and Hiller, E. (1986) Critical evaluation of platelet aggregation in whole human blood. *Am. J. Clin. Pathol.* **85,** 50–56.
5. Sweeney, J. D., Labuzzetta, J. W., Michielson, C. E., and Fitzpatrick, J. E. (1989) Whole blood aggregation using impedance and particle counter methods. *Am. J. Clin. Pathol.* **92,** 794–797.
6. Cardinal, D. C. and Flower, R. J. (1980) The electronic aggregometer: a novel device for assessing platelet behavior in blood. *J. Pharmacol. Methods* **3,** 135–158.
7. Gordge, M. P., Dodd, N. J., Rylance, P. B., and Weston, M. J. (1984) An assessment of whole blood impedance aggregometry using blood from normal subjects and haemodialysis patients. *Thromb. Res.* **36,** 17–27.

8. Bevan, J. and Heptinstall, S. (1985) Serotonin-induced platelet aggregation in whole blood and the effects of ketanserin and mepyramine. *Thromb. Res.* **38,** 189–194.

9. Fox, S. C., Burgess-Wilson, M., Heptinstall, S., and Mitchell, J. R. (1982) Platelet aggregation in whole blood determined using the Ultra-Flo 100 Platelet Counter. *Thromb. Haemost.* **48,** 327–329.

10. Storey, R. F., Sanderson, H. M., White, A. E., May, J. A., Cameron, K. E., and Heptinstall, S. (2000) The central role of the P_{2T} receptor in amplification of human platelet activation, aggregation, secretion and procoagulant activity. *Br. J. Haematol.* **110,** 925–934.

7

Secretion From Dense Granules

Luminescence Method for Adenine Nucleotides

M. Fred Heath

1. Introduction

1.1. Summary of Method

In this procedure, modified from Lundin et al. *(1)*, the firefly luciferin-luciferase system is used to produce a light output proportional to the ATP concentration in the extracellular medium from platelet preparations. This output is measured in a luminometer to estimate the ATP concentration. The subsequent addition of pyruvate kinase/phosphoenolpyruvate (PK/PEP) converts the ADP present to ATP, allowing estimation of ADP from the increase in light output. The further addition of adenylate kinase/CTP converts the AMP present to ADP, which is transformed into ATP by the PK/PEP and estimated from the further increase in light output *(2)*. The detection limit is approx 20 nM for each nucleotide in the original preparation. The range is up to approx 10 µM total nucleotides. This technique therefore provides a sensitive method for the measurement of the secretion of ADP and ATP from platelet dense granules.

1.2. Outline of Theory

1.2.1. Stable Light Output

The firefly luciferin-luciferase system enables continuous monitoring of the ATP concentration if the intensity of the light emission can be measured.

$$\text{ATP} + \text{D-luciferin} + O_2 \rightarrow \text{AMP} + PP_i + \text{oxyluciferin} + CO_2 + \text{light}$$

The firefly catalytic cycle can be regulated to minimize product inhibition and so obtain a stable light emission, rather than a transient peak light emission. Only a negligible proportion of the ATP is consumed by the luciferase reaction.

From: *Methods in Molecular Biology, vol. 272:*
Platelets and Megakaryocytes, Vol. 1: Functional Assays
Edited by: J. M. Gibbins and M. P. Mahaut-Smith © Humana Press Inc., Totowa, NJ

1.2.2. Internal Standardization

With stable light emission, each individual assay can be calibrated by the addition at the end of the assay of a known amount of ATP (e.g., 100 pmol) as an internal standard, to compensate for any variation of firefly luciferase activity resulting from, for example, the conditions of sample preparation.

1.2.3. Conversion of ADP to ATP

The method used by Lundin et al. *(1)* uses pyruvate kinase to convert ADP to ATP in the presence of an excess of phosphoenolpyruvate (PEP).

$$ADP + PEP \rightarrow ATP + pyruvate$$

Potassium ions are a required cofactor of pyruvate kinase, and are added to the reaction buffer.

1.2.4. Conversion of AMP to ADP

The method used is a two-addition procedure to convert AMP to ADP with adenylate kinase and CTP *(1,2)*. CTP is used in great excess, as it drives the adenylate kinase reaction but not the luciferase reaction.

$$AMP + CTP \rightarrow ADP + CDP$$

ADP is then converted to ATP by the PK/PEP reaction. Traces of ATP in CTP preparations are allowed for by adding CTP first and noting the baseline before addition of adenylate kinase.

1.3. Outline of Major Procedures

There are three steps: (1) extraction of nucleotides; (2) luminometry; (3) calculation.

2. Materials

2.1. Extraction Procedure

1. 100 mM EDTA: 372 mg Na$_2$EDTA in 10 mL water. Store at 4°C. Stable.
2. Ethanol (absolute).

2.2. Luminometry

1. ATP monitoring reagent (AMR): Bio-Orbit Kit (Turku, Finland) (1243-107) component (contains firefly luciferase, D-luciferin, bovine serum albumin—50 mg/vial, magnesium acetate—500 µmol/vial, inorganic pyrophosphate—0.1 µmol/vial). Reconstituted just before use with 5 mL water/vial. Use at room temperature. May be stored frozen for 2 mo. Similar kits are available from BioThema (Haninge, Sweden) ATP Kit SL (144-041).
2. Tris buffer with potassium acetate (Tris-KAc buffer): Bio-Orbit/BioThema kit buffer (100 mM Tris-acetate, 2 mM EDTA, pH 7.75 ± 0.05 at 25°C) augmented with 25 mM potassium acetate (*see* **Subheading 1.2.3.**). 2 M potassium acetate (1.963 g/10 mL water), stable if stored frozen. Add 625 µL to 50 mL of buffer. Store at 4°C.
3. Pyruvate kinase/phosphoenolpyruvate (PK/PEP): The first component is pyruvate kinase, 10 mg/mL in 50% glycerol (Roche 109045; 200 U/mg) (*see* **Note 1**). Stable at 4°C. The second component is 200 mM phosphoenolpyruvate, prepared by dissolving 500 mg

phospho-(enol)pyruvate tri(cyclohexylammonium) salt (Sigma P7252) in 4.5 mL water plus 0.62 mL 100 mM acetic acid. Stable frozen. The working reagent consists of equal volumes of the two components, mixed as required and held on ice.

4. CTP: For stock (250 mM), dissolve 100 mg cytidine 5'-triphosphate disodium salt (Sigma C1506) in 400 µL 500 mM (60 g/L) Tris base and add 288 µL water. Store frozen. Prepare working reagent (25 mM) as 1 vol. CTP stock plus 1 vol Tris buffer (as Bio-Orbit kit component and without KAc) and 8 vol water.

5. Adenylate kinase (AK): Adenylate kinase is available as myokinase as a suspension in ammonium sulfate (Sigma M3003). As sulfate ions are inhibitory to the luciferase reaction, they must be removed by desalting. For a suspension of 1000 U myokinase, spin in microfuge 15 min. Prepare 1:9 Tris buffer (as Bio-Orbit kit component and without KAc):water. Dissolve pellet in diluted buffer. Wash a PD-10 desalting column (Amersham Biosciences, Chalfont, St. Giles, UK) with 25 mL diluted buffer. Load AK solution. Wash with 0.5 mL diluted buffer. Elute column with diluted buffer. Collect only 3 mL. Store frozen.

6. ATP standard (10 µM): Bio-Orbit/BioThema kit component (0.1 µmol ATP, 2 µmol magnesium sulfate). Reconstitute with 10 mL water/vial. Recommended to store frozen in 1-mL aliquots—stable 2 mo. Do not refreeze stored aliquots.

7. ADP standard (10 µM): Dissolve 67 mg adenosine 5'-diphosphate bis(cyclohexylammonium) salt (Sigma A4386) in 100 mL water. Dilute 100X in water and store frozen in 1-mL aliquots.

8. AMP standard (10 µM): Dissolve 41.5 mg adenosine 5'-monophosphate sodium salt (Sigma A1752) in 100 mL water. Dilute 100X in water and store frozen in 1 mL aliquots.

3. Methods

3.1. Extraction Procedure

1. To 1 mL of a preparation containing platelets, add 100 µL 100 mM EDTA.
2. Spin in microfuge 5 min to remove cells.
3. Take 500 µL supernatant and add to 500 µL ethanol to stabilize the nucleotide concentrations.
4. Spin in microfuge 5 min.
5. Store on ice (*see* **Note 2**).

3.2. Luminometry

1. Prepare luminometer and set to zero (*see* **Note 3**).
2. Prepare reagents: AMR, Tris-KAc buffer and AK at room temperature; PK/PEP, CTP, ATP, ADP, AMP on ice.
3. Place in luminometer cuvet: 810 µL Tris-KAc buffer, 100 µL of sample from extraction procedure, 100 µL AMR.
4. Place cuvet in luminometer and record reading when stable—reading A (*see* **Note 4**).
5. Add to cuvet in luminometer: 10 µL PK/PEP and record reading when stable—reading B (*see* **Note 5**).
6. Add to cuvet in luminometer: 10 µL CTP and record reading when stable—reading C (*see* **Subheading 1.2.4.**).
7. Add to cuvet in luminometer: 10 µL AK and record reading when stable—reading D.
8. Add to cuvet in luminometer: 10 µL ATP standard and record reading when stable—reading E.
9. For calibration:
   a. The sample is a control sample containing no platelets.
   b. Make two further additions, recording readings when stable: 10 µL ADP standard (reading F), then 10 µL AMP standard (reading G).

3.3. Calculation (see Note 6)

The first calculation is made on the calibration sample:

1. E-D is the signal that corresponds to 100 pmol ATP.
2. A is the apparent background signal in the ATP measurement. Corr(ATP) = 100 × A/(E-D) is the correction (to nearest pmol) to be subtracted from subsequent ATP measurements (*see* **Note 7**).
3. B-A is the apparent background signal in the ADP measurement. Corr(ADP) = 100 × (B-A)/(E-D) is the correction (to nearest pmol) to be subtracted from subsequent ADP measurements.
4. D-C is the apparent background signal in the AMP measurement. Corr(AMP) = 100 × (D-C)/(E-D) is the correction (to nearest pmol) to be subtracted from subsequent AMP measurements.
5. F-E is the signal for 100 pmol ADP. 100 × (F-E)/(E-D) gives the actual number of pmol measured, and must be considered as quality control (*see* **Note 8**).
6. G-F is the signal for 100 pmol AMP. 100 × (G-F)/(E-D) gives the actual number of pmol measured, and must be considered as quality control (*see* **Note 8**).

The calculations of nucleotide content for each sample are then:

1. ATP (pmol) = 100 × A/(E-D) – Corr(ATP)
2. ADP (pmol) = 100 × (B-A)/(E-D) – Corr(ADP)
3. AMP (pmol) = 100 × (D-C)/(E-D) – Corr(AMP)

See **Note 9** for variations on AMR methods.

4. Notes

1. If pyruvate kinase is purchased as a suspension in ammonium sulfate, it can be processed as AK (*see* **Subheading 2.2., step 5**).
2. Further precipitation may occur on standing. The sample must be cleared by recentrifugation before luminometry.
3. This work has been routinely performed on a Bio-Orbit 1250 luminometer, which contained a ^{14}C standard. The background and standard were checked against the specification to ensure proper function before each use. Consult the documentation for other luminometers.
4. If a Bio-Orbit 1250 luminometer is to be used, it should be set to print the integrated signal after each 10 s. A chart recorder could also be attached for continuous readout of the signal.
5. The Bio-Orbit 1250 printer was turned off during additions to the cuvet.
6. These calculations are best handled by a computer—e.g., on a spreadsheet.
7. This and the other corrections should be of the order of 1 pmol.
8. My view is that these numbers say more about the ADP and AMP preparations than about the system. I therefore accepted ADP values of 100 ± 10 pmol and AMP values of 90 ± 10 pmol.
9. Variations: There is widespread use of AMRs alone for ATP-only measurements, including measurements with live platelets in lumiaggregometers (e.g. Chronolog). Beigi et al. (*3*) have attached luciferase to living platelets *via* a protein A-luciferase construct and monitored the cell-surface ATP.

References

1. Lundin, A., Hasenson, M., Persson, J., and Pousette, A. (1986) Estimation of biomass in growing cell lines by adenosine triphosphate assay. *Meth. Enzymol.* **133,** 27–42.
2. Jarvis, G. E., Evans, R. J., and Heath, M. F. (1996) The role of ADP in endotoxin-induced equine platelet activation. *Eur. J. Pharmacol.* **315,** 203–212.
3. Beigi, R., Kobatake, E., Aizawa, M., and Dubyak, G. R. (1999) Detection of local ATP release from activated platelets using cell surface-attached firefly luciferase. *Am. J. Physiol.* **276,** C267–C278.

8

Platelet Dense-Granule Secretion

The [³H]-5-HT Secretion Assay

David Crosby and Alastair W. Poole

1. Introduction

Thrombus generation is supported and enhanced by the release of a number of substances from the α and dense granules stored within platelets. The secreted granular contents are critical to the recruitment of platelets and to the stabilization of the aggregate. Dense granules contain a nonmetabolic adenine nucleotide pool of ATP and ADP, calcium, pyrophosphate, and 5-hydroxytryptamine (5-HT). Here, a method for studying the secretion of 5-HT is detailed, based on detection of secretion of [³H]-5-HT from prelabeled platelets.

Platelets express a plasma membrane 5-HT active transporter that takes 5-HT up into the cells, where it is repackaged into dense granules. When platelets are incubated with exogenous [³H]-5-HT, this will be taken up and incorporated into the stored pool of 5-HT, ready for secretion. The percentage of 5-HT released upon stimulation may be calculated from the amount released by stimulation, as a fraction of the total 5-HT content of the cells.

2. Materials

1. 5-Hydroxy [γ-³H]-tryptamine.
2. Creatinine sulfate (Amersham Biosciences, Buckinghamshire, UK).
3. Indomethacin 10 M in DMSO.
4. PGI_2 0.1 µg/mL in ethanol.
5. Tyrode's buffer (145 mM NaCl, 2.9 mM KCl, 10 mM HEPES, 1 mM $MgCl_2$, 5 mM glucose, pH 7.3).
6. 6% glutaraldehyde in Tyrode's.

3. Methods

1. Add 0.5 µCi [³H]-5-HT per 1 mL of platelet-rich plasma (PRP) and incubate at 37°C for 1 h (*see* **Note 1**).

From: *Methods in Molecular Biology, vol. 272:*
Platelets and Megakaryocytes, Vol. 1: Functional Assays
Edited by: J. M. Gibbins and M. P. Mahaut-Smith © Humana Press Inc., Totowa, NJ

2. Add PGI$_2$, 1 µL per 1 mL PRP, then immediately pellet by centrifugation at 1000g for 10 min.
3. Resuspend platelet pellet in Tyrode's buffer to a density of 4×10^8 platelets/mL.
4. Add indomethacin, 1 µL per 1 mL platelet suspension. Allow a 30-min rest period before stimulation.
5. Carry out experiment using 400-µL platelet suspension samples. Samples should be assayed at least in triplicate.
6. To terminate stimulation, at the appropriate time, add 400 µL glutaraldehyde solution and place on ice until all samples can be collected together at the end of the experiment (*see* **Note 2**).
7. Set aside three 200-µL samples of unstimulated labeled platelet suspension for estimation of total 5-HT labeling. Include a set of unstimulated samples as basal controls.
8. Centrifuge all samples including basals, but excluding the total samples, at 13,000g for 1 min to pellet platelets.
9. Remove 400 µL supernatant from each sample, add to 4 mL scintillation fluid, and measure radioactivity by liquid scintillation counting.
10. Add the three 200-µL samples of uncentrifuged totals directly to scintillation fluid for counting. This will give a figure for total 5-HT incorporation into platelets.
11. Determine the percentage release for each sample using the following equation:

$$\frac{(\text{sample} - \text{mean basal})}{(\text{mean total} - \text{mean basal})} \times 100 = \% \text{ 5-HT released}$$

Triplicated sample data may then be pooled for determination of mean and standard errors.

4. Notes

1. This is a standard protocol for determination of 5-HT secretion. We routinely use ^{3}H-labeled 5-HT, although it is also possible to use ^{14}C-labeled 5-HT.
2. It is preferable to stop reactions using glutaraldehyde, which rapidly quenches the release reaction. It is, however, also possible to avoid this step by rapidly centrifuging samples for 10 s at 13,000g immediately after stimulation and taking off 200 µL of supernatant to add to scintillation fluid. The time involved in undertaking these steps means, however, that this approach is unsuitable for accurate determination of time courses.

9

Analysis of the Releasable Nucleotides of Platelets

Joachim Jankowski, Lars Henning, and Hartmut Schlüter

1. Introduction

In platelets, two pools of nucleotides have been demonstrated: one is utilized for the metabolic needs of the platelets (*1*) and the second stores nucleotides in a metabolically inert form in dense granules. Upon activation of platelets, nucleotides are released from the dense granules into the extracellular space (*2*). The nucleotides, stored in the dense granules of platelets, can be divided into two subgroups—the mononucleotides and the dinucleotides. The mononucleotides comprise adenosine mono-, di-, and triphosphates (AMP, ADP, and ATP) as well as guanosine mono-, di-, and triphosphates (GMP, GDP and GTP). D'Souza and Glueck determined the following total amounts of mononucleotides in platelets (μmol/10^{-11} platelets): AMP, 0.7; ADP, 4.4; ATP, 5.5; GMP, 0.3; GDP, 0.75; and GTP, 0.7 (*1*). The dinucleotides comprise dinucleoside polyphosphates with adenosine (A) and/or guanosine (G) as nucleosides (Ap$_n$A, Ap$_n$G, Gp$_n$G) with phosphate chain lengths of $n = 2$ to $n = 7$ (*3–6*). The total content of the diadenosine polyphosphates was determined by Jankowski et al. (*7*) (μmol/10^{-11} platelets): Ap$_3$A, 0.78; Ap$_4$A, 0.96; Ap$_5$A, 0.38; and Ap$_6$A, 0.12. The concentrations of Ap$_n$G and Gp$_n$G are estimated to be a factor of 2 to 3 lower than those of the diadenosine polyphosphates.

Diverse responses to extracellular purines and pyrimidines have been documented in a wide range of biological systems, from single cells to whole organisms, and include smooth muscle contraction (*8*), neurotransmission in the peripheral (*9*) and central nervous systems (*10*), the immune response (*11*), platelet aggregation (*5,12*), pain (*13*), and modulation of cardiac function (*14*).

The emphasis of this chapter is on the determination of releasable nucleotides and total nucleotides of platelets, including mononucleotides and dinucleotides. The determination of nucleotides from platelets includes a deproteinization step to inactivate and remove nucleotide-hydrolyzing enzymes, a concentration step via a reversed-phase column, a separation step of mononucleotides and dinucleotides via affinity chromatography, and a determination step via analytical HPLC reversed-phase chromatography. In addition, a MALDI-mass-spectrometric method is given to

From: *Methods in Molecular Biology, vol. 272:*
Platelets and Megakaryocytes, Vol. 1: Functional Assays
Edited by: J. M. Gibbins and M. P. Mahaut-Smith © Humana Press Inc., Totowa, NJ

confirm the identity of the nucleotides, which elute from the analytical HPLC reversed-phase chromatography.

2. Materials

HPLC water (gradient grade) and acetonitrile are purchased from Merck (Germany); all other substances are from Sigma-Aldrich (Germany).

2.1. Extraction of Nucleotides From Platelets

1. Platelet concentrates (2 × 200 mL) from transfusion medicine unsuitable for transfusion.
2. 0.9% NaCl (3 × 600 mL): solution for washing and resuspension of platelets.
3. 0.05 units/mL thrombin for stimulation of the platelets.
4. Ap_4 (100 µg): internal standards for the quantification of mononucleotides. Ap_4 must be purified before use. P(1),P(2):P(2),P(3)-*bis*-methylene diadenosine triphosphate (100 µg): internal standard for quantification of dinucleotides *(15)*.

2.2. Deproteination of the Platelet Extract

1. Perchloric acid 70% (v/v) for deproteinization.
2. KOH (5 *M*) for neutralization of the perchloric-acid-treated supernatant.

2.3. Concentration of Nucleotides by Reversed-Phase Chromatography

1. Reversed-phase chromatography column (Lichroprep®; 310 × 65 mm, 40–65 µm, Merck, Germany) for concentration of nucleotides.
2. Triethylammonium acetate (TEAA, 40 m*M*) in water: eluent A.
3. 80/20 (v/v) acetonitrile/water: eluent B.

2.4. Separation of Mononucleotides and Dinucleotides by Affinity Chromatography

1. For affinity chromatography phenyl boronic acid is coupled to a cation-exchange resin (BioRex70™, BioRad, Hercules, CA) *(16,17)*. BioRex70 resin (200–400 mesh, Na⁺-form) is obtained from BioRad Laboratories and is suspended in 0.25 *M* sodium acetate (pH 5.0). The resin is conjugated with m-aminophenylboronic acid hemisulfate in the presence of 1-ethyl-3-(3-dimethylaminopropyl)-carbodiimide. The resin is initially washed in sodium acetate and sodium bicarbonate, and then is sequentially washed with 0.85 *M* ammonium acetate (pH 9.0) in 15% (v/v) ethanol, next with 1 *M* ammonium acetate (pH 9.8) and 50 m*M* ammonium acetate (pH 4.5), and finally with 1 *M* ammonium acetate (pH 4.5) in water. The affinity resin is packed into a glass column (Superperformance™, 15 × 300 mm, Merck, Germany).
2. Aqueous 1 *M* NH₄Ac (pH 9.5): eluent A.
3. Aqueous 10 *M* HCl: eluent B.

2.5. Desalting and Concentration of Nucleotides by Reversed-Phase Chromatography

1. Analytical reversed-phase chromatography column (Supersphere™, 210 × 4.1 mm, 4 µm, Merck, Germany) for desalting and concentration of nucleotides.
2. Triethylammonium acetate (TEAA, 40 m*M*) in water: eluent A.
3. 80/20 (v/v) acetonitrile/water: eluent B.

2.6. Determination of Nucleotides by Reversed-Phase Chromatography

1. Analytical reversed-phase chromatography column (RP-18e; Chromolith SpeedROD™; 50–4.6 mm; macropore size 2 μm; Merck, Germany) for determination of nucleotides.
2. 2 mM tetrabutylammonium hydrogensulfate (TBA) in a phosphate buffer (10 mM) K_2HPO_4, pH 6.8: eluent A.
3. 20/80 (v/v) acetonitrile/water: eluent B.
4. Ap$_n$A (with n = 3–6; each 3 μg) as standard mixture.
5. For dinucleotides: Ap$_n$A (with n = 3–6); for mononucleotides: AMP, ADP ATP (each about 20 μg) for spiking experiments if necessary.

2.7. Separation of the Ion-Pair Reagent TBA From the Nucleotides

2.7.1. Cation-Exchange Chromatography

1. Analytical cation-exchange column (Mini-S PC 3.2 mm × 30 mm; Amersham Biosciences, Buckinghamshire, UK).
2. Eluent A: 20 mM sodium acetate in water, pH 4.8.

2.7.2. Reversed-Phase Chromatography

1. Analytical reversed-phase chromatography column (μRPC2/18, 3.2 × 30; Amersham Biosciences) for desalting the fraction from the cation-exchange chromatography (*see* **Subheading 2.7.1.**), containing the nonbinding substances (the nucleotides).
2. Eluent A: Triethylammonium acetate (TEAA, 40 mM) in water.
3. Eluent B: 80/20 (v/v) acetonitrile/water.

2.8. Identification of Nucleotides by MALDI Mass Spectrometry

1. 50 mg/mL 3-hydroxy-picolinic acid in water: MALDI-matrix.
2. Cation-exchange beads (AG 50 W-X12, 200–400 mesh, Bio-Rad) equilibrated with NH_4^+ as counter-ion, are added to this mixture to remove Na^+ and K^+ ions.

3. Methods

3.1. Extraction of Nucleotides From Platelets

The strategy for the determination of releasable nucleotides from human platelets stimulated with thrombin is shown in **Fig. 1**. The method is also applicable for the determination of the total nucleotide pool of human platelets. In this case the experimenter is referred to **Subheading 3.1.1.** (*see* **Note 1**).

3.1.1. Extraction of Nucleotides From a Platelet Pool

1. The platelet concentrate is washed twice with an aqueous 0.9% NaCl solution.
2. The platelets are isolated from the aqueous 0.9% NaCl solution by centrifugation (2500g; 10 min).
3. After washing the platelet pellets are resuspended and centrifuged (2500g; 4°C; 5 min) and the platelet pellet is stored at –20°C for 12 h.

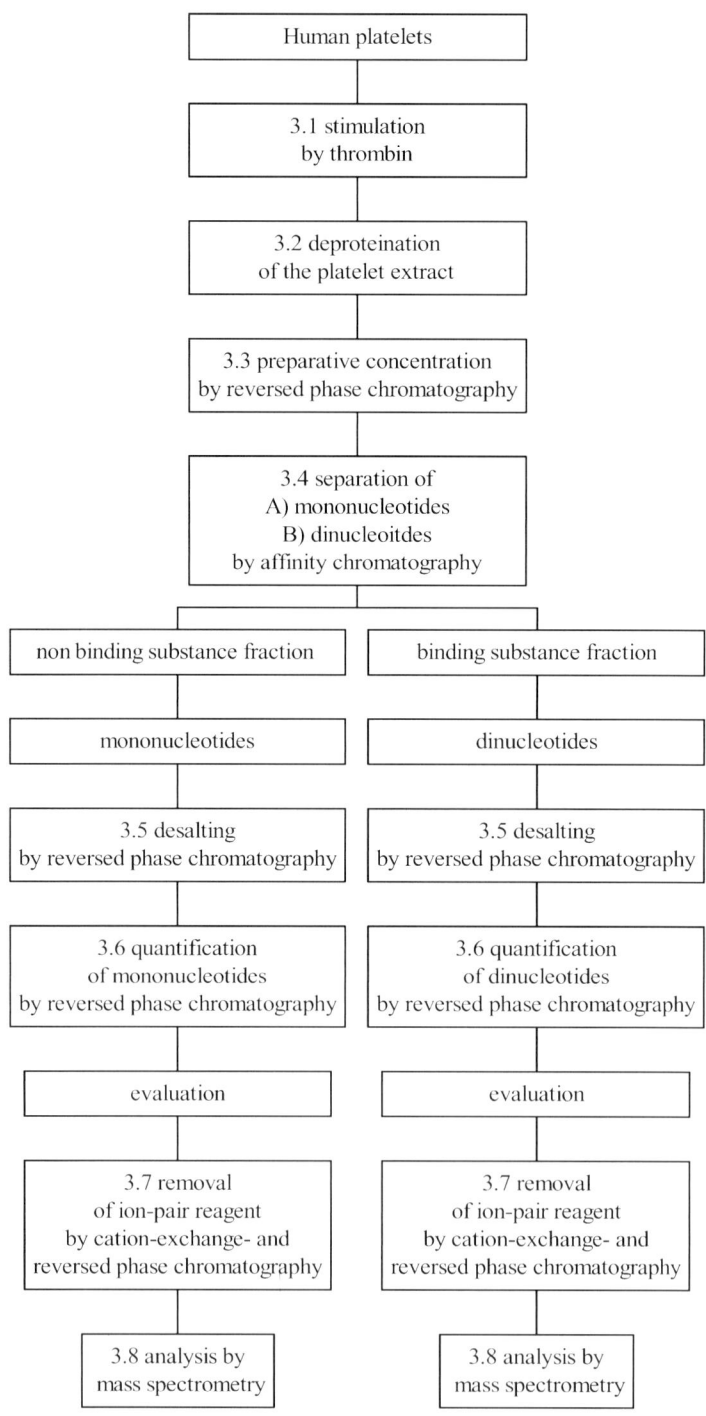

3.1.2. Extraction of Nucleotides From the Supernatant of Stimulated Platelets

1. The platelet concentrate is washed twice with an aqueous 0.9% NaCl solution. The platelets are isolated from the solution by centrifugation ($2500g$; 10 min).
2. After washing, the platelet concentrate is resuspended and centrifuged ($2500g$; 4°C; 5 min).
3. The washed and resuspended platelet concentrate is divided into two parts. One part is incubated with thrombin (0.05 unit/mL) for 2 min to release the nucleotides. As a control the second aliquot is not incubated with thrombin.

3.2. Deproteination of the Platelet Extract

1. The stimulated and the unstimulated platelet suspensions are centrifuged ($2500g$; 4°C; 10 min) to remove platelet residues.
2. Perchloric acid is added to the supernatants (final concentration: $0.6\ M$) and intensively mixed for 20 s.
3. The precipitated proteins are removed by centrifugation ($2500g$; 4°C; 5 min).
4. The pH is adjusted with $5\ M$ KOH to pH 7.0. Precipitated $KClO_4$ and proteins are removed by centrifugation ($2500g$; 4°C; 5 min) (*see* **Note 2**).

3.3. Concentration of Nucleotides by Reversed-Phase Chromatography

1. A C18 reversed-phase column is equilibrated with 40 mM TEAA in water (flow: 2 mL/min).
2. Triethylammonium acetate (TEAA) is added as ion-pair reagent to each supernatant (final TEAA concentration 40 mM).
3. By passing the supernatant through a C18 reversed-phase column using 40 mM TEAA in water (flow: 2 mL/min) the nucleotides are concentrated on the reversed-phase column. Nonbinding substances (salts, carbohydrates, etc.) are removed with aqueous 40 mM TEAA (flow: 2 mL/min).
4. The nucleotide fraction is eluted with 20% acetonitrile in water. The elution is detected by measuring the UV absorption at 254 nm.
5. The eluate is lyophilized and stored frozen at –80°C (*see* **Note 3**).

3.4. Separation of Mononucleotides and Dinucleotides by Affinity Chromatography

1. The affinity resin is packed into a glass column and equilibrated with $1\ M$ NH$_4$Ac (pH 9.5; flow: 2 mL/min). The chromatography is monitored by measuring the UV absorption at 254 nm.
2. The lyophilized eluate of the reversed-phase chromatography (*see* **Subheading 3.3.**) is dissolved in $1\ M$ ammonium acetate (pH 9.5); the pH is adjusted to pH 9.5.
3. The dissolved sample is loaded to the affinity column (2 mL/min) and the column is washed with 1 mol/L NH$_4$Ac (pH 9.5) with a flow rate of 2 mL/min to remove nonbinding substances (mononucleotides).
4. The fraction containing the nonbinding substances (mononucleotides) with a significant UV absorption is collected.

Fig. 1. *(see opposite page)* Scheme for the determination of mononucleotides and dinucleotides from human platelets.

5. Binding substances (dinucleotides) are eluted with 10 mM HCl in water and the eluting fraction collected (*see* **Note 4**).

3.5. Desalting and Concentration of Nucleotides by Reversed-Phase Chromatography

1. The reversed-phase column is equilibrated with aqueous 40 mM TEAA solution.
2. TEAA is added to the eluate of the affinity-chromatography (final concentration: 40 mM). The pH is adjusted to 6.5.
3. The sample is pumped at a rate of 0.5 mL/min onto the column.
4. After washing the column with 15 mL aqueous 40 mM TEAA solution, the fraction of interest is eluted with 20% acetonitrile in water.
5. The resulting fractions are stored at –80°C (*see* **Note 5**).

3.6. Determination of Nucleotides by Reversed-Phase Chromatography

1. The desalted mononucleotide and dinucleotide fractions from **Subheading 3.5.** are divided equally in two. To one of the two parts the mononucleotide mixture or the dinucleotide mixture is added for spiking experiments.
2. The reversed-phase column is equilibrated with eluent A. Samples (standard mixture, one part of desalted mononucleotide and dinucleotide fractions from **Subheading 3.5.**) are chromatographed by using the following gradient: 0–30 min: 0–40% B; 30–33 min: 40–100% B; 33–36 min: 100% B; flow: 1 mL/min.
3. The flow rate is 1.0 mL/min; absorption is measured at 254 nm.
4. The lyophilized eluates of the reversed-phase column (*see* **Subheading 3.5.**) are dissolved in eluent A and then injected into the HPLC system.
5. The resulting fractions are stored at –80°C (*see* **Note 6**).
6. Nucleotides are identified by retention time comparison with authentic substances and by MALDI-mass spectometry analysis (*see* **Subheading 3.7.**). Moreover, the nucleotides can be identified by spiking the nucleotides with authentic substances.

In **Fig. 2**, characteristic reversed-phase chromatograms of the mononucleotide fraction from the affinity gel of a platelet supernatant before (**Fig. 2A**) and after stimulation (**Fig. 2B**) with thrombin are given. In **Fig. 3** characteristic reversed-phase chromatograms of the dinucleotide fraction from the affinity gel of a platelet supernatant before (**Fig. 3A**) and after stimulation (**Fig. 3B**) with thrombin are presented.

3.7. Identification of the Nucleotides Eluting From the Analytical Reversed-Phase Column by MALDI-Mass Spectometry

3.7.1. Separation of the Ion-Pair Reagent From the Nucleotides: Cation-Exchange Chromatography

1. The cation-exchange column is equilibrated with eluent A. The absorption is measured at 254 nm.
2. The lyophilized eluate of the reversed-phase column is dissolved in eluent A and injected to the cation exchanger. The flow rate is 0.1 mL/min.
3. Nucleotides elute in the fraction containing the nonbinding substances. This fraction is collected.

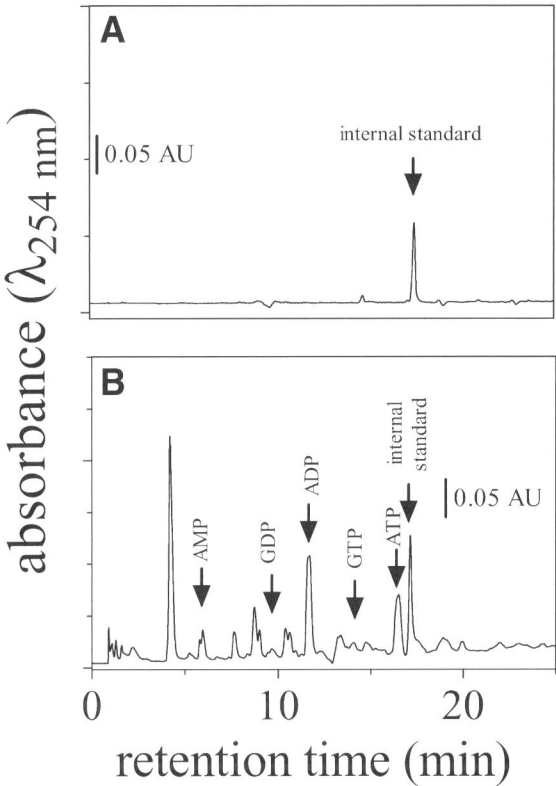

Fig. 2. Reversed-phase chromatogram of the mononucleotide-containing fraction from the affinity chromatography of a platelet supernatant before (**A**) and after stimulation (**B**) with thrombin (column: RP-18e Chromolith SpeedROD™; 50–4.6 mm; macropore size 2 μm; Merck, Germany; eluent A: 2 mM tetrabutylammonium hydrogensulfate in 10 mM K$_2$HPO$_4$, pH 6.8; eluent B: 80% (v/v) ACN in water; gradient: 0–30 min: 0–40% (v/v) B; 30–33 min: 40–100% (v/v) B; 33–36 min: 100% (v/v) B; flow: 1 mL/min).

3.7.2. Reversed-Phase Chromatography

1. The reversed-phase column is equilibrated with aqueous 40 mM TEAA solution.
2. TEAA is added to the eluate of the cation exchanger (*see* **Subheading 3.7.1.**) (final concentration: 40 mM). This sample is pumped at a rate of 0.1 mL/min onto the column.
3. After washing the column with 1 mL aqueous 40 mM TEAA solution, the fraction of interest is eluted with 20% acetonitrile in water. The resulting fractions are lyophilized and stored at –80°C.

3.8. Identification of Nucleotides by MALDI-Mass Spectometry

1. Authentic dinucleotides such as Ap$_6$A (10^{-5} M) should be used to test the performance of the mass spectrometer and for calibration purposes.

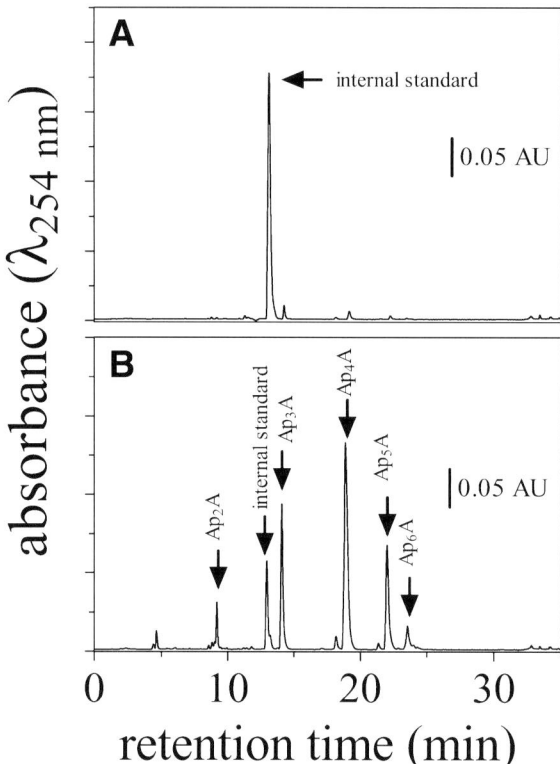

Fig. 3. Reversed-phase chromatogram of the dinucleotide-containing fraction to the affinity gel of a platelet supernatant before **(A)** and after stimulation **(B)** with thrombin conditions (as in **Fig. 2**).

2. The isolated nucleotide-containing fractions are each dissolved in 10 μL double-distilled water.

3. To the dissolved nucleotide-conatining samples a 5-μL suspension of cation-exchange beads (AG 50 W-X12, 200–400 mesh, Bio-Rad) equilibrated with NH_4^+ as counter-ion are added to remove Na^+ and K^+ ions.

4. 1 μL of the analyte solution is mixed with 1 μL of the matrix solution (50 mg/mL 3-hydroxy-picolinic acid in water [HPA] on the MALDI target).

5. The mixture must be dried gently before the introduction into the mass spectrometer.

6. 10–20 single spectra should be accumulated for a better signal-to-noise ratio.

7. For measurement of PSD-MALDI spectra, several hundred spectra are accumulated. In **Fig. 4** a typical MALDI mass spectrum **(Fig. 4A)** and PSD-MALDI mass spectrum **(Fig. 4B)** is given (*see* **Note 7**).

4. Notes

1. The method described here uses platelet concentrates for the determination of releasable nucleotides from platelets. Nevertheless, the method is also suitable for the determination of

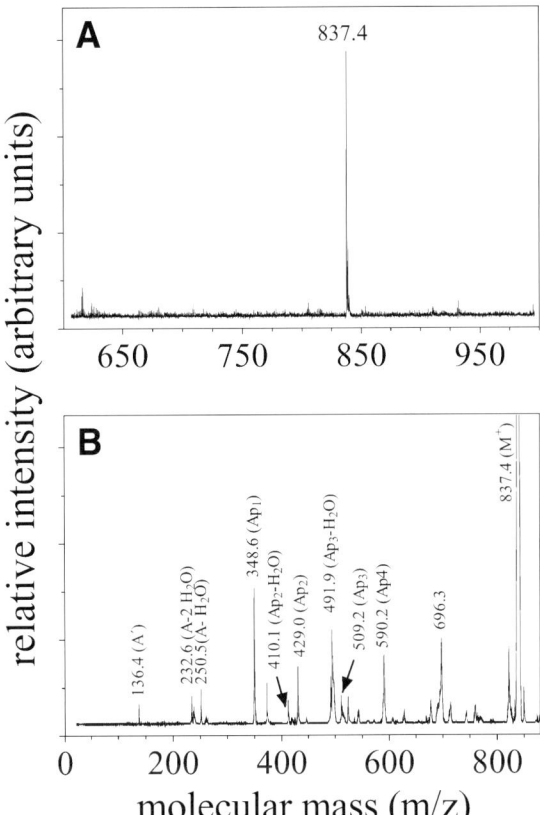

Fig. 4. Positive-ion MALDI mass spectrum (**A**) and PSD-MALDI mass spectrum (**B**) of the fraction eluting at 19 min (**Fig. 3B**). The masses of the labeled signals correspond to the non-protonated molecular ions. The mass of the signal in **A** corresponds with the molecular weight of diadenosine tetraphosphate (Ap$_4$A). In the PSD-MALDI spectrum, interpretation of the fragment ions are given in the figure. (A': adenine; A: adenosine; Ap$_1$: adenosine monophosphate; Ap$_2$: adenosine diphosphate; Ap$_3$: adenosine triphosphate; Ap$_4$: adenosine tetraphosphate).

nucleotides from platelets directly prepared from human blood. For the isolation of the platelets, 20 mL heparinized blood is centrifuged at 160g for 10 min. The resulting platelet-rich plasma is centrifuged at 2500g. The resulting platelet pellet is resuspended 1:1 with aqueous 0.9% NaCl and washed twice as described above (*see* **Subheading 3.1.1.**). The volumes of the solutions, as well as dimension of the column, have to be adjusted to account for the lower number of platelets and therefore decreased concentration of nucleotides. A detailed description is reported in Jankowski et al. (**7**). In contrast to Jankowski et al., we now recommend using a RP-18e Chromolith SpeedROD™ column instead of the reversed-phase column Poros R2/H (100 × 2.1 mm i.d., Perseptive Biosystems, Wiesbaden,

Germany). The Chromolith SpeedROD™ column separates nucleotides with a significantly higher resolution.

The release of platelet nucleotides by thrombin-induced aggregation has long been established *(18)*. Upon aggregation with thrombin, approx 50% of ADP and 40% of ATP is released *(1)*. If total nucleotide contents in platelets shall be determined, the cell membranes of platelets must be broken by freezing them. After thawing the platelet content is released into the supernatant.

2. The extraction step of nucleotides appears to be rather critical, as underlined by several authors *(19–21)*. It has to be harsh enough to allow an efficient release of the nucleotides but should not be too drastic to avoid the degradation of the labile mononucleotides. If the extraction is too mild, it may lead to an incomplete release of the pool of cellular nucleotides, because of a poor permeabilization of the cell walls or because it allows enzymatic degradation activities to persist; but it may also lead to artifactually high values of nucleotides, as observed by Meyer et al. *(21)*. It should be emphasized that weak acids (like formic acid) should be used cautiously, since they are susceptible to inducing an increase in the level of nucleotides, as described by Garrison et al. *(20)*.

The most suitable extraction reagents are probably trichloroacetic and perchloric acid; the reliability of the extraction step can be further enhanced by combining with the acidic extraction a mechanical disruption of the cells (sonication), as recommended by Garrison et al. *(20)*. Alcohols are probably not satisfactory extraction reagents, even at high concentration (70% for ethanol), since their use results in a marked increase in the level of nucleotides during the extraction steps (for periods of at least 30 to 60 min) as shown by Meyer et al. *(21)*.

3. To remove the $KClO_4$ as well as low-molecular-weight hydrophilic substances (such as carbohydrates) and also hydrophobic substances (such as proteins and lipids) from the sample and to concentrate the nucleotides, preparative reversed-phase chromatography is necessary. TEAA is added as ion-pair reagent to allow the nucleotides to bind to the stationary phase.

4. Mononucleotides and dinucleotides can be separated with self-prepared affinity chromatography medium. The gel is based on a cation-exchange gel to which a phenyl boronic acid is coupled covalently. It is most important to use a ammonium acetate buffer (pH 9.5), which is exactly 1 *M*, to achieve the separation of mononucleotides from dinucleotide with the boronate affinity column *(22)*.

5. The desalting of the nucleotide-containing fraction prior to the determination by reversed-phase chromatography is recommended because the presence of salts may result in poor peak shapes *(7)*.

6. Before chromatography of the nucleotide-containing fractions from platelets, the performance of the reversed-phase column must be tested with a nucleotide standard mixture. Only in the case of a sufficient resolution of the nucleotides of the standard mixture the nucleotide containing fractions from platelets should be analyzed by the reversed-phase chromatography. A spiking experiment may be useful if there is no mass spectrometer available in the laboratory.

In comparison to other commercially available reversed-phase columns, the reversed-phase column RP-18e Chromolith SpeedROD™ is characterized by high resolution for nucleotides and high chemical stability. Moreover, the column seems to be very stable toward contamination. Nevertheless, after frequent use of the column, treatment with a mixture of acetonitrile/formic acid (50/50 v/v) is recommended. Avoid the mixture coming into contact with water within the HPLC system including the column. Therefore, pump 100% acetonitrile through the system before and after you use the acetonitrile/formic acid mixture.

7. Prior to the MALDI-mass spectroscopy (MS) analysis of individual fractions from the reversed-phase chromatography (*see* **Subheading 3.6.**) the ion-pair reagent TBA must be removed, because this reagent suppresses the signals of the nucleotides in the MALDI-MS spectra. As a result, in these spectra only the signal of the protonated TBA ion can be observed. In this protocol TBA is captured by the cation exchanger, whereas nucleotides do not bind to the cation exchanger. Before the MALDI analysis, sodium acetate has to be removed from the nucleotide fraction by reversed-phase chromatography using TEAA as ion-pair reagent. In constrast to TBA, the ion-pair reagent TEAA is removable from nucleotides by lyophilization. After lyophilization the isolated nucleotides are analyzable by MALDI-MS.

References

1. D'Souza, L. and Glueck, H. I. (1977) Measurement of nucleotide pools in platelets using high pressure liquid chromatography. *Thromb. Haemost.* **38**, 990–1001.
2. Daniel, J. L., Molish, I. R., and Holmsen, H. (1980) Radioactive labeling of the adenine nucleotide pool of cells as a method to distinguish among intracellular compartments. Studies on human platelets. *Biochim. Biophys. Acta* **632**, 444–453.
3. Schlüter, H., Offers, E., Brüggemann, G., van der Giet, M., Tepel, M., Nordhoff, E., et al. (1994) Diadenosine phosphates and the physiological control of blood pressure. *Nature* **367**, 186–188.
4. Schlüter, H., Gross, I., Bachmann, J., Kaufmann, R., van der Giet, M., Tepel, M., et al. (1998) Adenosine(5′) oligophospho-(5′) guanosines and guanosine(5′) oligophospho-(5′) guanosines in human platelets. *J. Clin. Invest.* **101**, 682–688.
5. Jankowski, J., Tepel, M., van der Giet, M., Tente, I. M., Henning, L., Junker, R., et al. (1999) Identification and characterization of P(1), P(7)-Di(adenosine-5′)-heptaphosphate from human platelets. *J. Biol. Chem.* **274**, 23,926–23,931.
6. Jankowski, J., Hagemann, J., Tepel, M., van der Giet, M., Stephan, N., Henning, L., et al. (2001) Dinucleotides as growth promoting extracellulary mediators: Presence of dinucleoside diphosphates Ap_2A, Ap_2G and Gp_2G in releasable granlues of platelets. *J. Biol. Chem.* **276**, 8904–8909.
7. Jankowski, J., Potthoff, W., van der Giet, M., Tepel, M., Zidek, W., and Schlüter, H. (1999) High-performance liquid chromatographic assay of the diadenosine polyphosphates in human platelets. *Anal. Biochem.* **269,** 72–78.
8. Ralevic, V. and Burnstock, G. (1991) Effects of purines and pyrimidines on the rat mesenteric arterial bed. *Circ. Res.* **69**, 1583–1590.
9. Burnstock, G. and Wood, J. N. (1996) Purinergic receptors: their role in nociception and primary afferent neurotransmission. *Curr. Opin. Neurobiol.* **6**, 526–532.
10. Fredholm, B. B. (1995) Purinoceptors in the nervous system. *Pharmacol. Toxicol.* **76,** 228–239.
11. Dubyak, G. R. and el-Moatassim, C. (1993) Signal transduction via P2-purinergic receptors for extracellular ATP and other nucleotides. *Am. J. Physiol.* **265,** C577–C606.
12. Lüthje, J. and Ogilvie, A. (1984) Diadenosine triphosphate (Ap_3A) mediates human platelet aggregation by liberation of ADP. *Biochem. Biophys. Res. Commun.* **118,** 704–709.
13. Pintor, J., Diaz-Hernandez, M., Gualix, J., Gomez-Villafuertes, R., Hernando, F., and Miras-Portugal, M. T. (2000) Diadenosine polyphosphate receptors from rat and guinea-pig brain to human nervous system. *Pharmacol. Ther.* **87**, 103–115.

14. Olsson, R. A. and Pearson, J. D. (1990) Cardiovascular purinoceptors. *Physiol. Rev.* **70,** 761–845.
15. Klein, E., Mons, S., Valleix, A., Mioskowski, C., and Lebeau, L. (2002) Synthesis of enzymatically and chemically non-hydrolyzable analogues of dinucleoside triphosphates Ap₃A and Gp₃G. *J. Org. Chem.* **67,** 146–153.
16. Wielckens, K., Bredehorst, R., Adamietz, P., and Hilz, H. (1981) Protein-bound polymeric and monomeric ADP-ribose residues in hepatic tissues. Comparative analyses using a new procedure for the quantification of poly(ADP-ribose). *Eur. J. Biochem.* **117,** 69–74.
17. Barnes, L. D., Robinson, A. K., Mumford, C. H., and Garrison, P. N. (1985) Assay of diadenosine tetraphosphate hydrolytic enzymes by boronate chromatography. *Anal. Biochem.* **144,** 296–304.
18. Holmsen, H. and Day, H. J. (1971) The platelet release reaction and its role in platelet aggregation. *Acta Med. Scand. Suppl.* **525,** 75–78.
19. Baker, J. C. and Jacobson, M. K. (1986) Alteration of adenyl dinucleotide metabolism by environmental stress. *Proc. Natl. Acad. Sci. USA* **83,** 2350–2352.
20. Garrison, P. N., Mathis, S. A., and Barnes, L. D. (1989) Changes in diadenosine tetraphosphate levels in *Physarum polycephalum* with different oxygen concentrations. *J. Bacteriol.* **171,** 1506–1512.
21. Meyer, D., Moris, G., Wolff, C. M., Befort, N., and Remy, P. (1990) Significance of dinucleoside tetraphosphate production by cultured tumor cells exposed to the presence of ethanol. *Biochimie* **72,** 57–64.
22. Garrison, P. N. and Barnes, L. D. (1984) Assay of adenosine 5′-P1-tetraphospho-P4-5′-adenosine and adenosine 5′-P1-tetraphospho-P4-5′-guanosine in *Physarum polycephalum* and other eukaryotes. An isocratic high-pressure liquid-chromatography method. *Biochem. J.* **217,** 805–811.

10

Studies of Secretion Using Permeabilized Platelets

Tara W. Rutledge and Sidney W. Whiteheart

1. Introduction

Exocytosis from the three granules of platelets (dense-core, alpha, and lysosome) is a key event in normal hemostasis. Defects in these processes lead to bleeding-time disorders, such as Hermansky-Pudlak and gray platelet syndromes (*1–4*). Conversely, hyperactive secretion causes inappropriate clot formation, leading to the occurrence of stroke or heart attack (*5,6*). These two examples of hypo- and hyperactive platelets underline the need to understand the molecular mechanisms that are required for the platelet-release reaction. Recent advances by several groups have elucidated at least some of the proteins required for platelet exocytosis. Soluble NSF attachment protein receptor (SNARE) proteins mediate platelet granule-plasma membrane fusion (reviewed in *7–9*). These integral membrane proteins form heterotrimeric (or hetero-tetrameric) complexes that span the two bilayers of a membrane fusion junction (reviewed in *10,11*). Proteins of the t-SNARE class (target membrane SNAREs), such as syntaxin 2 and SNAP-23, have been shown to be required for all three granule-release events (*12–15*). Syntaxin 4, however, participates only in alpha-granule and lysosome release (*12–14*). v-SNAREs (vesicle SNAREs), such as VAMP-3/hceb and VAMP-8/endobrevin, have been shown to be present in platelets (*16,17*) and have been implicated in alpha-granule and dense-core exocytosis (*17,18*). With the estab-lishment of the SNAREs as the basic membrane fusion machinery for granule release, the focus now turns to SNARE regulatory molecules that control how the t- and v-SNAREs interact with each other. Molecules such as Munc18, DOC2, Munc13, Rab, and members of the synaptophysin/pantophysin families are present in platelets (T. W. Rutledge and S. W. Whiteheart, unpublished observations; T. D. Schraw and A. M. Bernstein, personal communications; *19–21*) and may hold the key to the distinct regulation of each of the three platelet-secretion events.

In vitro assays using permeabilized cells have long been important tools for dis-secting cellular functions. For platelets, this approach was initially used to assess the importance of intracellular signaling molecules (e.g., *22,23*). Subsequently, our group

From: *Methods in Molecular Biology, vol. 272:*
Platelets and Megakaryocytes, Vol. 1: Functional Assays
Edited by: J. M. Gibbins and M. P. Mahaut-Smith © Humana Press Inc., Totowa, NJ

and others have used this approach to dissect the molecular events that mediate granule release *(12,15,20,21)*. Several reagents have been used to permeabilize platelets, such as digitonin *(24,25)*, saponin *(26)*, alpha toxin *(27,28)*, and streptolysin-*O* (SLO). Permeabilization has also been achieved through electroporation *(29)*. Streptolysin-*O*, a pore-forming bacterial toxin, has advantages over other permeabilizing methods as it specifically binds to cholesterol in the plasma membrane, forming pores in a temperature-sensitive manner. The pores formed allow diffusion of proteins with molecular weights ranging up to 150–200 kDa *(30)*, which permits the passage of many recombinant proteins, peptides, and antibody molecules. Secretion is triggered by increasing the free Ca^{2+} concentration or in response to the addition of GTPγS. Using this scheme, it is possible to determine the role of various proteins in the platelet-release reaction. While the assay system described here has been extensively used to study granule release, other platelet events, such as calpain activation *(31)*, protein phosphorylation *(21)*, and cytoskeletal rearrangements *(14)*, are seen.

2. Materials

1. *Platelets:* Both freshly prepared and banked platelets have been used as a source of cells. In our experience *(15)*, the two preparations of cells differ little in their capacity to be permeabilized and to secrete granule components (*see* **Note 1**). Platelets used for the assays described below are obtained as citrated units from the Central Kentucky Blood Center (Lexington, KY). Expired platelet units are not recommended for this assay.
2. *Permeabilizing Agent:* Streptolysin-*O* (Sigma, St. Louis, MO or Corgenix, Peterborough, UK) is reconstituted in Buffer A as an 8 U/mL stock solution. Aliquots (400 μL) are frozen at –20°C and discarded after use (*see* **Note 2**).
3. *Antibodies:* Platelet factor 4 (PF4) antibody is purchased from Accurate Chemical Co. (Westbury, NY) and secondary, donkey anti-sheep IgG horseradish peroxidase conjugate is purchased from Sigma Chemical Co. (A-3415, St. Louis, MO). Other antibodies used as potential assay inhibitors are either commercial monoclonal antibodies or polyclonal antibody reagents produced by our laboratory. Generally, the antibodies are dialyzed against phosphate-buffered saline (PBS) prior to their use as inhibitors in the assay (*see* **Note 3**).
4. *PBS:* 137 mM NaCl, 2.7 mM KCl, 4.3 mM Na_2HPO_4, 1.47 mM KH_2PO_4, pH 7.4 (NaOH).
5. Apyrase, type VII (Sigma): 3 mg/mL (~340 U/mL) stock in calcium-free Tyrode's buffer is stored as 25-μL aliquots at –20°C. The remainder of a thawed aliquot is discarded after use.
6. Prostaglandin I_2 (PGI_2) (Sigma): 1 mg/mL stock in calcium-free Tyrode's buffer is stored as 10-μL aliquots at –20°C. The remainder of a thawed aliquot is discarded after use.
7. Calcium-free Tyrode's buffer: 154 mM NaCl, 2.7 mM KCl, 1 mM $MgCl_2$, 5.6 mM D-glucose, 7 mM $NaHCO_3$, 0.6 mM NaH_2PO_4, 0.35% bovine serum albumin (BSA, fraction V), 5 mM EGTA, 5 mM sodium PIPES, pH 6.5 (KOH).
8. Buffer A: 120 mM sodium glutamate, 5 mM potassium glutamate, 2.5 mM EDTA, 2.5 mM EGTA, 3.15 mM $MgCl_2$, and 1 mM dithiothreitol, 20 mM HEPES, pH 7.4 (NaOH).
9. ATP (Roche Molecular Biochemicals, Indianapolis, IN): 200 mM stock solution in Buffer A; aliquots stored at –20°C.
10. ABTS developing solution: 1.06 mM 2,2′-azino-di[3-ethyl-benzthiazoline-6-sulfonic acid] (ABTS) (Roche Molecular Biochemicals) in 0.05 M Na_2HPO_4, 0.1 M citric acid, pH 4.2, 0.03% H_2O_2. This solution can be stored at –20°C without H_2O_2, which should be added just before use.

11. Hydroxytryptamine creatinine sulfate, 5-[1,2-^{3}H(N)]-(serotonin) ([^{3}H]-serotonin), is available from PerkinElmer Life Sciences (Boston, MA) and stored as aliquots at –80°C for several months (*see* **Note 4**).
12. High-binding, polystyrene 96-well plates (EIA/RIA 3369) (Costar, Corning, NY).
13. ELISA binding buffer: 50 mM CAPS, pH 11.5 (HCl).
14. ELISA wash buffer: 0.035 mM NaH$_2$PO$_4$, 0.165 mM Na$_2$HPO$_4$, 1.54 mM NaCl, and 0.5% (v/v) Tween-20.
15. Blocking buffer: 5% (w/v) nonfat dry milk in Tris-buffered saline.
16. Citrate-phosphate buffer: 93.2 mM Na$_2$HPO$_4$, 53.4 mM citric acid, pH 4.2.
17. 10 mM p-nitrophenyl-N-acetyl-β-D-glucosaminide (Sigma): Stock is reconstituted in 150 mM NaCl; 10-mL aliquots can be stored at –20°C.
18. 0.08 N NaOH.
19. Electron microscopy fixative solution: 6% (v/v) glutaraldehyde (Electron Microscopy Sciences, Fort Washington, PA) and 80 mM lysine (Sigma) in 0.1 M Sorenson's phosphate buffer.
20. 0.1 M Sorenson's phosphate buffer: 8.1 mg/mL KH$_2$PO$_4$, 1.88 mg/mL Na$_2$HPO$_4$.
21. Osmium tetroxide (OsO$_4$) (Electron Microscopy Sciences: 1% (v/v) in 0.1 M Sorenson's phosphate buffer.
22. Uranyl acetate (Electron Microscopy Sciences): 4% (w/v) aqueous solution.
23. Absolute ethanol.
24. Propylene oxide (Electron Microscopy Sciences).
25. Spurr's resin: Mix 26 g nonenyl succinic anhydride (NSA), 6 g DER, and 10 g vinyl cyclohexene dioxide (VCD). Prior to use, add 0.4 g dimethylaminoethanol (DMAE) and mix well. All chemicals are available from Electron Microscopy Sciences.
26. Scintillation cocktail: Econo-Safe Counting Cocktail (Research Products International, Mount Prospect, IL).

3. Methods

3.1. Platelet Preparation

1. Freshly banked platelets (no more than five days old) are obtained as units from the Central Kentucky Blood Center (Lexington, KY). The following discussion assumes that only one unit of platelets will be used.
2. Gently pour the citrated, platelet-rich plasma (PRP) into two 50-mL conical tubes (~50 mL total volume) and incubate for 5 min at 25°C in the presence of 10 ng/mL PGI$_2$ and 3 µg/mL apyrase (~340 mU/mL).
3. Recover the platelets by centrifugation (Beckman GS-6R, 450g) for 5 min at room temperature (at least 25°C) with the centrifuge brake set at low.
4. After removal of the platelet-poor plasma by aspiration, gently resuspend the cells by swirling the cell pellet in 7–10 mL of calcium-free Tyrode's buffer and 3 µg/mL apyrase.
5. Remove the suspended platelets by pouring into a new conical tube and discard the remaining tightly pelleted red blood cells.
6. Repeat the washing steps two additional times, avoiding the use of both glass pipets and small-bore pipet tips; this limits inadvertent activation.
7. Finally, gently resuspend the cells by swirling the cell pellet in 1–2 mL of Buffer A. This generates a sufficient concentration for 20–40 × 50-µL aliquots (~10^7–10^8 platelets per reaction) to be used in the secretion reactions. Once in Buffer A, the cells are stable for approx 60 min; however, for best results, they should be used as soon as possible.

3.2. Permeabilization of Platelets

It is important to test conditions for each preparation of SLO to assure that the platelet plasma membrane is permeabilized but the granule membranes remain intact.

1. To test the extent of SLO permeabilization, increasing concentrations of SLO (0.2–1.2 U/mL final concentration) are incubated with the platelets under assay conditions (as described in **Subheading 3.4.1.**). Generally, 0.8 U/mL SLO has proven to be ideal for platelet permeabilization (*see* **Note 5**).
2. After incubation, the platelets are cleared from the reaction by centrifugation and the level of lactate dehydrogenase (LDH) in the supernatant is measured using a photometric assay with lactate and NADPH *(15)*. LDH, a 140 kDa cytoplasmic protein, is a valid indicator of toxin pore formation. If the SLO test assay uses [^{3}H]-serotonin-labeled cells (*see* **Subheading 3.4.1.**), the appearance of the radiolabel will assess the degree to which the dense-core granule membranes have been permeabilized (*see* **Note 5**).

3.3. Agents for Stimulation of Granule Release

In our experience, permeabilized platelets can be stimulated to secrete 50–80% of alpha and dense-core granule contents and 20–40% of lysosomal content. Secretion of permeabilized platelets can be stimulated through several different methods, although the most effective is to increase the concentration of free calcium. A concentration of 10–100 µ*M* CaCl$_2$ is generally sufficient to induce release from each of the intracellular granules. All reported calcium concentrations are calculated as free calcium (*see* **Note 6**). Other divalent cations, such as Mn^{2+}, Pb^{2+}, Zn^{2+}, and Sr^{2+}, can be used to stimulate platelet granule exocytosis (D. Chen, personal communication). The most potent cation, Pb^{2+}, stimulates both dense-core granule and lysosome secretion at 1 n*M*, though the extent of release is only half that of 10 µ*M* Ca^{2+}. Divalent cations, Sr^{2+}, Mn^{2+}, and Zn^{2+}, also stimulate secretion when present at concentrations of 100 µ*M* (D. Chen, personal communication).

GTPγS has been shown to activate both trimeric and small G proteins and can be used to stimulate permeabilized platelet secretion. GTPγS (25–100 µ*M*) stimulates release from each of the granules in permeabilized platelets; however, the time course of release demonstrates a distinct lag (100–300 s) relative to the release induced by Ca^{2+} *(13)*.

3.4. Assays for Released Granule Cargo

3.4.1. Dense Core Granules

Platelets incorporate radiolabeled serotonin into their dense core granules, which then can be a measure of granule release.

1. Platelets are metabolically labeled with [^{3}H]-serotonin by incubating platelet-rich plasma (PRP, obtained in **step 1, Subheading 3.1.**) with 0.4 µCi/mL [^{3}H]-serotonin at 37°C for 45 min.
2. After labeling, the platelets are incubated for 5 min at 25°C in the presence of 3 µg/mL apyrase (~340 mU/mL) and 10 ng/mL PGI$_2$, washed in calcium-free Tyrode's buffer, and are resuspended in 1–2 mL Buffer A (as described in **Subheading 3.1., steps 2–7**).

3. During incubation, prepare a set of reaction tubes each containing 2 μL of 200 m*M* ATP (for a final reaction concentration of 4 m*M* ATP), the appropriate amount of SLO (as determined by the titration in **step 1, Subheading 3.2.**), and sufficient Buffer A to achieve a total volume of 50 μL. For most preparations of SLO, 10 μL of 8 U/mL SLO (for a final reaction concentration of 0.8 U/mL SLO) is sufficient, thereby requiring the addition of 38 μL of Buffer A.

4. Add 50 μL of the labeled platelet suspension to each reaction tube (final reaction volume of 100 μL) and incubate the reactions at room temperature for 10 min to permeabilize the cells. To avoid dilution of platelet reactions, the total volume should be maintained at 100–130 μL by adjusting the volume of Buffer A added to the assay, in accordance with the volume of effector to be added.

5. Once the platelets are permeabilized, transfer the cells to ice for 30 min. This temperature shift effectively inactivates SLO and allows time for effector molecules that are being tested to diffuse into the platelet.

6. Warm the samples to 25°C for 5 min, stimulate by adding an appropriate concentration of CaCl$_2$ (e.g., 4.31 μL of 100 m*M* CaCl$_2$, per 100 μL assay in Buffer A is used to achieve a free calcium concentration of 100 μ*M*), or other secretion-inducing agent (*see* **Subheading 3.3.**) and incubate at 25°C for 5 min. If GTPγS is used as a stimulus, a longer incubation time (15–30 min) is required.

7. Clear the reactions by centrifugation for 1 min in a microfuge set at maximum speed.

8. The postreaction supernatants are removed and retained for analysis of release from all three granule pools (dense granules, this section; alpha granules, **Subheading 3.4.2.**; lysosomes, **Subheading 3.4.3.**).

9. The pellets are resuspended in 100 μL of Buffer A and the platelets are disrupted via five successive cycles of freezing and thawing on dry ice and at 37°C, respectively.

10. Add aliquots (30–60 μL) of supernatants and platelet pellets to 3 mL of scintillation cocktail and assay for the presence of [^{3}H]-serotonin. Release of dense-core granule contents is determined by measuring the appearance of radiolabeled serotonin in the supernatants and a reduction of retained serotonin in the platelet pellets. Detection of [^{3}H]-serotonin is the most sensitive and convenient method; however, a fluorimetric assay for serotonin can also be used *(32)*.

3.4.2. Alpha Granules

Release of alpha-granule contents can be measured by one of several different methods. Surface expression of P-selectin, measured by fluorescence-activated cell sorting (FACS), has been effectively used *(12)*. The release of von Willebrand's factor has also been used to assess alpha-granule secretion *(20)*; however, we have found it difficult to measure due to high background levels, presumably from residual plasma. We use the chemokine, platelet factor 4 (PF4), as a secretion marker since it is a soluble, alpha-granule protein whose normal plasma levels are low *(33)*. PF4 is released into the supernatant upon granule secretion; therefore, it can be measured along with serotonin and β-hexosaminidase. To measure PF4 release, a standard ELISA assay is used with an anti-PF4 antibody from Accurate Chemical Co. (*see* **Note 7**). The ELISA assay for PF4 detection is as follows:

1. In a 96-well plate, add 100 μL of ELISA binding buffer and 1–2 μL of antigen (either supernatant or disrupted pellet obtained from the assay as described in the dense-core granule assay, end of **steps 8–9, Subheading 3.4.1.**) and incubate at 37°C for 2 h.

2. Wash the wells twice with 200 µL of ELISA wash buffer.

3. Add 200 µL of blocking buffer to each well and incubate at 37°C for 1 h.

4. Wash the plate again twice with ELISA wash buffer.

5. For detection of bound PF4, add 100 µL of 10 ng/mL sheep anti-human PF4 antibody in blocking buffer to each well and incubate at 25°C for 1–2 h.

6. Wash the wells four times with ELISA wash buffer prior to the addition of 100 µL donkey, anti-sheep peroxidase conjugate diluted 1:500 in blocking buffer.

7. Incubate the plate at 25°C for 1 h, wash four times with ELISA wash buffer, and then incubate with 175 µL of developing solution.

8. Incubate at 37°C for 20–30 min, periodically checking the ELISA plates for color development in an ELISA plate reader at 405 nm. Maximal color development (OD_{405} of 0.8 for stimulated secretion samples) can take up to 1 h, but is usually complete after 20–30 min. Important controls to include in this assay are: no antigen blanks (samples generally have an OD_{405} of 0.05); no primary blanks; and untreated, solubilized platelets to determine the maximum signal possible.

3.4.3. Lysosomes

Lysosome release is determined by measuring the β-hexosaminidase present in the postsecretion supernatants. The colorimetric assay used is based on the release of *p*-nitrophenol from *p*-nitrophenyl-acetyl-β-D-glucosaminide and is typically done in a 96-well plate format and read with an ELISA plate reader at 405 nm.

1. Mix 5 mL of citrate-phosphate buffer and 2.5 mL of 10 m*M p*-nitrophenyl-N-acetyl-β-D-glucosaminide (hexosaminidase substrate solution).

2. Add 100 µL of the hexosaminidase substrate solution to each well with 5 µL of the secretion assay supernatants or disrupted platelet pellets (from **steps 8–9, Subheading 3.4.1.**).

3. Incubate the assays at 37°C for 18 h.

4. The reactions are stopped by the addition of 60 µL of 0.08 *N* NaOH (*see* **Note 8**).

5. The plate can be analyzed immediately following the addition of NaOH. Typically, OD_{405} readings of 0.30–0.70 are obtained from the supernatants of stimulated control samples, while resting platelet supernatants are expected to have OD_{405} readings of 0.01–0.05.

3.5. Test Assay

Although all release events can be measured from the same sample, [³H]-serotonin-labeled cells offer a fast and convenient test of reaction conditions before the more laborious assays for alpha-granule and lysosome release are performed. Initially, it is recommended that a quick test assay be performed to determine the quality of the platelet preparation. Five samples are required: a total reaction to determine the maximum extent of serotonin uptake, an unstimulated reaction to determine the level of background release (or leakage), and three Ca^{2+}-stimulated reactions to determine the appropriate amount of calcium required for maximal granule release.

1. In a total volume of 50 µL of Buffer A, add 2 µL of 200 m*M* ATP and 10 µL of 8 U/mL SLO to each assay tube.

2. Add 50 µL of the labeled platelet suspension (end of **step 2, Subheading 3.4.1.**), and incubate reaction at room temperature for 5 min to allow permeabilization.

3. To the three calcium titration reactions, add increasing amounts of free calcium (10^{-5}–10^{-3} *M* Ca^{2+}) to stimulate granule release.

4. After incubation for 5 min clear the unstimulated reaction and the three calcium titration reactions by centrifugation for 1 min in a microfuge set at maximum speed.
5. Analyze supernatant aliquots (30–50 μL) by scintillation counting to determine whether the calcium stimulus was adequate.
6. Disrupt the total sample via at least five freeze-thaw cycles (*see* **step 9, Subheading 3.4.1.**) and assay a similar aliquot by scintillation counting. Typically, the total level of [^{3}H]-serotonin should be approximately 2500–3000 cpm in a 40 μL aliquot and the levels in the supernatant of the unstimulated reaction and the maximal calcium sample should be 100–300 cpm and 1000–2500 cpm, respectively (*see* **Note 9**). The concentration of calcium that elicits the greatest [^{3}H]-serotonin release should be used in subsequent assays.

3.6. Data Analysis

Following platelet activation, secretion is measured by sedimenting the permeabilized platelets and retaining both the platelet pellets and the supernatants. The supernatants can be analyzed for secreted granule markers ([^{3}H]-serotonin, hexosaminidase, and PF4) as described in **Subheading 3.4.** The pellets are disrupted by five successive freeze-thaw cycles and are analyzed for content of granule markers. The sum of these two values for any reaction is the total marker present per reaction. For any given reaction, percent secretion is calculated as follows:

$$(\text{supernatant value} / \text{total marker present in reaction}) \times 100$$

3.7. Secretion Assay With Secretory Machinery Effectors

Several inhibitory reagents, such as recombinant proteins, antibodies, and peptides, can be used to probe the role of SNAREs and SNAPs in platelet exocytosis. Since t- and v-SNAREs are generally type II membrane proteins, their cytosolic domains can be used to inhibit membrane-trafficking events; however, care must be taken to assess the specificity of the inhibition since these domains undergo spurious interactions with noncognate SNAREs *(34,35)*. Use of SNARE-specific antibodies has also been effective, although it must be demonstrated that the antibodies are truly isoform-specific. Due to the similarity within the classes of SNARE proteins *(36)*, there is frequent cross-reactivity of antibodies, which can confuse interpretation of results. Additionally, an immunoglobulin control should be included in these experiments to ensure that the observed effects are specific to the molecule(s) of interest. Finally, peptides, based on regions of SNAREs *(13,15,37)* and SNARE-interacting proteins *(38–41)*, have been effectively used to demonstrate that a particular protein is involved in secretion (*see* **Note 10**).

3.8. Electron Microscopy of Permeabilized Platelets

Platelets that have been permeabilized, incubated with various reagents, and stimulated as described for the platelet exocytosis assay can be prepared for ultrastructural analysis by electron microscopy (*see* **refs. 14** and **31** for examples).

1. To fix the platelet reactions (end of **step 6, Subheading 3.4.1.**), add an equal volume of fixative solution and incubate at room temperature for 1.5 h.
2. Wash the platelets three times for 15 min each with 0.1 *M* Sorenson's phosphate buffer.

3. Osmicate with 1% OsO_4 in 0.1 *M* Sorenson's on ice for 10 min.
4. Following two brief washes in ice-cold H_2O, add 4% aqueous uranyl acetate to the fixed platelets and incubate at 4°C for 1–2 h. (Caution: Uranyl acetate is a radioactive product. Therefore follow appropriate guidelines for use.)
5. Wash the platelets in 0.1 *M* Sorenson's phosphate buffer and dehydrate in the following graded series of ethyl alcohols for 5 min each: 50%, 70%, 80%, 90%, 100%, and a previously unopened absolute ethanol.
6. Wash twice with propylene oxide and incubate overnight in a 1:1 mixture of propylene oxide and Spurr's resin to allow infiltration of the resin into the sample.
7. Embed samples in Spurr's resin, and polymerize by incubation at 50°C for 48 h.
8. Section the polymerized blocks, mount on copper grids, and examine by transmission electron microscopy following optional counterstaining with uranyl acetate and lead citrate.

3.9. Further Comments on the Secretion Assay

With any in vitro assay, the challenge is to determine how well it recapitulates the processes that occur in intact cells. For this system, the time course of secretion is slightly slower than in intact cells; however, it maintains the same temporal difference between early dense-core granule release and late lysosome release *(42)*. Additionally, secretion in permeabilized platelets is dependent on both ATP *(15)* and cytosol (T. W. Rutledge, unpublished observations). Other platelet functions are recapitulated by this assay system. By including γ-[^{32}P]-ATP into Buffer A, one can demonstrate calcium-, cAMP-, and GTPγS- stimulated phosphorylation of proteins. The spectra of phosphoproteins mimic that seen in intact, activated platelets (T. D. Schraw, personal communications). In addition, calcium-dependent cytoskeletal rearrangements *(14)* and activation of calpain *(31)* can be clearly demonstrated in permeabilized cells. This assay system has also been able to recapitulate calcium-dependent activation of the small GTP-binding proteins Ral and Rap (T. W. Rutledge, unpublished observations). Though the fibrinogen receptor is activated to its high-affinity state, as indicated by increased fibrinogen binding (P. P. Lemons, personal communication), the permeabilized platelet system does not recapitulate all the events required for aggregation, possibly due to the lack of plasma factors ultimately required for aggregation and clot formation. In short, this rather robust assay system is not only useful for the analysis of platelet secretion, but may also prove useful in dissecting other platelet functions.

4. Notes

1. One subtle difference between freshly obtained and banked platelets is that banked cells tend to incorporate higher levels of labeled serotonin into their dense-core granules. This increases the raw signal resulting from dense core granule release.
2. The quality of the SLO reagent is important for the success of the subsequent secretion assays. Of the preparations we have tested, reduced SLO from Corgenix and Sigma are of the highest quality and appear to work effectively. SLO can also be purified using the methods outlined in **ref. 43**.
3. Protein preparations should be as pure as possible and can be added to the reactions during SLO incubation. While antibody and protein reagents are frequently prepared in glycerol to maintain their stability, higher levels of glycerol (>5%) are inhibitory. This assay system

can also tolerate 1.1% (v/v total) DMSO and 1.4% (v/v total) ethanol. Care should be taken to ensure that any observed effects are specific to the molecule introduced and are not due to buffer constituents, such as high salt concentrations and organic solvents. This problem can easily be avoided with the inclusion of a buffer alone control.

4. The stability of the [^{3}H]-serotonin should be monitored. A consistent increase in the background levels of [^{3}H] in the supernatant of unstimulated control reactions is often an indication that the labeled compound is degraded.

5. Two variables are most relevant: temperature and SLO concentrations. At 37°C, leakage of dense-core contents is detected when cells are permeabilized with 0.8 U/mL SLO; however, this is almost eliminated when the platelets are incubated at 25°C. Ideally each lot of SLO should be tested, though we have generally found that 0.8 U/mL SLO at 25°C for 10 min permeabilizes the cells to the highest extent (55–60%), with little effect on granule membranes *(15)*.

6. Several websites can be used to conveniently make these calculations. *See also* **ref. 44**. We currently employ the ion concentration calculator MaxChelator at http://www.stanford.edu/~cpatton/maxc.html. A version of this program is also available for PDAs at http://www.stanford.edu/~cpatton/palm/index.html.

7. Care must be taken to assure that any inhibitors added to the secretion assay or the platelets do not affect the ELISA assay. Heparin and Triton X-100 are specific examples of compounds that interfere with this assay. When a potential inhibitor is either a protein or an antibody, the ELISA plate's protein binding capacity should not be exceeded. Another issue of concern is the stability of PF4. Measurement of PF4 release should be performed without delay, but if necessary, samples can be stored up to one week at –80°C without significant degradation of signal.

8. Up to a total of 100 μL of 0.08 *N* NaOH can be added to further intensify the color.

9. A significant deviation from these values could be an indication that the calcium stock solution is incorrect or that the SLO is nonfunctional. A lack of radiolabel in the total sample indicates potential degradation of the serotonin radiolabel or a lack of response to stimuli due to premature activation of the platelet preparation during the workup.

10. When applying this technology, it is important to include peptides with a scrambled amino acid sequence as a specificity control. This assures that the effects observed are due to the linear sequence of the inhibitory peptide and not just its bulk chemistry.

References

1. Huizing, M., Anikster, Y., and Gahl, W. A. (2001) Hermansky-Pudlak syndrome and Chediak-Higashi syndrome: Disorders of vesicle formation and trafficking. *Thromb. Haemost.* **86,** 233–245.
2. Huizing, M., Anikster, Y., and Gahl, W. A. (2000) Hermansky-Pudlak syndrome and related disorders of organelle formation. *Traffic* **1,** 823–835.
3. Rendu, F. and Brohard-Bohn, B. (2001) The platelet release reaction: Granules' constituents, secretion and functions. *Platelets* **12,** 261–273.
4. Smith, M. P., Cramer, E. M., and Savidge, G. F. (1997) Megakaryocytes and platelets in alpha-granule disorders. *Baillieres Clin. Haematol.* **10,** 125–148.
5. Islim, I. F., Bareford, D., Ebanks, M., and Beevers, D. G. (1995) The role of platelets in essential hypertension. *Blood Press.* **4,** 199–214.
6. Andrioli, G., Ortolani, R., Fontana, L., Gaino, S., Bellavite, P., Lechi, C., et al. (1996) Study of platelet adhesion in patients with uncomplicated hypertension. *J. Hypertens.* **14,** 1215–1221.

 7. Reed, G. L., Fitzgerald, M. L., and Polgar, J. (2000) Molecular mechanisms of platelet exocytosis: Insights into the "secrete" life of thrombocytes. *Blood* **96,** 3334–3342.
 8. Furie, B., Furie, B. C., and Flaumenhaft, R. (2001) A journey with platelet P-selectin: The molecular basis of granule secretion, signaling and cell adhesion. *Thromb. Haemost.* **86,** 214–221.
 9. Yoshioka, A., Horiuchi, H., Shirakawa, R., Nishioka, H., Tabuchi, A., Higashi, T., et al. (2001) Molecular dissection of alpha- and dense-core granule secretion of platelets. *Ann. N.Y. Acad. Sci.* **947,** 403–406.
10. Hay, J. C. and Scheller, R. H. (1997) SNAREs and NSF in targeted membrane fusion. *Curr. Opin. Cell Biol.* **9,** 505–512.
11. Jahn, R. and Sudhof, T. C. (1999) Membrane fusion and exocytosis. *Annu. Rev. Biochem.* **68,** 863–911.
12. Flaumenhaft, R., Croce, K., Chen, E., Furie, B., and Furie, B. C. (1999) Proteins of the exocytotic core complex mediate platelet alpha-granule secretion. Roles of vesicle-associated membrane protein, SNAP-23, and syntaxin 4. *J. Biol. Chem.* **274,** 2492–501.
13. Chen, D., Lemons, P. P., Schraw, T., and Whiteheart, S. W. (2000) Molecular mechanisms of platelet exocytosis: Role of SNAP-23 and syntaxin 2 and 4 in lysosome release. *Blood* **96,** 1782–1788.
14. Lemons, P. P., Chen, D., and Whiteheart, S. W. (2000) Molecular mechanisms of platelet exocytosis: Requirements for alpha-granule release. *Biochem. Biophys. Res. Commun.* **267,** 875–880.
15. Chen, D., Bernstein, A. M., Lemons, P. P., and Whiteheart, S. W. (2000) Molecular mechanisms of platelet exocytosis: Role of SNAP-23 and syntaxin2 in dense core granule release. *Blood* **95,** 921–929.
16. Bernstein, A. M. and Whiteheart, S. W. (1999) Identification of a cellubrevin/vesicle associated membrane protein 3 homologue in human platelets. *Blood* **93,** 571–579
17. Polgar, J., Chung, S. H., and Reed, G. L. (2002) Vesicle-associated membrane protein 3 (VAMP-3) and VAMP-8 are present in human platelets and are required for granule secretion. *Blood* **100,** 1081–1083.
18. Feng, D., Crane, K., Rozenvayn, N., Dvorak, A. M., and Flaumenhaft, R. (2002) Subcellular distribution of 3 functional platelet SNARE proteins: Human cellubrevin, SNAP-23, and syntaxin 2. *Blood* **99,** 4006–4014.
19. Fitzgerald, M. L. and Reed, G. L. (1999) Rab6 is phosphorylated in thrombin-activated platelets by a protein kinase C-dependent mechanism: Effects on GTP/GDP binding and cellular distribution. *Biochem. J.* **342,** 353–360.
20. Shirakawa, R., Yoshioka, A., Horiuchi, H., Nishioka, H., Tabuchi, A., and Kita, T. (2000) Small GTPase Rab4 regulates Ca^{2+}-induced alpha-granule secretion in platelets. *J. Biol. Chem.* **275,** 33,844–33,849.
21. Reed, G. L., Houng, A. K., and Fitzgerald, M. L. (1999) Human platelets contain SNARE proteins and a Sec1p homologue that interacts with syntaxin 4 and is phosphorylated after thrombin activation: Implications for platelet secretion. *Blood* **93,** 2617–2626.
22. Coorssen, J. R. and Haslam, R. J. (1993) GTPγS and phorbol ester act synergistically to stimulate both Ca^{2+}-independent secretion and phospholipase D activity in permeabilized human platelets. Inhibition by BAPTA and analogues. *FEBS Lett.* **316,** 170–174.
23. Sloan, D. C. and Haslam, R. J. (1997) Protein kinase C-dependent and Ca2+-dependent mechanisms of secretion from Streptolysin O-permeabilized platelets: Effects of leakage of cytosolic proteins. *Biochem. J.* **328,** 13–21.

24. Marcu, M. G., Zhang, L., Nau-Staudt, K., and Trifaro, J. M. (1996) Recombinant scinderin, an F-actin severing protein, increases calcium-induced release of serotonin from permeabilized platelets, an effect blocked by two scinderin-derived actin-binding peptides and phosphatidylinositol 4,5-bisphosphate. *Blood* **87,** 20–24.

25. Elzagallaai, A., Rose, S. D., Brandan, N. C., and Trifaro, J. M. (2001) Myristoylated alanine-rich C kinase substrate phosphorylation is involved in thrombin-induced serotonin release from platelets. *Br. J. Haematol.* **112,** 593–602.

26. Authi, K. S., Rao, G. H., Evenden, B. J., and Crawford, N. (1988) Action of guanosine 5′-[beta-thio]diphosphate on thrombin-induced activation and Ca^{2+} mobilization in saponin-permeabilized and intact human platelets. *Biochem. J.* **255,** 885–893.

27. Arvand, M., Bhakdi, S., Dahlback, B., and Preissner, K. T. (1990) *Staphylococcus aureus* alpha-toxin attack on human platelets promotes assembly of the prothrombinase complex. *J. Biol. Chem.* **265,** 14,377–14,381.

28. Flaumenhaft, R., Furie, B., and Furie, B. C. (1999) Alpha-granule secretion from alpha-toxin permeabilized, MgATP-exposed platelets is induced independently by H^+ and Ca^{2+}. *J. Cell. Physiol.* **179,** 1–10.

29. Knight, D. E. and Scrutton, M. C. (1993) Electropermeabilized platelets: A preparation to study exocytosis. *Methods Enzymol.* **221,** 123–138.

30. Ahnert-Hilger, G., Mach, W., Föhr, K. J., and Gratzl, M. (1989) Poration by α-toxin and Streptolysin-*O*: An approach to analyze intracellular process. *Methods in Cell Biol.* **31,** 63–90.

31. Rutledge, T. W. and Whiteheart, S. W. (2002) SNAP-23 is a target for calpain cleavage in activated platelets. *J. Biol. Chem.* **277,** 37,009–37,015.

32. Holmsen, H. and Dangelmaier, C. A. (1989) Measurement of secretion of serotonin. *Methods Enzymol.* **169,** 205–210.

33. Harrison, P. and Cramer, E. M. (1993) Platelet alpha-granules. *Blood Rev.* **7,** 52–62.

34. Fasshauer, D., Antonin, W., Margittai, M., Pabst, S., and Jahn, R. (1999) Mixed and non-cognate SNARE complexes. Characterization of assembly and biophysical properties. *J. Biol. Chem.* **274,** 15,440–15,446.

35. Yang, B., Gonzalez, L., Jr., Prekeris, R., Steegmaier, M., Advani, R. J., and Scheller, R. H. (1999) SNARE interactions are not selective. Implications for membrane fusion specificity. *J. Biol. Chem.* **274,** 5649–5653.

36. Bock, J. B., Matern, H. T., Peden, A. A., and Scheller, R. H. (2001) A genomic perspective on membrane compartment organization. *Nature* **409,** 839–841.

37. Guo, Z., Turner, C., and Castle, D. (1998) Relocation of the t-SNARE SNAP-23 from lamellipodia-like cell surface projections regulates compound exocytosis in mast cells. *Cell* **94,** 537–548.

38. Polgar, J. and Reed, G. L. (1999) A critical role for N-ethylmaleimide-sensitive fusion protein (NSF) in platelet granule secretion. *Blood* **94,** 1313–1318.

39. DeBello, W. M., O'Connor, V., Dresbach, T., Whiteheart, S. W., Wang, S. S., Schweizer, F. E., et al. (1995) SNAP-mediated protein-protein interactions essential for neurotransmitter release. *Nature* **373,** 626–630.

40. Schweizer, F. E., Dresbach, T., DeBello, W. M., O'Connor, V., Augustine, G. J., and Betz, H. (1998) Regulation of neurotransmitter release kinetics by NSF. *Science* **279,** 1203–1206.

41. Dresbach, T., Burns, M. E., O'Connor, V., DeBello, W. M., Betz, H., and Augustine, G. J. (1998) A neuronal Sec1 homolog regulates neurotransmitter release at the squid giant synapse. *J. Neurosci.* **18,** 2923–2932.

42. Greenberg-Sepersky, S. M. and Simons, E. R. (1985) Release of a fluorescent probe as an indicator of lysosomal granule secretion by thrombin-stimulated human platelets. *Anal. Biochem.* **147,** 57–62.

43. Bhakdi, S., Roth, M., Sziegoleit, A., and Tranum-Jensen, J. (1984) Isolation and identification of two hemolytic forms of streptolysin-O. *Infect. Immun.* **46,** 394–400.

44. Patton, C., Thompson, S., and Epel, D. (2004) Some precautions in using chelators to buffer metals in biological solutions. *Cell Calcium.* **35,** 427–431.

11

Measurement of Platelet Arachidonic Acid Metabolism

Richard W. Farndale, Philip G. Hargreaves, Joanna L. Dietrich, and Rosemary J. Keogh

1. Introduction

Platelets respond to low levels of agonists such as collagen or thrombin with primary signals that, although small, are functionally significant because they are amplified by autocrine and paracrine pathways such as the secretion of ADP and ATP from the dense granules. An important mediator of the action of low-dose collagen, especially, which is not dependent on granule secretion, is thromboxane A_2, a prostanoid that is a potent platelet agonist in its own right, binding to G-protein-linked receptors on the cell surface to stimulate calcium signals via phospholipase $C\beta$. The precursor of the prostanoids is arachidonic acid (AA), liberated from platelet membrane lipids by the action of phospholipase A_2. AA is processed in two stages by cyclooxygenase to yield prostaglandin (PG) H_2. This process is aspirin-sensitive, as the drug irreversibly acetylates and inhibits cyclooxygenase, providing the basis for the old and effective antithrombotic use for aspirin, which itself underscores the involvement of collagen in arterial thrombosis. Thromboxane synthase then consumes a proportion of PGH_2 to generate thromboxane (Tx) A_2. Other products of platelet arachidonate metabolism include PGD_2, which exercises an inhibitory role on platelet function as a consequence of its capacity to activate adenylate cyclase, like its homolog, PGI_2 (prostacyclin). PGI_2 in circulation, however, is largely produced by the vascular endothelial cells rather than the platelets.

This chapter will deal with the measurement of the activity of the prostanoid pathway, detailing a method to measure AA release from metabolically labeled platelets, a thin-layer chromatography procedure for AA-containing lipids, and an ELISA assay for TxA_2.

Together, these methods provide a means of measuring the activity of the thromboxane pathway at its initiation (phospholipase A_2 activity), intermediate metabolism (cyclooxygenase activity), and endpoint (thromboxane production). A platelet-preparation section provides details which are applicable to each of these methods.

From: *Methods in Molecular Biology, vol. 272:*
Platelets and Megakaryocytes, Vol. 1: Functional Assays
Edited by: J. M. Gibbins and M. P. Mahaut-Smith © Humana Press Inc., Totowa, NJ

Different forms of phospholipase (PL) A_2 exist in a variety of tissues and, indeed, species. Secreted forms of PLA_2 are a component of snake and insect venoms (which may be relevant where these materials are used to modify platelet function) and may also have a role in mammalian physiology since leukocytes in particular may release such enzymes at sites of inflammation. Although platelets contain several PLA_2 isoforms *(1,2)*, the platelet PLA_2 isoform of major interest here is the cytoplasmic enzyme, a 95-kDa protein *(3–5)* whose structure has been solved *(6–9)* but whose regulation remains the subject of study and debate. The enzyme has a calcium-binding domain, like that of protein kinase C, and it requires calcium for activity *(10)*. It is not clear that the ligand-dependent activation of cytoplasmic (c) PLA_2 is calcium-driven, however, as activation of $cPLA_2$ can be achieved despite buffering of cytoplasmic Ca^{2+} levels, although Ca^{2+}-binding may be involved in targeting the enzyme to the plasma membrane where its substrate resides *(11)*. The enzyme exists in several phosphorylated forms, and phosphorylation on serine residues, as a consequence of various MAP kinase activities, or possibly a combination of such events, has been linked with the activation process *(10,12,13)*.

1.1. PLA₂ Activity

A simple method for measuring the activity of the PLA_2 pathway in platelets, based on the method of Joseph et al. *(14)*, consists of three steps:

- Platelet preparation,
- Radiolabeling with [³H]arachidonic acid,
- Treatment of platelets with ligand, and sampling the supernatant.

The overall time taken for the assay is around 4 h, not including liquid scintillation counting. Each sample tube contains about 50 µL of platelets, so that 2–3 mL of platelet suspension will be sufficient for up to 20 different assay conditions, each sampled in triplicate. Small numbers of platelets, even as few as 10^7 per tube, may be used successfully, potentially allowing the method to be applied to limited supplies of blood, such as from laboratory animals. Since the authors have not used the method in this context, however, it will be important to test these more demanding applications using experimental parameters derived from study of human platelets. Guidance for this is provided below.

1.1.1. Platelet Preparation

Several different sources of platelets have been used successfully, starting either from whole blood blood as a source of platelet-rich plasma (PRP) or from platelet concentrates or apheresis platelets. Any method that yields platelets in single-cell suspension is likely to be acceptable. It may be prudent for detailed signaling studies to avoid the use of PGI_2, PGE_1, or their analogs, which interfere with the pathway *(15)*, for example by inhibiting calcium signaling as a consequence of elevation of cyclic AMP levels *(16)*. However, since the platelets are incubated for 1 h subsequent to their isolation, there may be sufficient time for recovery from the inclusion of PGs during the preparation process.

1.1.2. Radiolabeling

Platelets turn over arachidonate-containing lipids quite quickly, enabling exogenous radiolabeled AA to be incorporated into phospholipid pools rapidly enough to support the assay procedure described below. AA is incorporated by acyltransferases into lysophospholipids using arachidonylCoA as an intermediate. Each of the major phospholipids, phosphatidyl -choline, -ethanolamine, -serine, and -inositol, contains significant pools of AA at the *sn*2 position, which may be mobilized during activation *(17,18)*. It is not clear that AA is incorporated into each at equal rate, however, and in the procedure described below, phosphatidylcholine may be the major repository for [^{3}H]AA.

The requirements for radiolabeling are not stringent, the main consideration being that the platelet suspension should not be entirely free of protein; otherwise, loss of AA from the medium may substantially be a consequence of adsorption by the vessel wall rather than uptake by platelets. This is the reason for leaving some plasma behind at the preparation stages described below. Polystyrene tubes are particularly subject to this problem. Polypropylene centrifuge tubes have generally proved satisfactory, however, and the presence of residual plasma proteins is sufficient to prevent adsorption whichever tube is used. Should there be a need to use more carefully washed platelets, it is important to include in the medium low levels (0.35%, w/v) of bovine serum albumin (BSA), which binds AA and prevents it being adsorbed by the vessel wall. The suitability of tubes for both radiolabeling and the assay itself can readily be verified by measuring recovery of a known amount of [^{3}H]AA after incubating in the appropriate medium for 1 h.

Similarly, platelet count during the labeling procedure is not a pressing concern: The platelets at 5×10^8/mL will take up >90% of the radiolabel during 60 min, and the amount of [^{3}H]AA release in the subsequent assay depends on its concentration during labeling rather than the platelet count during labeling: a 30-fold increase in platelet count gives rise to less than 2-fold increase in AA release (*see* **Fig. 1**). Thus, a given level of platelets, say 5×10^8/mL, will incorporate the radiolabel readily using [^{3}H]AA 1 µCi/mL; and a 45-µL aliquot of these platelets will yield a good, measurable response, up to about 100% of the background level, and counts of around 5000 dpm. Radiolabeling at this level is therefore ample to produce good signals from platelets at 1×10^8/mL, but should higher levels of [^{3}H]AA labeling be required it should be borne in mind that ethanol concentrations approaching 1% (v/v), equivalent to 10 µCi/mL, might activate platelets. Should higher levels of incorporation be required, the radioactive concentration of the stock [^{3}H]AA may first be increased by evaporation under a stream of nitrogen. It is also possible, though more expensive, to use [^{14}C]AA, e.g., as used in **Subheading 3.2.3.**, as an alternative to [^{3}H]AA.

For these various practical reasons, therefore, the protocol given in **Subheading 3.1.2.** is recommended.

1.1.3. AA Release Assay

The release assay is time-dependent, as would be anticipated, but reaches a plateau after a few minutes (*see* **Fig. 2**). The assay is useful for times as short as a few seconds, and using thrombin as agonist, no delay can be detected between start of the reaction

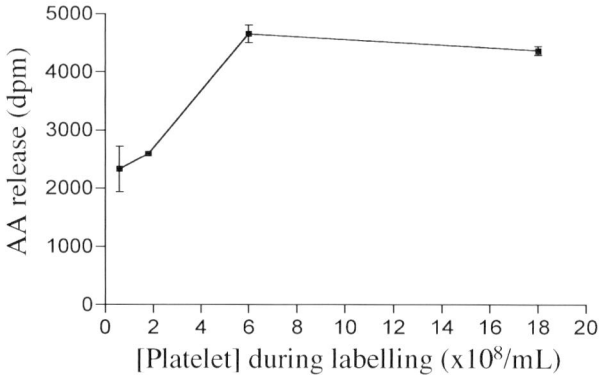

Fig. 1. Platelets were prepared according to **Subheading 3.1.1.**, resuspended to concentrations from 0.6×10^8/mL to 1.8×10^9/mL, then labeled using 1.0 µCi [^{3}H]AA/mL as described in **Subheading 3.1.2.** After centrifugation to remove excess [^{3}H]AA, the platelets were resuspended to the same volume of LB, and the release assay run for 5 min as described in **Subheading 3.1.3.**, using collagen (100 µg/mL) as agonist. The graph shows AA release (dpm) of triplet determinations, basal activity having been subtracted. Thus, across a concentration range during the radiolabeling process in excess of one order of magnitude, the AA release varies by about twofold.

and release of AA, whereas with collagen, a delay of about 20 s is observed *(19)*. Under the conditions described, agonist-stimulated release is substantially complete after 2 min. Surprisingly, the peak level of release, as well as its initial rate, is dependent on the concentration of the activator, implying that release is balanced by re-incorporation into lipids. The endpoint reflects the concentration of agonist, and the assay can be allowed to run for a time beyond that required to reach plateau levels. Thus, the assay becomes more robust, because it is insensitive to minor variations in incubation time. To stop the reaction, a solution of EDTA containing formaldehyde is added.

1.1.4. Thin-Layer Chromatography for AA-Containing Lipids

The release assay described above measures AA turnover directly in platelets after ligand stimulation. It is possible to measure the depletion of AA from lipids, either *in situ* using platelets radiolabeled as above, or in vitro using purified enzyme (or possibly permeabilized platelets) to which radiolabeled lipid has been added. Many methods exist in the literature for chromatography of membrane phospholipids. A good description of a two-dimensional separation is provided by Holub and Watson *(20)*, which might readily be adapted to study AA metabolism. Amersham Bioscience datasheets also provide details of a solvent system to separate AA from hydrophilic breakdown products (principally ^{3}H$_2$O) and which can be used to verify the purity of the radiolabel, or indeed to purify it should the need arise. **Subheading 3.2.1.** provides a rapid

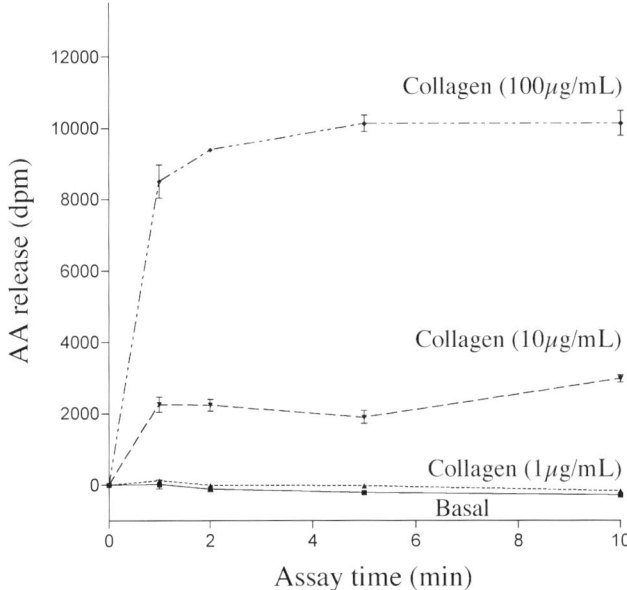

Fig. 2. Platelets were prepared according to **Subheading 3.1.1.**, resuspended to 10^9/mL, then labeled using 1.0 μCi [^{3}H]AA/mL. The release assay was run for the indicated times, as described in **Subheading 3.1.3.**, stimulating the platelets with collagen fibers at the indicated level. The graph shows AA release (dpm), initial basal levels having been subtracted. Thus, the release process is virtually complete after 2 min, with the level of release varying with the agonist concentration.

one-dimensional method that can readily be used for multiple small samples and can thus provide the basis for a quantitative assay. A preparative method using larger sample volumes (and poorer resolution of individual lipids) is described in **Subheading 3.2.3.**

1.1.5. In Vitro Measurement of PLA$_2$ Activity

Thin-layer chromatography can be adapted to study PLA$_2$ activity directly, which requires access to purified enzyme. In principle, platelet lysates or PLA$_2$ immunoprecipitates from such lysates are usable *(21)*, although we have not applied the method in this mode. For recombinant or purified cPLA$_2$, 200 ng per assay tube is ample. For the assay itself, based on the method of Cross et al. *(22)*, stearoyl,[^{14}C]arachidonoylphosphatidylcholine (14C-SAPC) is a suitable substrate, which is mixed with stearoyl,arachidonoyldiacylgylcerol as vehicle.

1.2. Measurement of Thromboxane Generation

It may be preferable to measure the production of thromboxane rather than AA release for a number of reasons. In platelet activatory studies, the principle prostanoid involved in amplifying the primary stimulus is TxA$_2$. Thus, TxA$_2$ represents the ultimate product of the pathway, although if the investigator is more interested in the regulation of the start of the pathway, measurement of AA release may be more appropriate. A key difference between the two measurements is in their sensitivity: at best, the AA release assay yields about a two-fold increase in [^{3}H]AA in the assay supernatant, and gains in utility from its high reproducibility. In marked contrast, the levels of thromboxane, measured as TxB$_2$, to which the active product, TxA$_2$, is rapidly converted, may increase 1000-fold (from about 0.5 to over 100 ng/10^8 platelets over a few minutes) after modest stimulation of platelets by primary agonists such as collagen *(23)*. This property alone makes the assay awkward to use if it is intended to measure basal levels of TxB$_2$ accurately, since it may be impossible to apply the same dilution to all samples to arrive within the rather narrow sensitivity range of the assay. Another consideration may be expense. Commercially available kits provide the most obvious recourse, but cost around \$3.70 per sample. (In marked contrast, the plasticware used for the AA release assay will prove more expensive than the radiolabel consumed.) If many samples are to be measured, however, then a procedure for derivatizing TxB$_2$ has been described in detail by McNicol *(24)*, which will allow an ELISA to be constructed at modest expense using commercially available antibodies.

Once established, the TxB$_2$ assay can be used to measure the activity of cyclo-oxygenase, measured as TxB$_2$ production in the presence of a high level of exogenous AA. This is described in **Subheading 3.3.2.**

Similar kits are available to measure PGD$_2$ (e.g., from Cayman Chemical Co.) allowing one to measure the proportional flux through other branches of the AA pathway—for example, after treatments that modify thromboxane synthase activity.

2. Materials

1. Loading buffer (LB): 145 mM NaCl, 5 mM KCl, 1 mM MgSO$_4$, 10 mM glucose, 10 mM HEPES, 500 μM EGTA, pH 7.4. Filter-sterilize and store at 4°C.
2. Release assay stopping reagent: 40 mM EDTA in 0.38% (v/v) formaldehyde. Stable at room temperature indefinitely.
3. In vitro assay buffer: 290 mM KCl, 14 mM CaCl$_2$, 145 mM Tris-HCl, pH 7.4, to which 6 mM DTT is added immediately before use. Store frozen in aliquots.
4. In vitro assay stopping reagent: Ethanol containing 2% (v/v) acetic acid and 1% arachidonic acid (v/v), the latter added immediately before use. Store at room temperature, tightly stoppered.
5. TLC solvent A: Chloroform : methanol : acetic acid : water (75 : 25 : 8 : 3, v/v). Make up fresh.
6. TLC solvent B: Ethylacetate : iso-octane : water : acetic acid (55 : 75 : 100 : 8, v/v). Make up fresh.
7. Tx assay stopping reagent: 100 mM EDTA containing 25 μM indomethacin (used ice-cold, with indomethacin added immediately before use). Store EDTA solution at room temperature.
8. Apyrase (Sigma Grade VII).
9. [^{3}H] arachidonic acid (*see* **Note 1**).
10. Bovine serum albumin (BSA).
11. Chloroform.
12. Methanol.
13. 1 M hydrochloric acid.

14. Stearoyl,[^{14}C]arachidonoylphosphatidylcholine (14C-SAPC)—Amersham Biosciences (Bucks, UK) CFA 504, 50 mCi/mmol).
15. Stearoyl,arachidonoyldiacylgylcerol (DAG)—Sigma (S6389).
16. Stearoyl,arachidonoylphosphatidylcholine (nonlabeled standard).
17. Arachidonic acid (nonlableled standard).
18. Whatman LK6DF silica gel TLC plates.
19. TxB$_2$ immunoassay kit (e.g., [DE0700] R&D systems Abingdon, UK, Amersham Biosciences BioTrak range [RPN220] and Cayman Chemical Co. [#519031, available in the UK through Alexis Biochemicals Nottingham, UK]).

3. Methods

3.1. Arachidonate Release Assay

3.1.1. Platelet Preparation

3.1.1.1. PLATELETS FROM POOLED CONCENTRATES OR APHERESIS PACKS

Each pack (which is anticoagulated with an ACD-based formulation) contains up to 10^{11} platelets, at a concentration of about 5×10^8/mL. Allow 2 mL of concentrate for every 1 mL suspension required finally. Process platelets using 15 mL polypropylene centrifuge tubes.

1. Pellet the platelets from 6 mL concentrate by centrifuging at 2000 rpm (G$_{max}$ ~700g) for 15 min using an MSE Mistral benchtop centrifuge or equivalent. Remove and discard 5.5 mL plasma.
2. Resuspend by adding 500 µL LB and pipetting briskly, but avoiding any packed red cells at the base of the pellet. Transfer platelets to a clean tube, and make up to 3 mL with LB (*see* **Subheading 2., step 1**).
3. Sample for counting platelet numbers, and adjust to 5×10^8 platelets/mL using LB. Add apyrase (Sigma Grade VII) to 0.1 U/mL.

[Yield: 3–5 mL]

3.1.1.2. PLATELETS FROM WHOLE BLOOD

Platelet concentration is much lower in PRP than in therapeutic concentrates or pools, and the yield of platelets will be correspondingly lower. Allow 3 mL of blood for every 1 mL suspension required.

1. Centrifuge 6 mL of whole blood (anticoagulation with ACD or other citrate) at 1200 rpm (G$_{max}$ ~200g) for 15 min. For more information on blood collection and anticoagulation, refer to Chapters 1 and 2, vol. 1.
2. Remove PRP, maximizing the recovery of platelets. Add apyrase (Sigma Grade VII) to 0.1 U/mL.
3. Centrifuge PRP (~2.5 mL) at 2000 rpm (G$_{max}$ ~700g) for 15 min. Remove and discard 2.25 mL plasma.
4. Resuspend by adding 500 µL LB and pipetting as above. Transfer platelets to a clean tube, and make up to 1 mL with LB.
5. Sample for counting, and adjust to 5×10^8 platelets/mL using LB. Add apyrase to 0.1 U/mL.

[Yield: ~2 mL]

3.1.2. Radiolabeling for AA Release Assay *(see **Notes 1** and **2**)*

1. To 1 mL platelets at, typically, 5×10^8/mL (range 0.1 to 1×10^9/mL) in LB containing apyrase (0.1 U/mL) and either residual plasma or 0.35% (w/v) BSA, add 1 μCi [^{3}H]AA. Incubate in a water bath at 37°C for 1 h (*see **Notes 3–5***).
2. Add 4 mL LB containing apyrase (0.1 U/mL), and centrifuge at 2000 rpm for 10 min (G_{max} ~700g).
3. Remove and discard as much supernatant as possible (*see **Note 2*** concerning disposal of radioactivity) and resuspend platelets in 1 mL LB containing apyrase (0.1 U/mL) and 0.35 % (w/v) BSA. Hold at 37°C for up to 2 h before use.

3.1.3. AA Release Assay

1. Dispense activators (e.g., collagen or thrombin) in a volume of 5 μL into 500-μL polypropylene microfuge tubes. Prewarm the tubes to 37°C in a water bath.
2. Begin the reaction by pipetting 45 μL of labeled, prewarmed platelet suspension (*see **Note 5***) into each tube, whirlimixing briefly and returning to the water bath. The reaction should be timed, so begin dispensing each set of triplet tubes at no shorter than 20-s intervals.
3. 5 min later, begin to stop the reaction by adding 50 μL of release assay stopping reagent (*see **Subheading 2., step 2***), capping each tube and whirlimixing vigorously. Preserve the timing when each triplet of tubes is stopped, so that each is incubated for exactly 5 min (*see **Note 6***).
4. Microfuge the assay tubes (10,000g, 1 min), now containing 100 μL of fluid, as soon as possible (*see **Note 7***), and carefully sample up to 75 μL of the supernatant into liquid scintillation tubes (*see **Note 8***). Add scintillant, cap and shake well, then estimate radioactivity using an instrument that provides dpm. Count a 45-μL portion of the labeled platelet suspension, allowing the percentage of ^{3}H released from the platelets to be estimated. This lies in the range 5 to 10% of the platelet-associated radioactivity.

3.2. Measurement of Turnover of AA-Containing Lipids

3.2.1. Lipid Extraction and Thin-Layer Chromatography (TLC)

Platelets should be radiolabeled and handled as for the AA release assay. After treatment with ligand, AA-containing lipids are extracted with a mixture of chloroform and methanol, to rupture and solubilize membranes, followed by further chloroform and finally HCl *(25,26)*. The latter ensures that phospholipids and AA itself are neutral and thus fully enter the hydrophobic solvent.

1. After incubation of 45 μL [^{3}H]AA-labelled platelets with 5 μL ligand, preferably in a screw-cap microfuge tube, add 50 μL CHCl$_3$:CH$_3$OH (1:2, v/v), cap, and whirlimix vigorously.
2. Add 50 μL CHCl$_3$, 50 μL water, then 15 μL 1 *M* HCl. Whirlimix vigorously.
3. Centrifuge at 10,000g for 1 min, then carefully remove the lower phase (about 100 μL) into a clean microfuge tube. Avoid the denatured proteins at the interface, and especially do not transfer any of the aqueous upper phase, which will distort the running of the chromatogram.
4. Load the lower phase onto the origin of a plastic-backed silica gel thin-layer chromatography plate (Macherey Nagel, obtained from Camlab, Cambridge, UK), drying between

10-μL additions so that the lipid is constrained in a small-diameter spot. The sample volume may be reduced by evaporation under a stream of N_2 to speed the handling of multiple samples. The chromatogram is run in TLC solvent A (*see* **Subheading 2., step 5**). Separation will take about 25 min for a 10-cm plate, and up to about 1 h if greater resolution is achieved by using a 20-cm plate.

3.2.2. Detection of Lipids

Lipids can be identified with reference to appropriate unlabeled standards, run in control lanes. The TLC solvent will adequately resolve phosphatidylcholine, phosphatidylinositol and phosphatidylserine, from arachidonic acid, which runs close to the solvent front. Lipids can be stained either as described by Holub and Watson *(20)*, or by the simple expedient of placing the chromatogram in a chamber containing a few iodine crystals. The vapor will color the lipids yellow-brown after a few minutes.

The simplest method of quantitation is to cut each lane of the dry chromatogram into strips about 5 mm in length, place each in a scintillation vial, cover with scintillant, and allow lipids to desorb overnight before liquid scintillation counting (lsc). This is less of a problem if toluene-based scintillant, or other formulation designed for nonaqueous samples, is used, e.g., Quickszint 501 (Zinsser Analytic UK) (*see also* **Note 9**).

3.2.3. In Vitro Measurement of PLA₂ Activity

The following procedure may be valuable in testing the effect of inhibitors or other species, such as protein kinases, that may regulate the activity of PLA_2. Pretreatment of the enzyme will be necessary, to be determined by experiment.

1. Add to assay tubes (e.g., 1.5-mL microfuge tubes) 4×10^4 dpm 14C-SAPC (1 μL of CFA504), and 170 pmol DAG (20 μL of 8.5 μ*M* solution in ethanol).
2. Evaporate the organic solvents to dryness under nitrogen and store tubes at –80°C (for several weeks) until required.
3. Reconstitute sufficient tubes for the assay by adding 20 μL water and placing in a sonicator bath (e.g., Decon F5 Minor) for 2×4 min.
4. Dispense 35 μL in vitro assay buffer to each tube, and warm to 30°C in a water bath.
5. Begin the assay by adding PLA_2 preparation (45 μL containing 200 ng enzyme) to each tube, vortexing well.
6. After suitable times, e.g., 20 min, stop the reaction with 100 μL of stopping reagent.
7. Pipet all of the sample in a fume hood, 50 μL at a time, onto the pre-adsorbent area of the tracked Whatman LK6DF silica-gel plates, drying under a cool airstream between additions, allow to dry fully, and develop in TLC solvent B. Run AA and unreacted SAPC in control lanes. When the solvent front has advanced at least 15cm, remove the plate and allow to dry in a fume hood. The AA-containing region should be located by placing the plate over iodine crystals, as in **Subheading 3.2.2.**
8. Moisten the segment of the track containing the AA by pipetting 20 μL water, and carefully lift or scrape that region using a spatula into a scintillation vial. Determine the amount of $[^{14}C]AA$ by lsc.

3.3. AA Metabolites Measured Using 96-Well Kits

3.3.1. Measurement of Thromboxane B₂

The procedure will use washed platelets prepared as described above, omitting the radiolabeling step, and resuspending finally in protein-free LB to a concentration of 1×10^8/mL. The sensitivity of the assay makes it useful where limited numbers of platelets are available (*see* **Note 10**).

1. Dispense ligand into 500-µL polypropylene microfuge tubes in a volume of 5 µL in triplicate. Prewarm the tubes to 37°C in a water bath.
2. Begin the reaction by pipetting 45 µL of labeled, prewarmed platelet suspension into each tube, whirlimixing briefly and returning to the water bath. The reaction should be timed, so begin dispensing each set of triplet tubes at no shorter than 20-s intervals.
3. After suitable time, e.g., 5 min, stop the reaction by adding 50 µL of ice-cold EDTA/indomethacin, preserving the timing of the assay as described for AA release. Whirlimix thoroughly and hold the sample tubes on ice until the assay is complete.
4. Centrifuge the samples for 1 min at 10,000g and remove the supernatant to a clean microfuge tube, either for immediate assay or for storage. In our hands, the stopped samples are stable for months at –80°C.

Precise details for the assay are provided with each supplier's kit, so that protocols will not be given here. In the R&D Systems ImmunoAssay kit (DE0700), TxB_2 from the sample competes with alkaline phosphatase-conjugated TxB_2 for an anti-TxB_2 antibody, the latter being captured on a 96-well plate. A color reaction ensues, in which color decreases with $[TxB_2]$. Other suitable similar kits are from Amersham Biosciences BioTrak range (RPN220) and Cayman Chemical Co (#519031, available in the UK through Alexis Biochemicals). Of these, the R&D Systems kit claims a rather wider range, operating from about 10 pg/mL to about 10,000 pg/mL, whereas the others mentioned extend only as far as 1000 pg/mL, with similar initial sensitivity. The assay using the Amersham Biosciences and the R&D Systems kits can be completed within a working day, where longer incubation (18 h) is needed for the Cayman kit. Each uses a sample volume of 50 to 100 µL.

3.3.2. Measurement of Cyclooxygenase Activity

An important use for the TxB_2 assay is to measure cyclooxygenase activity. In this instance, the activatory stimulus is arachidonic acid itself, applied in high dose (30 µM) for 6 min. Thus, the TxB_2 generated represents flux through the synthetic pathway rather than physiological stimulus. This parameter may be useful in measuring the function of cyclooxygenase/thromboxane synthase in the study of inhibitors such as aspirin or in investigating the regulation of these enzymes.

4. Notes

1. [³H]arachidonic acid is available from several manufacturers. The Amersham product ([5,6,8,9,11,12,14,15-³H]-arachidonic acid, initial specific activity 200 Ci/mmol) is

supplied in ethanol at a higher and more convenient concentration (1 mCi/mL) than the ICN Flow product, at one tenth of this concentration, although in other respects, the latter product is suitable.

2. It is important to observe the necessary safety precautions and local rules when using radioactivity. ^{3}H presents no external hazard, but internalization by ingestion or any other route should be avoided. When experimentation is complete, ensure that your workplace is free of contamination by swabbing and liquid scintillation counting. The levels of radioactivity used here will not under any circumstances approach current safe-exposure limits.

3. The uptake of [^{3}H]AA by the platelets can be monitored by sampling the supernatant after the centrifugation step, and comparing with the level of radioactivity in an equal volume of resuspended platelets. The majority should be associated with the platelets. If not, or if background levels in the subsequent assay are high, the radiochemical purity of the AA may be suspect, especially if it is more than a few months old. This may be verified by thin-layer chromatography (*see* **Subheading 3.2.**).

4. For platelets at low levels (0.1×10^9/mL or lower) it will be useful to establish that uptake of [^{3}H]AA is complete during the 60-min incubation. Extend the incubation time accordingly. Uptake is more rapid with occasional whirlimixing.

5. Where effects of inhibitors are to be investigated, after labeling and resuspension, the stock of platelets can be divided into different pre-incubations to which inhibitors or their solvent vehicles are added. Each of these should be sampled under control conditions to establish that the basal turnover of AA is not compromised by either the inhibitor or its solvent.

6. This timing allows 15 conditions to be accommodated within a 5-min assay. Since beyond 3 or 4 min, AA release is essentially independent of time, the assay can safely be extended up to about 10 min to increase the number of conditions under test in a single run. Include control replicates toward the beginning and end of each run to confirm constancy within the experiment.

7. The stopped reaction mixture is stable for up to 30 min after the reaction, allowing several runs to be completed before processing if necessary.

8. After the stopped samples are centrifuged, a pellet of packed platelets will just be visible at one side of the tip of the microfuge tube. Be sure to avoid this pellet when sampling the supernatant for liquid scintillation counting, since it will typically contain 50,000 dpm of tritium, nine times as much as the supernatant. Such a pellet will be clearly visible when using platelets at 1×10^9/mL, but very much less obvious at 10% of this level of platelets.

9. [^{3}H]-labeled lipids may also be visualized using [^{3}H]-sensitive fluors with a PhosphorImager (Molecular Dynamics Inc.) or by direct detection using a Berthold Inc. linear scanner. Ultimately, lsc provides the most sensitive method, and despite the labor involved, may prove to be the most rapid.

10. The key question here is of dilution: a working platelet suspension of 10^8/mL will yield a TxB$_2$ concentration of perhaps 200,000 pg/mL when maximally stimulated over 5 min, from a 500 pg/mL basal level. The stimulated samples should be diluted, say, 200-fold for assay in the buffer provided with the kit. Basal samples may need no dilution at all, which should be established by preliminary experiment. However, given the different buffer concentration that will result, it is important that platelet-free LB is used as a control for basal samples in the assay. Dilution of samples activated with threshold levels of stimulus will need to be investigated as they arise, so that perhaps a 10-fold dilution will be suitable for these as well as for basal samples.

References

1. Mounier, C., Faili, A., Vargaftig, B. B., Bon, C., and Hatmi, M. (1993) Secretory phospholipase A$_2$ is not required for arachidonic acid liberation during platelet activation. *Eur. J. Biochem.* **216,** 169–175.
2. Mounier, C., Vargaftig, B. B., Franken, P. A., Verheij, H. M., Bon, C., and Touqui, L. (1994) Platelet secretory phospholipase A$_2$ fails to induce rabbit platelet activation and to release arachidonic acid in contrast with venom phospholipases A$_2$. *Biochim. Biophys. Acta* **1214,** 88–96.
3. Leslie, C. C., Voelker, D. R., Channon, J. Y., Wall, M. A., and Zelarney, P. T. (1988) Properties, and purification of an arachidonoyl-hydrolyzing phospholipase A$_2$ from a macrophage cell line, RAW 2647. *Biochim. Biophys. Acta* **963,** 476–492.
4. Leslie, C. C. (1991) Kinetic properties of a high molecular mass arachidonoyl-hydrolyzing phospholipase A$_2$ that exhibits lysophospholipase activity. *J. Biol. Chem.* **266,** 11,366–11,371.
5. Kramer, R. M., Roberts, E. F., Manetta, J., and Putnam, J. E. (1991) The Ca^{2+}-sensitive cytosolic phospholipase A$_2$ is a 100-kDa protein in human monoblast U937 cells. *J. Biol. Chem.* **266,** 5268–5272.
6. Perisic, O., Fong, S., Lynch, D. E., Bycroft, M., and Williams, R. L. (1998) Crystal structure of a calcium-phospholipid binding domain from cytosolic phospholipase A$_2$. *J. Biol. Chem.* **273,** 1596–1604.
7. Xu, G.-Y., McDonagh, T., Yu, H.-A., Nalefski, E. A., Clark, J. D., and Cumming, D. A. (1998) Solution structure, and membrane interactions of the C2 domain of cytosolic phospholipase A$_2$. *J. Mol. Biol.* **280,** 485–500.
8. Bittova, L., Sumandea, M., and Cho, W. (1999) A structure-function study of the C2 domain of cytosolic phospholipase A$_2$. Identification of essential calcium ligands, and hydrophobic membrane binding residues. *J. Biol. Chem.* **274,** 9665–9672.
9. Dessen, A., Tang, J., Schmidt, H., Stahl, M., Clark, J. D., Seehra, J., et al. (1999) Crystal structure of human cytosolic phospholipase A$_2$ reveals a novel topology, and catalytic mechanism. *Cell* **97,** 349–360.
10. Leslie, C. C. (1997) Properties, and regulation of cytosolic phospholipase A$_2$. *J. Biol. Chem.* **272,** 16,709–16,712.
11. Channon, J. Y. and Leslie, C. C. (1990) A calcium-dependent mechanism for associating a soluble arachidonoyl-hydrolyzing phospholipase A$_2$ with membrane in the macrophage cell line RAW 264 7. *J. Biol. Chem.* **265,** 5409–5413.
12. Borsch-Haubold, A. G., Ghomashchi, F., Pasquet, S., Goedert, M., Cohen, P., Gelb, M. H., et al. (1999) Phosphorylation of cytosolic phospholipase A$_2$ in platelets is mediated by multiple stress-activated protein kinase pathways. *Eur. J. Biochem.* **265,** 195–203.
13. Gijon, M. A., Spencer, D. M., Kaiser, A. L., and Leslie, C. C. (1999) Role of phosphorylation sites, and the C2 domain in regulation of cytosolic phospholipase A2. *J. Cell. Biol.* **145,** 1219–1232.
14. Joseph, S., Krishnamurthi, S., and Kakkar, V. V. (1988) Differential effects of the diacylglycerol kinase inhibitor R59022 on thrombin versus collagen-induced human platelet secretion. *Biochim. Biophys. Acta* **969,** 9–17.
15. Xing, M., Post, S., Ostrom, R. S., Samardzija, M., and Insel, P. A. (1999) Inhibition of phospholipase A$_2$-mediated arachidonic acid release by cyclic AMP defines a negative feedback loop for P$_{2Y}$ receptor activation in madin-darby canine kidney D$_1$ cells. *J. Biol. Chem.* **274,** 10,035–10,038.

16. Moos, M. and Goldberg, N. D. (1988) Cyclic AMP opposes IP$_3$-induced calcium release from permeabilised human platelets. *Second Messengers and Phosphoproteins* **12,** 163–170.

17. Bills, T. K., Smith, J. B., and Silver, M. J. (1977) Selective release of arachidonic acid from the phospholipids of human platelets in response to thrombin. *J. Clin. Invest.* **60,** 1–6.

18. Broekman, M. J. (1986) Stimulated platelets release equivalent amounts of arachidonate from phosphatidylcholine, phosphatidylethanolamine, and inositides. *J. Lipid Res.* **27,** 884–891.

19. Hargreaves, P. G., Licking, E. F., Sargeant, P., Sage, S. O., Barnes, M. J., and Farndale, R. W. (1994) The tyrosine kinase inhibitors, genistein, and methyl 2,5-dihydroxycinnamate, inhibit the release of (^{3}H)arachidonate from human platelets stimulated by thrombin or collagen. *Thromb. Haemost.* **72,** 634–642.

20. Holub, B. J. and Watson, S. P. (1996) Methods for measuring agonist-induced phospholipid metabolism in intact human platelets, in *Platelets: A Practical Approach* (Watson, S. P. and Authi, K. S., eds.), IRL Press at Oxford University Press, Oxford, pp. 235–257.

21. Kramer, R. M., Checani, G. C., Deykin, A., Pritzker, C. R., and Deykin, D. (1986) Solubilization, and properties of Ca2+-dependent human platelet phospholipase A2. *Biochim. Biophys. Acta* **878,** 394–403.

22. Cross, M. J., Stewart, A., Hodgkin, M. N., Kerr, D. J., and Wakelam, M. J. O. (1995) Wortmannin, and its structural analogue demethoxyviridin inhibit stimulated phospholipase A2 activity in Swiss 3T3 cells: wortmannin is not a specific inhibitor of phosphatidylinositol 3-kinase. *J. Biol. Chem.* **270,** 25,352–25,355.

23. Hargreaves, P. G., Jenner, S., Merritt, J. E., Sage, S. O., and Farndale, R. W. (1996) Ionomycin-stimulated arachidonic acid release in human platelets: a role for protein kinase C, and tyrosine phosphorylation. *Thromb. Haemost.* **76,** 248–252.

24. McNicol, A. (1996) Platelet preparation, and estimation of functional responses, in *Platelets: A Practical Approach* (Watson, S. P. and Authi, K. S., eds.), IRL Press at Oxford University Press, Oxford, pp. 1–26.

25. Bligh, E. G. and Dyer, W. J. (1959) A rapid method of total lipid extraction, and purification. *Can. J. Biochem. Phys.* **37,** 911–918.

26. O'Neill, L. A. N. and Lewis, G. P. (1988) Effect of interleukin-1 on free arachidonic acid levels in human synovial cells. *Biochem. Soc. Trans.* **16,** 286–287.

12

Measurement of the Platelet Procoagulant Response

**Johan W. M. Heemskerk, Paul Comfurius,
Marion A. H. Feijge, and Edouard M. Bevers**

1. Introduction

Platelets play a dual role in the normal hemostatic process. Injury of a vessel wall causes exposure of structural elements such as collagen that will trap platelets circulating in the blood. This initiates two processes, which occur simultaneously, resulting in formation of a stable thrombus. Adhesion and subsequent activation of platelets, achieved through various ligand-receptor interactions, will cause platelets to clump at the site of injury, thus forming a physical barrier to prevent further blood loss. The primary platelet aggregate thus formed is consolidated by a network of fibrin, the end product of blood coagulation. The latter process involves a cascade of enzymatic reactions, several of which are localized on and strongly enhanced by the presence of a suitable phospholipid surface. This procoagulant phospholipid surface is provided mainly by platelets activated in such a way as to expose anionic phospholipids, in particular phosphatidylserine (PS) *(1,2)*. The thrombin that is produced as a result of the coagulation process is also a potent platelet-activating agonist. Accordingly, it is widely recognized that the processes of platelet activation and coagulation are strongly interacting and mutually dependent *(3)*.

Platelet-collagen interaction, particularly through the signaling collagen receptor, glycoprotein VI, is a main trigger of PS exposure. Activation of isolated platelets adhering to immobilized collagen, mimicking a damaged vessel wall, causes a prominent, prolonged rise in cytosolic $[Ca^{2+}]_i$, which precedes both exposure of PS and formation of membrane blebs at the cell surface *(4)*. Similarly, treatment of platelets with Ca^{2+} ionophores, such as ionomycin or A23187, elicits PS exposure and bleb formation, demonstrating that these responses require a substantial elevation in $[Ca^{2+}]_i$ *(1)*. Procoagulant, PS-exposing platelets are also formed in platelet-rich plasma or whole blood, when the coagulation process is initiated (for review, *see* **ref. 3**).

In quiescent, nonactivated platelets, the various phospholipid classes are asymmetrically distributed over both leaflets of the plasma membrane. Whereas the outer leaflet consists predominantly of choline-containing phospholipids, the aminophospholipids,

From: *Methods in Molecular Biology, vol. 272:*
Platelets and Megakaryocytes, Vol. 1: Functional Assays
Edited by: J. M. Gibbins and M. P. Mahaut-Smith © Humana Press Inc., Totowa, NJ

including PS, are almost exclusively located in the cytoplasmic leaflet. An aminophospholipid translocase is held responsible for keeping PS localized at the cytoplasmic site of the plasma membrane of quiescent platelets *(2)*. Upon platelet activation, where intracellular Ca^{2+} levels are raised, membrane phospholipid asymmetry can readily be lost due to the activation of a scramblase, which facilitates bidirectional movement of the major plasma membrane phospholipids. Concomitant inhibition of an aminophospholipid translocase under these conditions prevents surface-exposed PS from being pumped back to the inner membrane leaflet. This process of PS exposure is generally referred to as the *platelet procoagulant response*, because it generates platelets that provide a suitable surface for assembly and catalysis of two sequential reactions of the coagulation cascade, the activation of factor X by the tenase complex (factors IXa and VIIIa) and the subsequent activation of prothrombin to thrombin by the prothrombinase complex (factors Xa and Va). The precise mechanisms and activation pathways required to evoke the procoagulant response remain to be elucidated *(3)*.

This chapter provides a number of techniques and protocols aimed at further elucidating the environmental and intracellular factors involved in the platelet procoagulant response. We first describe a simple and rapid procedure to prepare washed, plasma-free platelet suspensions on small scale. Subsequently, for such platelets in suspension, methods are given to measure the procoagulant activity—i.e., PS exposure—as well as to determine the transbilayer movements of phospholipids underlying PS exposure using a fluorescent-labeled PS analogue. Since Ca^{2+} ions play a major role in the initiation of the procoagulant response, we also provide protocols for simultaneous measurement of elevated $[Ca^{2+}]_i$ and PS exposure, either in platelet suspensions by flow cytometry or in single platelets by microscopic multifluorescence video imaging. This approach uses a combination of fluorescent-labeled calcium indicators to monitor free $[Ca^{2+}]_i$ and fluorescent-labeled annexin V as a probe, which preferentially binds to PS-exposing platelets at physiological Ca^{2+} concentrations *(5)*.

2. Materials

2.1. Rapid Small-Scale Preparation of Washed Platelets

1. Anticoagulant acid-citrate-dextrose (ACD) solution: 52 mM citric acid, 80 mM trisodium citrate, 180 mM glucose.
2. Buffer A, HEPES buffer, pH 6.6: 137 mM NaCl, 10 mM HEPES, 5 mM glucose, 2.7 mM KCl, 2 mM MgCl$_2$, 0.05% (w/v) fatty-acid-free bovine serum albumin (BSA), adjusted with NaOH at pH 6.6 (store buffer without BSA and glucose at 4°C; glucose and BSA should be added prior to use).
3. Buffer B: same as buffer A, but at pH 7.4.
4. Buffer C: same as buffer B, but without BSA (for analysis of phospholipid scrambling; *see* **Subheading 2.3.**).
5. Acetoxymethyl esters of the fluorescent Ca^{2+} probes, Fura-2, Fluo-3, or Oregon Green-488 (OG488) Bapta-1 (Molecular Probes, Eugene, OR).

2.2. Prothrombinase Activity of Washed Platelets in Suspension

1. Bovine coagulation proteins, factor Xa, factor Va, and prothrombin, may be obtained commercially (e.g., Enzyme Research Labs Inc., USA), or may be purified from bovine blood according to published methods *(6)*.

2. Suspension of washed platelets in buffer B, diluted to 5×10^6 platelets/mL (for preparation, *see* **Subheading 3.1.**).
3. 195 m*M* $CaCl_2$ in buffer B.
4. Horm-type collagen (Nycomed, Munich, Germany), diluted to 320 µg/mL with collagen dilution buffer, supplied by the manufacturer.
5. Purified human α-thrombin (e.g., Enzyme Research Labs Inc., South Bend, IN) at 256 n*M* in buffer B (note: 1 unit/mL α-thrombin corresponds to 11.4 n*M*).
6. Stop buffer: 120 m*M* NaCl, 50 m*M* Tris-HCl, 2 m*M* EDTA, and 0.05% (w/v) BSA, pH 7.4.
7. Thrombin-specific chromogenic substrate, H-D-Phe-Pip-Arg-para-nitroaniline (S2238, Chromogenix, Mölndal, Sweden), dissolved in water at 1.4 m*M*.

2.3. Continuous Analysis of Phospholipid Scrambling in Washed Platelets

1. 1-Oleoyl-2-(6-7-nitrobenz-2-oxa-1,3-diazol-4-yl)amino)caproyl-*sn*-glycero-3-phosphoserine (NBD-PS) (Avanti Polar Lipids, Alabaster, AL), 1 m*M* in chloroform (kept at –20°C). Prior to addition of NBD-PS to the platelets, an aliquot from the stock solution in chloroform is flushed with nitrogen to evaporate the solvent; the dried probe is dissolved in buffer C (*see* **Subheading 2.1.**) at a concentration of 1 m*M*.
2. Phenylmethane sulfonyl fluoride (PMSF), dissolved in dimethylsulfoxide (DMSO) at a concentration of 200 m*M*.
3. Sodium dithionite, 1 *M* in a solution of 1 *M* Tris-HCl (no pH adjustment) (*see* **Note 10**).
4. 10% (w/v) Triton X-100 in water.

2.4. Flow-Cytometric Measurement of Activated, PS-Exposing Platelets

1. Flow cytometer equipped with conventional Argon laser (488 nm) and additional red diode laser (633 nm).
2. Suspension of Fluo-3 (or OG488-Bapta-1) (Molecular Probes Inc., Eugene, OR) labeled, washed platelets. Dilute the suspension to 5×10^7 platelets/mL in buffer B (for preparation, *see* **Subheading 3.1.**).
3. Alexa Fluor 647-labeled annexin V (AF647-annexin V) or Oregon Green 488-labeled annexin V (OG488-annexin V), obtained from NeXins Research (Kattendÿke, the Netherlands) or Molecular Probes.
4. 190 m*M* $CaCl_2$.
5. Solutions of 320 µg/mL collagen and human 256 n*M* α-thrombin, prepared as indicated in **Subheading 2.2.**
6. Polystyrene tubes for flow cytometry.

2.5. Microscopic Measurement of Activated, PS-Exposing Platelets

1. Inverted fluorescence microscope with UV-transparent optics, equipped with 60X UV-transparent oil objective and two dichroic mirrors that can easily be inserted into the fluorescence light path.
2. Sensitive camera-based fluorescence digital imaging system, connected to the microscope, capable of rapidly detecting changes in fluorescence of two different probes (changeable excitation and emission prisms or filters). Systems provided by Visitech (Sunderland, Tyne & Wear, UK) provide these facilities.
3. Horm-type collagen (Nycomed, Munich, Germany), diluted to 320 µg/mL with collagen dilution buffer, supplied by the manufacturer.
4. Fibrinogen (Enzyme Research Labs Inc.), dissolved in buffer B at 5 mg/mL.

5. Collagen- or fibrinogen-coated cover slips. Cover slips are cleaned by a treatment with 2 *M* HCl in 50 vol% ethanol, followed by repeated rinsing with saline. Incubate cover slip with collagen suspension (320 µg/mL) or fibrinogen solution (5 mg/mL) for 30 min. Rinse with saline, and incubate for 10 min with buffer B, supplemented with 5% BSA to block uncovered glass. For buffers and other media, *see* **Subheadings 2.1.** and **2.2.**

6. Cover slip chamber to hold a collagen- or fibrinogen-coated cover slip.

7. For (quasi-) simultaneous detection of Fura-2 and Oregon Green-488 (or fluorescein) fluorescence, the following filter sets give well-separated bright signals. Fura-2 fluorescence: alternating 340- and 380-nm excitation filters (15-nm half-bandwidths), 400-nm long-pass dichroic mirror, and 510-nm emission filter (half-bandwidth 40 nm). Oregon Green-488 (or fluorescein) fluorescence: 485-nm excitation filter (half bandwidth 22 nm), 505-nm long-pass dichroic mirror, and 530-nm emission filter (half-bandwidth 30 nm).

8. Platelets loaded with Fura-2 in buffer B (5×10^7 platelet/mL) (*see* **Subheading 3.1.**)

9. Annexin V labeled with Oregon Green 488 (OG488-annexin V) or with fluorescein isothiocyanate (FITC-annexin V) (NeXins Research), at a concentration of 300 µg/mL.

3. Methods

3.1. Rapid Small-Scale Preparation of Washed Platelets

This section provides a method to rapidly prepare washed platelets from small volumes of blood, for use in measurements described hereafter. Because traces of plasma may cause artifact procoagulant activity, it is important to remove plasma components by extensive washing.

1. Human blood (10 mL) is collected in a polystyrene tube using one volume of ACD solution for each 5 volumes of blood. To avoid platelet activation, free flow of blood from the forearm vein is preferred, and the first two milliliters of blood are discarded. A lightly applied tourniquet is recommended; use of a vacuum system often causes increased numbers of procoagulant platelets.

2. Erythrocytes are spun down at 200*g* for 15 min using a bench-top centrifuge (no brake). Approximately 4 mL platelet-rich plasma (PRP) is collected in microfuge tubes (1 mL per tube); avoid contamination with buffy coat material or erythrocytes. If contaminating erythrocytes are present, the centrifugation step may be repeated.

3. In experiments where platelets are to be labeled with a Ca^{2+}-sensitive fluorescent probe, incubate the PRP (approx 2×10^8 platelets/mL) at 37°C for 30 min with the acetoxymethyl ester of either Fluo-3 (5 µ*M*), OG488 Bapta-1 (5 µ*M*) or Fura-2 (3 µ*M*), as desired.

4. Centrifuge the PRP at 15,000*g* for 2 min; remove supernatant and resuspend platelet pellet in 1 mL buffer A. Add 100 µL ACD solution and centrifuge at 15,000*g* for 1 min. Repeat this step twice.

5. Resuspend the final platelet pellet in 0.25 mL buffer B. Collect contents of all tubes and allow the platelets to recover by incubation at 37°C for 10 min after preparation (*see* **Note 1**). Measure the platelet count using a suitable cell counter (refer to Chapter 3, vol. 1 for further details on platelet counting). Alternatively, measure the optical density at 405 nm, using buffer B as a blank. An optical density of 0.025 corresponds to approx 10^6 platelets/mL.

3.2. Prothrombinase Activity of Washed Platelets in Suspension

Described below is a procedure to measure prothrombin-converting activity by the prothrombinase complex assembled on the surface of washed platelets in suspension. In the protocol, the platelets are pre-activated with a mixture of collagen and thrombin, but other activating agents may also be used (*see* **Note 2**).

1. Prepare a mixture of 5.0 n*M* factor Xa and 10.0 n*M* factor Va in buffer B. Add CaCl$_2$ to a concentration of 3 m*M*. Keep this mixture on ice.
2. Prepare solution of 10 µ*M* prothrombin in buffer B, supplied with 3 m*M* CaCl$_2$. Keep on ice.
3. Prepare polystyrene tubes with 490 µL stop buffer.
4. Preincubate 150 µL of washed platelets in buffer B (5 × 10^6 platelets/mL) for 3 min at 37°C in a flat-bottom polystyrene tube (*see* **Subheading 3.1.**). Stir the suspension gently (about 100 rpm) with a small Teflon-coated magnetic stirring bar (7 × 2 mm) (*see* **Note 3**).
5. To activate the platelets, add successively 2.5 µL of CaCl$_2$ solution, 5 µL of collagen suspension and 2.5 µL of α-thrombin solution, while stirring. Final activation conditions are 3 m*M* CaCl$_2$, 10 µg/mL collagen and 4 n*M* α-thrombin (*see* **Notes 4–5**).
6. After 10 min of activation, add 20 µL of factor Va/Xa solution, and allow the mixture to equilibrate for 1 min (continue stirring).
7. Add 20 µL of prothrombin solution to start the prothrombinase reaction (start stopwatch). Final prothrombinase-activating conditions are thus 3 m*M* CaCl$_2$, 1.0 n*M* factor Va, 0.5 n*M* factor Xa, and 1.0 µ*M* prothrombin (*see* **Note 6**).
8. Exactly 1 min after prothrombin addition, transfer a sample of 10 µL of the mixture to a polystyrene tube containing 490 µL stop buffer.
9. To check for linearity of the reaction in time, take another sample at 2 min after prothrombin addition.
10. After collecting the samples (taken at different time points) from various assay tubes, determine the amount of thrombin in each polystyrene tube by transferring fractions of 200 µL to a microtiter well plate. Then add 50 µL of chromogenic substrate solution to each well on the plate (final concentration of 280 µ*M* S2238), and read the change in absorbance at 405 nm with a microtiter plate reader equipped with a program for enzyme kinetics.
11. To determine the concentration of thrombin from the measured change in absorbance, construct a calibration curve with serial dilutions of thrombin (*see* **Note 7**).

3.3. Continuous Analysis of Phospholipid Scrambling in Washed Platelets

This assay aims to measure the progression and rate of activity of the phospholipid-scrambling process in suspensions of activated platelets. It relies on the principle that the fluorescence signal of each molecule of internalised NBD-PS probe that migrates from the inner to the outer leaflet during the scrambling process will be abolished instantaneously by the action of dithionite *(7,8)*. A slightly different washing procedure from that described in **Subheading 3.1.** is used for experiments with NBD-PS-labeled platelets. After the washing step, the platelet suspension is incubated with 200 µ*M* PMSF for 15 min at 37°C. Platelets are subsequently washed as described in **Subheading 3.1.**, but finally resuspended in buffer C (albumin-free buffer B) (*see* **Note 8**).

1. Add 2 µL NBD-labeled PS (1 m*M* in buffer C) to 2 mL of platelets (2 × 10^8/mL), and allow the fluorescent phospholipid to be translocated to the inner membrane leaflet

(the final concentration of probe is 1 μM, which corresponds to approx 1.25% of the endogenous phospholipid). Incubation for 45 min at 37°C will result in 80–90% internalization of the probe.

2. To remove noninternalized probe, add 100 μL of 10% (w/v) BSA solution per mL platelet suspension, in addition to 100 μL ACD solution. Centrifuge at 15,000g for 1 min and resuspend the pellet in buffer C. This suspension is then kept at room temperature for analysis of the phospholipid scrambling (use within 2 h).

3. Place a cuvet containing 2 mL of a dilution of the NBD-PS-labeled platelet suspension (10^7 platelets/mL) in a spectrofluorometer (at defined temperature). Gently stir the suspension using a Teflon-coated magnetic stirring bar. Sample fluorescence intensity at λ_{em} 534 nm (λ_{ex} 472 nm) at 0.5-s intervals.

4. Add $CaCl_2$ at the desired concentration (usually 3 mM). Activate the platelets by adding agonist (e.g., thrombin, ionomycin, thapsigargin) and monitor the fluorescence signal continuously (*see* **Note 9**).

5. After the desired time interval of activation, add 10 μL dithionite solution (1 M, freshly prepared), and resume monitoring the fluorescence signal. Upon initiation of the scramble process the signal decreases, as exposed fluorescent lipid probe will be immediately quenched (*see* **Notes 10–12**).

6. To verify whether the amount and quality of the dithionite solution added is sufficient to quench all the probe that has been externalized, add 20 μL of 10% (w/v) Triton X-100, which will lyse the platelets, thus making all NBD label susceptible to dithionite.

3.4. Flow-Cytometric Measurement of Activated, PS-Exposing Platelets

A double-labeling, flow cytometry method is described to measure fractions of vital, activated platelets that have undergone the procoagulant response, i.e., have PS exposed in the outer leaflet of the plasma membrane *(4)*. To identify the state of activation, platelets are loaded with a fluorescent probe that monitors elevated $[Ca^{2+}]_i$. Bright Ca^{2+} probes, excited by the 488-nm line of an argon laser, are Fluo-3 and OG488 Bapta-1. Nonvital platelets will not load with these Ca^{2+} probes, as they will not metabolize the acetoxymethylester form in which these probes are added. Unstimulated platelets are able to hydrolyze the ester and therefore will accumulate the probe. To detect surface-exposed PS, annexin V is labeled with a fluorescent dye absorbing at the 630-nm line of a red diode laser. Alternatively, single-dye measurements can be performed, e.g., with only OG488-annexin V (*see* **Notes 13–15**).

1. Prepare (marked) polystyrene tubes with 25 μL buffer B supplemented with 3.0 mM $CaCl_2$ for flow cytometry.

2. Preincubate 150 μL of Fluo-3-loaded (or OG488 Bapta-1 loaded) platelets in buffer B (5×10^7/mL) for 3 min at 37°C in a flat-bottom polystyrene tube (*see* **Subheading 3.1.**). Stir the suspension gently (about 100 rpm) with a small Teflon-coated magnetic stirring bar (7×2 mm).

3. To activate the platelets, add successively 2.5 μL of $CaCl_2$ solution, 5 μL of collagen suspension, and 2.5 μL of α-thrombin solution. Stir for 1 min. Final activation conditions are 3 mM $CaCl_2$, 10 μg/mL collagen and 4 nM α-thrombin (*see* **Note 9**).

4. Add 2 μL AF647-annexin V to (marked) polystyrene tubes.

5. Transfer 25-μL samples of platelet suspension to polystyrene tubes, mix gently by pipetting up and down three times.

6. Incubate for 5 min, and add 200 µL buffer B, supplied with 3 mM CaCl$_2$.
7. Measure fluorescence at 488-nm and 630-nm excitation (2-channel fluorescence mode) in 10,000 platelets with flow cytometer.
8. For data analysis, select platelet events from forward and side scatter pattern. Then plot AF647 annexin V fluorescence as a function of Fluo-3 fluorescence. This will give two populations of AF647 annexin V-positive platelets: one without Fluo-3 fluorescence (non-vital platelets), and one with increased Fluo-3 fluorescence in comparison to unstimulated platelets (activated, PS-exposing platelets) (*see* **Notes 14** and **15**).

3.5. Microscopic Measurement of Activated, PS-Exposing Platelets

By high-resolution fluorescence video microscopy, the activation state of platelets can be monitored in time by measuring the rise in $[Ca^{2+}]_i$, for example using the ratiometric fluorescence probe Fura-2. With equipment allowing multiple probe measurements, for each individual cell, changes in $[Ca^{2+}]_i$ can even be compared with the corresponding surface appearance of PS, for example with OG488-annexin V *(9)*. Here, we describe a non-confocal, camera-based method that uses filter sets suited for optimal detection of both Fura-2 and OG488 (or fluorescein) fluorescence with washed platelets. Because of the small volume of platelets (only about 6 fL), highly transparent optics are required.

1. Prepare 8 nM α-thrombin solution in buffer B, supplemented with 1 mM CaCl$_2$.
2. Mount the chamber with collagen- or fibrinogen-containing cover slip on the stage of the inverted fluorescence microscope.
3. Transfer into the chamber 300 µL Fura-2-loaded platelets in buffer B (5×10^7 platelets/mL), supplemented with 1 mM CaCl$_2$ and 0.50 µg/mL OG488-annexin V (or FITC-annexin V).
4. Continuously record the changes in Fura-2 fluorescence (alternative excitation at 340 and 380 nm) of platelets that are in the optical plane of the collagen or fibrinogen on the cover slip (*see* **Note 16**).
5. At discrete time points, monitor the OG488 (or FITC) fluorescence of the same microscopic image.
6. After 10 min, add 300 µL of α-thrombin solution, and continue recording of the Fura-2 and OG488 images.
7. From the stored Fura-2 ratio and OG488 images, overlays are produced off-line to identify the platelets that are elevated in $[Ca^{2+}]_i$ and those that expose PS.

4. Notes

1. The method for preparing washed platelets can further be scaled down to allow isolation of platelets from mouse or rat blood. In case of human blood, the recovery of platelets amounts to approx 30%. The quality of the final platelet suspension may be judged from appearance of the swirling when the suspension is lightly shaken. Allowing this effect to occur may require incubation at 37°C for 10 min after preparation. Note that for the loading of rat or mouse platelets with Ca^{2+} probes, washed platelets should be used instead of PRP.
2. Because even trace amounts of plasma can profoundly interfere with the prothrombinase reaction, it is important to use platelets that are washed twice, as described in **Subheading 3.1.**
3. A device for stirring multiple tubes simultaneously in a water bath could be used. This will allow 4–6 prothrombinase assays to be performed at the same time. The stirring devices are not commercially available, but may be developed by a technical department.

4. Note that the platelet concentration during the activation amounts to 4.7×10^6 platelets/mL, while it is reduced in the prothrombinase assay to 3.75×10^6/mL. Under these conditions, the platelets, even when fully exposing PS, are the rate-limiting factor in the prothrombin conversion.

5. For the measurement of the procoagulant response with collagen fibers (or collagen plus α-thrombin), it is recommended that activation and subsequent prothrombinase measurements be performed in triplicate.

6. Factor Va is added in excess over factor Xa in order to avoid contribution of factor V released from the platelets. When desired, the prothrombinase assay conditions may be modified to determine the contribution of platelet factor V release to the thrombin-forming activity. In this case, exogenous factor Va is not added, and a tenfold higher concentration of factor Xa is recommended.

7. The assay conditions should fulfill two requirements: the reaction rate should be (linearly) dependent on the concentration of procoagulant phospholipid (i.e., PS-exposing platelets), and the substrate prothrombin should not become rate limiting (i.e., the amount of thrombin formed must be linear in time for at least 2 min). The prothrombinase activity of completely lysed platelets, which express maximal procoagulant activity, can be used to test the assay conditions. For this, the platelet suspension is sonicated for 3 min (intermittent with 30-s intervals) on ice. Prothrombinase activities should be linear for dilutions of the platelet sonicate between 0 and 20%. Note that maximal prothrombinase activity of platelets activated with ionomycin never exceeds that of a 20% sonicate of the platelet suspension. Upon changing the platelet concentration, the above requirements should be carefully checked.

8. To measure scramblase activity with NBD-labeled phospholipid probe, the final resuspension buffer should be albumin-free HEPES buffer pH 7.4 (buffer C). Note that albumin will extract the lipid probe from the outer leaflet of the platelet membrane. Although not described here, extraction of the probe by BSA can be used as a discontinuous procedure to measure transbilayer movement of the lipids *(8)*. PMSF treatment of the platelets before labeling is required, as this prevents degradation of NBD-PS after internalization. Pretreatment of the platelets with 200 μ*M* PMSF will, however, reduce the response to thrombin by approx 15% (unpublished observation), but allows the performance of fluorescence measurements for at least 2 h without appreciable loss of signal. Nevertheless, it is recommended that the effect of PMSF be verified for each agonist used.

9. As aggregation of platelets will disturb the fluorescence signal, specific inhibitors of aggregation may be applied (e.g., Arg-Gly-Asp peptides).

10. The dithionite reagent is not stable, due to spontaneous oxidation. Best results are obtained when the reagent is prepared in a narrow tube. After dissolving, the reagent (in 1 or 2 mL) is kept on ice without further agitation. When samples are taken, pipet from the bottom of the tube.

11. Eventually, bi-exponential curve fitting may be applied to quantify the decay of the fluorescence signal. For this, the following equation can be used:

$$I(t) = (I_0 - Blk)(Ae^{-k_1(t-t0)} + (1 - A)e^{-k_2(t-t0)}) + Blk$$

where $I(t)$ is the fluorescence intensity as function of time *(t)*, I_0 is the intensity at time 0 *(t_0)*, *Blk* is the residual (blank) fluorescence after addition of Triton X-100, and *A* and *(1–A)* are the fractions of the label in the two pools whose intensity decays at rates k_1 and k_2 (it should be emphasized that the physiological significance of the two pools has not been established).

12. In principle, dithionite can also be added prior to the agonist. However, one should realize that dithionite is a strong reducing agent, which may affect or destroy some agonists. The solution of dithionite is unstable under air and loses activity after 1 h. Therefore, make sure that all fluorescence is immediately quenched upon addition of dithionite to a preparation of lysed platelets (in the presence of 0.1% Triton X-100).

13. Oregon Green-488 Bapta-1 and also Fluo-4 are Ca^{2+} probes with absorption and emission spectra similar to Fluo-3, but with brighter fluorescence and decreased bleaching. Use the dye-loaded platelets within 2 h of isolation (store at room temperature to reduce probe leakage).

14. It should be emphasized that annexin V does not bind exclusively to PS. At elevated $[Ca^{2+}]$ (above 5 mM), annexin may also bind to PE. In addition, the presence of PE will increase the binding of annexin to lipid surfaces with a low (<5) mole% of PS *(10)*. At 3 mM Ca^{2+}, however, binding of annexin is rather specific for PS. Note also that apoptotic, necrotic, and lysed cells have exposed PS at their surface membrane and thus stain positive for annexin V.

15. For adequate detection of fluorescence with the flow cytometer, control incubations should be performed with single dyes, i.e., either Fluo-3-loaded platelets alone or unloaded platelets with added AF647-annexin V. Optimal sensitivity of photo-multiplier tubes should be determined by (single-dye) comparisons of unstimulated platelets and platelets stimulated with 10 μM ionomycin in the presence of 1 mM $CaCl_2$. The ionomycin-stimulated platelets should have at least a 2.5-fold increase in Fluo-3 fluorescence and about 90% should stain positively with AF647-annexin V.

16. We use Quanticell software (Visitech, Sunderland, UK) to store digital images to a 128 MB real-time image processor. For Fura-2 fluorescence, good results are obtained by hardware averaging of four 340- and 380-nm images, background subtraction, and calculation of ratio images. Sequences of ratio images (one per 2–5 s) are stored on hardware media, using Quanticell software. With respect to OG488 fluorescence, a threshold is set to suppress the fluorescence from the soluble, unbound annexin V. Using the collected sequences of images, and geometric regions, matching individual cells are analyzed off-line for changes in fluorescence.

Acknowledgment

We acknowledge an investment grant from the Netherlands Organization for Scientific Research NWO 902-68-241.

References

1. Bevers, E. M., Comfurius, P., and Zwaal, R. F. A. (1991) Platelet procoagulant activity, physiological significance and mechanisms of exposure. *Blood Rev.* **5,** 146–154.
2. Zwaal, R. F. A. and Schroit, A. J. (1997) Pathophysiological implications of membrane phospholipid asymmetry in blood cells. *Blood* **89,** 1121–1132.
3. Heemskerk, J. W. M., Bevers, E. M., and Lindhout, T. (2002) Platelet activation and coagulation. *Thromb. Haemost.* **88,** 186–193.
4. Siljander, P., Farndale, R. W., Feijge, M. A. H., Comfurius, P., Kos, S., Bevers, E. M., et al. (2001) Platelet adhesion enhances the glycoprotein VI-dependent procoagulant response. Involvement of p38 MAP kinase and calpain. *Arterioscler. Thromb. Vasc. Biol.* **21,** 618–627.
5. Thiagarajan, P. and Tait, J. F. (1991) Collagen-induced exposure of anionic phospholipids in platelets and platelet-derived microparticles. *J. Biol. Chem.* **266,** 24,302–24,307.

6. Rosing, J., van Rijn, J. L. M. L., Bevers, E. M., van Dieijen, G., Comfurius, P., and Zwaal, R. F. A. (1985) The role of activated human platelets in prothrombin and factor X activation. *Blood* **65,** 319–332.

7. McIntyre, J. C. and Sleight, R. G. (1991) Fluorescence assay for phospholipid membrane asymmetry. *Biochemistry* **30,** 11,819–11,827.

8. Williamson, P., Bevers, E. M., Smeets, E. F., Comfurius, P., Schlegel, R. A., and Zwaal, R. F. (1995) Continuous analysis of the mechanism of activated transbilayer lipid movement in platelets. *Biochemistry* **34,** 10,448–10,455.

9. Heemskerk, J. W. M., Vuist, W. M. J., Feijge, M. A. H., Reutelingsperger, C. P. M., and Lindhout, T. (1997) Collagen but not fibrinogen surfaces induce bleb formation, exposure of phosphatidylserine and procoagulant activity of adherent platelets. Evidence for regulation by protein tyrosine kinase-dependent Ca^{2+} responses. *Blood* **90,** 2615–2625.

10. Stuart, M. C. A., Reutelingsperger, C. P. M., and Frederik, P. M. (1998) Binding of annexin V to bilayers with various phospholipid compositions using glass beads in a flow cytometer. *Cytometry* **33,** 414–419.

13

Platelet Adhesion Assays Performed Under Static Conditions

Joanne M. Stevens

1. Introduction

The ability of platelets to recognize and adhere to sites of vascular damage in vivo is critical to their function in the cessation of bleeding. Upon damage to the vasculature, denudation of endothelial cells results in the exposure of extracellular matrix (ECM) proteins, the most thrombogenic and abundant of which is collagen. Adhesion to the exposed sub-endothelial ECM proteins is the first step in the formation of a hemostatic plug and involves the interplay of several cell-surface platelet receptors, the most important of which are probably the collagen-binding receptors.

The initial tethering interaction of platelets with the exposed ECM proteins involves a multimeric protein secreted by endothelial cells and stored within platelet alpha granules, von Willebrand factor (vWF). vWF interacts with collagen and also with the glycoprotein GPIbα, a constituent of the GPIb-V-IX complex on the surface of the platelet, thus acting as a bridging molecule between the two *(1)*. This initial weak interaction is closely followed by a higher-affinity interaction of collagen with the platelet cell surface by its ability to bind both GPVI and the integrin $\alpha_2\beta_1$. The importance of integrin $\alpha_2\beta_1$ in mediating tethering interactions between platelets and collagen was demonstrated by the fact that platelets isolated from patients lacking expression of the GPIa/α_2 integrin subunit, and therefore functional $\alpha_2\beta_1$, failed to bind or respond to collagen *(2)*. Recent studies involving glycoprotein VI (GPVI), $\alpha2$ and $\beta1$ knockout murine platelets have demonstrated a role for GPVI in tethering platelets to a collagen substrate in vitro *(3,4)*. While both of these collagen receptors are thought to be involved in platelet adhesion, activation of the platelet is believed to result largely through the induction of multiple intracellular signalling pathways through the GPVI-FcR γ chain complex *(5–8)*.

1.1. Methods for Assessing Platelet Adhesion Events

A number of non-adhesion systems exist to measure parameters involved in platelet adhesion. The direct interaction of platelets with collagen can readily be observed in aggregation experiments by measuring changes in turbidity of the platelet suspension

From: *Methods in Molecular Biology, vol. 272:*
Platelets and Megakaryocytes, Vol. 1: Functional Assays
Edited by: J. M. Gibbins and M. P. Mahaut-Smith © Humana Press Inc., Totowa, NJ

upon the addition of fibrillar collagen preparations, and in the presence of aggregation inhibitors such as the synthetic tetrapeptide arg-gly-asp-ser (RGDS). However, in such experiments, the contribution of either $\alpha_2\beta_1$ or GPVI in adhesion cannot be dissected unless inhibitors to either molecule are used. In static adhesion assays, the study of $\alpha2\beta1$ and GPVI in collagen adhesion can be determined either by assessing adhesion to monomeric collagen (a specific ligand for $\alpha_2\beta_1$), or collagen-related peptide (CRP) (both specific ligands for GPVI). Alternatively, cation-chelating agents can be included in fibrillar collagen adhesion assays, since cations are required for activation and ligand binding of the integrin $\alpha_2\beta_1$ but does not affect GPVI function and hence GPVI-mediated adhesion.

Similarly, vWF binding to GPIbα can also be assessed in the aggregometer. However, the shear stresses generated in a bench-top aggregometer are too low to induce the binding of vWF, so artificial tools such as the antibiotic ristocetin or the snake venom botrocetin are required. Alternatively, a modified viscometer has been developed to apply the high shear stresses needed to induce conformational changes in vWF such that it can interact directly with GPIbα and therefore avoid the need to use ristocetin or botrocetin to study vWF-GPIbα interactions *(9)*.

Static adhesion assays are useful tools in investigating the molecular basis of interactions between cell surface receptors and their ligands. They can also be used to investigate receptor-ligand interactions that are not necessarily required for adhesion, for example the interaction of the fibrinogen receptor and its ligands such as fibrinogen, thrombospondin, and vWF. Furthermore, since platelets are anucleate and not amenable to genetic manipulation, the use of specific pharmacological inhibitors of intracellular kinases and phosphatases is necessary for the dissection of the signaling pathways involved in platelet receptor-ligand interactions. As such, static adhesion assays provide a simple and cost-effective way of assessing the role of kinases, adaptor molecules, and receptors in mediating adhesion of platelets to different ECM components or peptides, before switching to more expensive techniques that assess adhesion under flow conditions. Such techniques often require expensive and complicated microscopy and imaging devices, whereas static-adhesion assays rely solely on the appropriate plate reader for the detection method employed.

1.2. Basic Principles of Static Adhesion Assays

Static adhesion assays are usually performed in microtiter plates coated with the protein or peptide of interest to which the binding molecule (e.g., receptor fragments, vWF, collagens) or cells expressing the binding protein (e.g., platelets, cell lines) are added, followed by the appropriate detection method. Adhesion assays can also be modified such that adhesion of platelets to a monolayer of endothelial cells rather than a substrate of purified protein or peptide is determined. In assays where the adhesion of isolated or recombinant receptors to their ligands is being measured, detection is usually facilitated either by directly radiolabeling the protein of interest (with ^{125}I, for example), or by ELISA with specific antibodies directed against the protein or a tag engineered onto the recombinant protein *(10,11)*. However, the variety of methods to label and detect whole cells that adhere to substrates are diverse and include:

- The use of horseradish peroxidase (HRP)-linked platelet-specific antibodies in ELISA-based assays. Substrate is added and absorbance measured at the appropriate wavelength *(4)*.
- Measurement of crystal violet staining of adherent cells by recording absorbance at 550 nm *(12)* or at 570 nm following lysis *(13)*.
- Measurement of intrinsic phosphatase activity following lysis *(14,15)* or hexose aminidase activity following lysis *(16)*.
- ^{51}Cr labeling or ^{14}C serotonin-loading platelets and subsequent detection following lysis *(16,17)*.
- Labeling platelets with fluorescent probes such as calcein-AM *(4)* and subsequent detection using a fluorimeter with excitation and emission wavelengths of ~494 nm and 517 nm, respectively.

1.3. Advantages and Considerations When Designing Fluorescent-Based Adhesion Assays

This chapter is concerned with assessing adhesion of platelets to substrata following labeling of the cells with a suitable fluorescent probe. In a typical fluorescence-based cell adhesion assay, labeled cells are incubated in wells of a microtiter plate that have been coated with the substrate of interest (e.g., ECM protein, peptide, endothelial cells). Cell adhesion is then determined after the unbound cells are removed by a series of washing steps. An ideal fluorescent label will retain proportionality between fluorescence and cell number, allowing numbers of adherent cells to be quantified. Furthermore, an ideal fluorescent marker should not interfere with the adhesion process. Since adhesion is a cell-surface phenomenon, cytoplasmic markers that can be passively loaded into cells are preferable to compounds that label cell surface molecules, provided that they are retained in the cell for the duration of the experiment or their leakage rate can be independently measured.

The method described in this chapter for measuring the adhesion of platelets to substrata is based on fluorescently labeling the cells with calcein-acetoxymethyl ester (AM) and the subsequent detection of adherent cells using a fluorimeter. Calcein-AM is a suitable fluorescent probe that is widely used in adhesion assays since it does not interfere with the adhesion process. Calcein-AM is a cell-permeable, nonfluorescent and hydrophobic compound that is rapidly hydrolyzed by cytoplasmic esterases inside the cell thus releasing the membrane-impermeable, hydrophilic, and intensely fluorescent calcein. While the fluorescent product calcein is retained by cells with intact plasma membranes, the unhydrolyzed calcein-AM rapidly leaks from dead or damaged cells with compromised membranes. The retention of calcein in cells over long periods is dependent on cell type; however, when choosing a fluorescent dye for labeling cells, the rate of dye loss over the course of the experiment should be considered. In our laboratory's experience, calcein leakage from platelets is minimal but can be accelerated by some agents—for example, flavonoid compounds. Fluorescence of extracellular calcein that has leaked from cells can be quenched by buffers containing Co^{2+} or Mg^{2+} ions and thereby provides a means of quantifying only intracellular fluorescence.

Many of the applications of calcein-AM—for example, cell-viability, cytotoxicity, and adhesion assays—have been demonstrated to closely parallel those of radiolabeling-based assays. However, the major advantage of using calcein-AM, or indeed any other suitable fluorescent probe, over radiolabeling techniques is that the labeling protocols are more rapid and these probes do not carry the risks or the disposal costs associated with the use of radioactive materials.

2. Materials

1. Coating buffer containing substrate of interest (*see* **Note 1**).
2. 96-well microtiter plate (we use white F-96 MaxiSorp plates, Nunc [Fisher Scientific, Loughborough, UK]).
3. Phosphate-buffered saline (PBS): 10 mM sodium phosphate, 27 mM potassium chloride, 137 mM sodium chloride, pH 7.4.
4. Blocking buffer: PBS containing 2% (w/v) bovine serum albumin (BSA).
5. Tyrode's buffer: 134 mM sodium chloride, 0.34 mM disodium hydrogen phosphate, 2.9 mM potassium chloride, 12 mM sodium bicarbonate, 20 mM HEPES, 5 mM glucose, 1 mM magnesium chloride, pH 7.3.
6. ACD: 85 mM sodium citrate, 71 mM citric acid, 110 mM glucose.
7. PGE$_1$ or PGI$_2$: stock solution at 125 μg/mL in ethanol stored at –20°C.
8. Calcein-AM: stock solution at 2 mg/mL in DMSO stored at –20°C.
9. Indomethacin: stock solution at 10 mM in DMSO stored at 4°C.
10. Apyrase: stock solution at 1000 U/mL in Tyrode's buffer, stored at –20°C.
11. Paraformaldehyde: 4% (w/v) diluted in PBS, pH 7.4.
12. Fluorimeter fitted with the appropriate filters for detection of calcein-labeled cells (we use a LS50B Luminescence Spectrometer, Perkin-Elmer [Boston, MA]).

3. Methods

3.1. Coating Microtiter Plates With Extracellular Matrix Proteins or Peptides

1. Dilute ECM protein/peptide to 5–20 μg/mL in a suitable buffer (*see* **Note 1**).
2. Add 50–100 μL protein solution to each well of a 96-well microtiter plate and incubate at room temperature (RT) or 37°C overnight (*see* **Note 2***)*.
3. Remove coating solution and wash wells twice in phosphate-buffered saline (PBS).
4. Aspirate any remaining PBS from the wells and fill completely with 2% (w/v) bovine serum albumin (BSA) diluted in PBS and incubate for at least 2 h at RT or 1 h at 37°C to block any uncoated surfaces (*see* **Note 3**).
5. Wash wells twice in PBS and air-dry before using for adhesion assay or storage at 4°C (*see* **Note 4**).

3.2. Fluorescent Labeling of Platelets

1. Isolate platelet-rich plasma (PRP) from 50 mL citrated whole blood by centrifugation at 200g for 20 min at RT.
2. Transfer PRP to a Falcon tube and add calcein-AM to a final concentration of 2 μg/mL. Mix gently by inversion and incubate for 1 h at 30°C protected from light (*see* **Note 5**).
3. Continue the preparation of washed platelets as described in Chapter 2, vol. 1 (*see* **Note 6**).
4. After the final wash of platelets, resuspend the platelet pellet in Tyrode's buffer to a density of 1–2 × 10^8 cells/mL (*see* **Note 7**).
5. Add indomethacin and apyrase to a final concentration of 10 μM and 1 U/mL respectively. Mix gently and rest at 30°C for 15–30 min in the dark before proceeding to the adhesion assay (*see* **Note 8**).

3.3. Adhesion Assay

1. If required, pre-incubate the labeled cells with pharmacological inhibitors, blocking antibodies, EGTA, RGDS peptide, and so on for 15–30 min at 37°C in the dark prior to addition to a substrate-coated microtiter plate.
2. Add agonist (if required to measure effect of activation of a particular signaling pathway on adhesion), mix gently by inversion (incubate in suspension if required), and add 50–100 µL of the cell suspension to each well ($1–2 \times 10^7$ cells/well), ensuring that each sample is added to individual wells in triplicate. Incubate for up to 1 h at 37°C protected from light.
3. Add 50 µL of 4% (w/v) paraformaldehyde, pH 7.4, to each well and incubate at RT for 15 min in the dark (*see* **Note 9**).
4. Read the plate using a fluorimeter to obtain values of total fluorescence per well (*see* **Note 10**).
5. Wash plates with PBS (150–250 µL/well) at least three to four times to remove loosely adherent cells.
6. Add 100 µL PBS or Tyrode's buffer to each well and read the plate again to obtain remaining fluorescence values representing the proportion of adherent cells. The proportion of adherent cells can be calculated as a proportion of the total fluorescence in an individual well before washing and removing unbound cells (*see* **Note 11**).

3.4. Modifications to Labeling and Adhesion Assay Protocol for Megakaryocytes and Megakaryocytic Cell Lines

Harvest cells and wash in media lacking serum and phenol red. Suspend the cell pellet to a density of 1×10^6 live cells/mL in media lacking serum and phenol red. Add calcein-AM to a final concentration of 2 µg/mL and incubate at 37°C for 1 h in the dark. Wash the cells in media lacking serum and phenol red and resuspend to 2×10^6 cells/mL. Add inhibitors, EGTA, RGDS peptide, and so forth and pre-incubate for 15–30 min. Add agonists if required, mix, and dispense 100 µL cell suspension per well (2×10^5 cells/well). Proceed with the adhesion assay as described above for platelets.

4. Notes

1. The concentration of peptide/protein used to coat plates should be optimized for each assay, usually in the range of 5–20 µg/mL. The choice of dilution buffer may also affect adhesion of the substrate to the microtiter plates. For example, Horm collagen (equine tendons, fibrils) is usually suspended in an 0.2 *M* sodium acetate buffer, pH 5.5, for the coating of plates; however, PBS is a suitable diluent for fibrinogen and pepsin-digested/acid soluble (monomeric) collagens.
2. The volume of coating solution can be reduced to 30 µL and reused several times if it is scarce. We use white F-96 MaxiSorp (Nunc) microtiter plates for our static-adhesion assays, although alternative sources and types of microtiter plate are available. Place plates in a sealed container with damp tissue at base to provide a humidified environment and prevent evaporation of coating buffer if coating plates overnight.
3. PBS containing 3% (w/v) nonfat milk protein can also be used to block plates.
4. Plates are stable for up to 6 mo after coating provided they are kept completely dry and stored at 4°C.
5. A stock of calcein-AM can be prepared at 2 mg/mL in DMSO and kept in small aliquots at –20°C. Such a stock solution will be stable for up to 3 yr. Wrap the tube containing the

platelet suspension in foil to prevent photo-bleaching of the calcein-labeled cells. Platelets are efficiently labelled in 30–60 min with no further labeling after 1 h.

6. Briefly, pellet the labeled cells in the presence of PGI_2 or PGE_1, aspirate the plasma, and wash once in Tyrode's/ACD buffer in the presence of PGI_2 or PGE_1. Pellet the platelets and suspend in Tyrode's buffer.

7. This allows the separation of adhesion and secretion/aggregation events and therefore the measurement of adhesion without the complication of secondary mediator pathways being activated that lead to aggregate formation and abnormally high fluorescence readings.

8. The Tyrode's buffer used to suspend the cells should be modified to include extra Mg^{2+}/Ca^{2+} ions if integrin-mediated adhesion is being assayed. For example, adhesion of platelets to fibrinogen requires supplementation with $CaCl_2$ (1 mM); adhesion to soluble collagens requires micromolar $CaCl_2$ (15 μM) and $MgCl_2$ (1 mM). Alternatively, GPVI-mediated adhesion to collagen can be separated from integrin-mediated collagen binding through the inclusion of EGTA (1 mM).

9. To prepare a 4% solution of paraformaldehyde, add 4 g to 100 mL of PBS and heat to ~60°C in a fume hood, adding a few drops of 1 N NaOH to help it dissolve. Once the solid has completely dissolved, allow the solution to cool to room temperature before adjusting to pH 7.4. Aliquots can be stored frozen and thawed in a 60°C water bath when needed. Cool to room temperature prior to use.

10. For detection of calcein-labeled cells, you will need a fluorimeter fitted with filters to excite at 494 nm and detect emission at 517 nm.

11. Alternatively, dilutions of labeled platelets of known density can be added to empty wells of the plate after the washing steps and read alongside the washed wells to obtain true values of the number of cells bound.

References

1. Hujdik, W. P. N., Sakariassen, K. S., Nievelstein, P. F. E. M., and Sixma, J. J. (1985) Role of factor VII-von Willebrand factor and fibronectin in the interaction of platelets in flowing blood with monomeric and fibrillar collagens types I and III. *J. Clin. Inv.* **75,** 531–540.
2. Nieuwenhuis, H. K., Akkerman, J. W. N., Houdijk, W. P. M., and Sixma, J. J. (1985) Human blood platelets showing no response to collagen fail to express surface glycoprotein-Ia. *Nature* **318,** 470–472.
3. Hotkotter, O., Nieswandt, B., Smyth, N., Muller, W., Hafner, M., Schulte, V., et al. (2002) Integrin $α_2$-deficient mice develop normally, are fertile, but display partially defective interaction with collagen. *J. Biol. Chem.* **277,** 10,789–10,794.
4. Nieswandt, B., Brakebusch, C., Bergmeier, W., Schulte, V., Bouvard, D., Mokhtari-Nejad, R., et al. (2001) Glycoprotein VI but not α2β1 integrin is essential for platelet interaction with collagen. *EMBO J.* **20,** 2120–2130.
5. Gibbins, J., Asselin, J., Farndale, R., Barnes, M., Law, C. L., and Watson, S. P. (1996) Tyrosine phosphorylation of the Fc receptor γ-chain in collagen-stimulated platelets. *J. Biol. Chem.* **271,** 18,095–18,099.
6. Asselin, J., Gibbins, J. M., Achison, M., Lee, Y.-H., Morton, L. F., Farndale, R. W., et al. (1997) A collagen-like peptide stimulates tyrosine phosphorylation of syk and phospholipase Cγ2 in platelets independent of the integrin α2β1. *Blood* **89,** 1235–1242.
7. Gibbins, J. M., Okuma, M., Farndale, R., Barnes, M., and Watson, S. P. (1997) Glyco-protein VI is the collagen receptor in platelets which underlies tyrosine phosphorylation of the Fc receptor γ-chain. *FEBS Lett.* **413,** 255–259.

8. Poole, A., Gibbins, J. M., Turner, M., van Vugt, M. J., van de Winkel, J. G. J., Saito, T., et al. (1997) The Fc receptor γ-chain and the tyrosine kinase Syk are essential for activation of mouse platelets by collagen. *EMBO J.* **16,** 2333–2341.

9. Depraetere, H., Ajzenberg, N., Girma, J. P., Lacombe, C., Meyer, D., Deckmyn, H., et al. (1998) Platelet aggregation induced by a monoclonal antibody to the A1 domain of von Willebrand factor. *Blood* **91,** 3792–3799.

10. Knight, C. G., Morton, L. F., Onley, D. J., Peachey, A. R., Messent, A. J., Smethurst, P. A., et al. (1998) Identification in collagen type I of an integrin $\alpha_2\beta_1$-binding site containing an essential GER sequence. *J. Biol. Chem.* **273,** 33,287–33,294.

11. Smith, C., Estavillo, D., Emsley, J., Bankston, L. A., Liddington, R. C., and Cruz, M. A. (2000) Mapping the collagen-binding site in the I domain of the glycoprotein Ia/IIa (integrin $\alpha_2\beta_1$). *J. Biol. Chem.* **275,** 4205–4209.

12. Huai, J. and Drescher, U. (2001) An ephrin-A-dependent signaling pathway controls integrin function and is linked to the tyrosine phosphorylation of a 120-kDa protein. *J. Biol. Chem.* **276,** 6689–6694.

13. Vossmeyer, D., Hofmann, W., Loster, K., Reutter, W., and Danker, K. (2002) Phospholipase Cγ binds $\alpha_1\beta_1$ integrin and modulates $\alpha_1\beta_1$ integrin-specific adhesion. *J. Biol. Chem.* **277,** 4636–4643.

14. Onley, D. J., Knight, C. G., Tuckwell, D. S., Barnes, M., and Farndale, R. W. (2000) Micromolar Ca^{2+} concentrations are essential for Mg^{2+}-dependent binding of collagen by the integrin $\alpha_2\beta_1$ in human platelets. *J. Biol. Chem.* **275,** 24,560–24,564.

15. Prevost, N., Woulfe, D., Tanaka, T., and Brass, L. F. (2002) Interactions between Eph kinases and ephrins provide a mechanism to support platelet aggregation once cell-to-cell contact has occurred. *PNAS* **99,** 9219–9224.

16. Santoro, S. A., Zutter, M. M., Wu, J. E., Staatz, W. D., Saelman, E. U. M., and Keely, P. J. (1994) Analysis of Collagen Receptors in *Extracellular Matrix Components* (Ruoslahti, E., ed.), Methods in Enzymology Vol. 245, Academic Press, San Diego, CA, pp. 147–183.

17. Haverstick, D. M., Cowan, J. F., Yamada, K. M., and Santoro, S. A. (1985) Inhibition of platelet adhesion to fibronectin, fibrinogen and von Willebrand factor substrates by a synthetic tetrapeptide derived from the cell-binding domain of fibronectin. *Blood* **66,** 946–952.

14

Platelet Adhesion Assays Under Flow
Using Matrix Protein-Coupled Adhesion Columns

Renata Polanowska-Grabowska and Adrian R. L. Gear

1. Introduction

The primary step in hemostasis after vascular injury is generally considered to be the adherence of circulating platelets to collagen exposed in the subendothelial connective tissues *(1,2)*. Such platelet adhesion is essential to limit bleeding and maintain blood vessel integrity. This process must occur extremely rapidly and involves a cascade of events including the initial platelet adhesion to the collagen surface and stabilization of the platelet-collagen bond, followed by spreading, activation of the glycoprotein (GP) IIb-IIIa fibrinogen receptor, and release of platelet granule contents. Platelet–platelet interactions then occur by platelet recruitment from the plasma, leading to the buildup of thrombi on the initial monolayer of adherent platelets.

A variety of methods have been developed to investigate the important initial platelet interactions with adhesive surfaces under static and flow conditions. These methods include platelet sedimentation onto a test surface *(3)*, pumping blood or platelet suspensions through annular *(4,5)* or parallel-plate perfusion chambers *(6–8)*; passing blood or platelet-rich plasma (PRP) through columns of glass beads *(9)*, polymer beads *(10)*, or polymer-coated beads *(11)*; filtration of collagen fibrils with adherent platelets on polycarbonate membranes *(12)*, and affinity binding of platelets on collagen-coated Sepharose beads *(13,14)*. The method to be described here is derived from that originally developed by Brass et al. *(13)*; where suspensions of washed radiolabeled platelets in a medium containing Tris-HCl and EDTA were passed slowly through a relatively long column of collagen-sepharose beads, with adhesion being measured by the difference in radioactivity of platelets applied and platelets eluted from the collagen-sepharose column. Our goal was to use affinity chromatography in the form of a microadhesion column of collagen-coated Sepharose beads incorporated in a continuous-flow system *(15)* (**Fig. 1**). This approach enables detailed study of rapid adhesion events to collagen or other adhesive proteins under flow conditions approaching those in the arterial microcirculation and before platelet secretion and aggregation occur *(16)*.

From: *Methods in Molecular Biology, vol. 272:*
Platelets and Megakaryocytes, Vol. 1: Functional Assays
Edited by: J. M. Gibbins and M. P. Mahaut-Smith © Humana Press Inc., Totowa, NJ

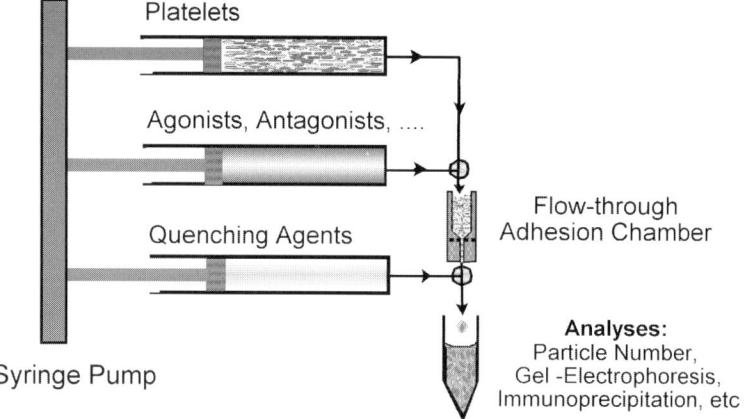

Fig. 1. Overall system for studying rapid platelet adhesion under flow conditions. A flow-through adhesion chamber/column forms the center of the system, which is illustrated in more detail in **Fig. 2**. Platelets are pumped through the adhesion chamber, which contains collagen-coated Sepharose beads or other beads with specific adhesive proteins of interest. The chamber is placed in line with the outflow of a 1-mL syringe in a controllable syringe pump *(15,18,21–25)*, and a second syringe can be used to pre-expose the platelets to an agonist, co-agonist, or other agent, before the cells enter the adhesion column. The effluent is analyzed for number of single platelets by a resistive-particle counter to assess the extent of adhesion at a given flow rate corresponding to a defined contact (adhesion) time. If necessary, a third syringe delivers quenching agent to the non-adherent (effluent) platelets emerging from the adhesion column. The simplest system only requires one syringe. Biochemical analyses can be performed on the adherent platelets as well as on the effluent cells, as described previously *(20,26–29)*.

2. Materials
2.1. Isolation of Washed Human Blood Platelets

1. Peripheral venous blood obtained from normal volunteers (*see* **Note 1**).
2. Anticoagulant: acid-citrate-dextrose (ACD): dissolve 15 g of citric acid monohydrate, 25 g of trisodium citrate dihydrate, and 20 g of dextrose per 1 L distilled water and store at 4°C for 2 wk. Other anticoagulants such as heparin or hirudin can also be used.
3. Inhibitors: apyrase grade VII (Sigma, St. Louis, MO; 250 U/mL), prostacyclin (PGI$_2$; Sigma; 1 mg/mL), indomethacin (Sigma; 1 mg/mL) in ethanol (*see* **Note 2**).
4. Washing buffer: ACD containing 0.3% (w/v) bovine serum albumin (BSA, fatty-acid-free; Sigma) and 2.5 U/mL apyrase.
5. Platelet resuspension buffer (modified HEPES-Tyrode's buffer): 137 mM NaCl, 2.7 mM KCl, 12 mM NaHCO$_3$, 0.36 mM Na$_2$HPO$_4$, 5.5 mM dextrose, 10 mM HEPES, pH 7.2–7.4, containing 2 mM Mg^{2+} (or other cations of interest), and 0.3% (w/v) BSA (*see* **Note 3**).
6. Shielded winged needles (Becton Dickinson, Franklin Lakes, NJ) 19-gauge, 30-mL syringes, 50-mL conical polypropylene centrifuge tubes, plastic pipets, 15-mL plastic round-bottom centrifuge tubes.

2.2. Preparation of Collagen-Coated Sepharose 4B Beads

1. Coupling buffer: 0.1 M NaHCO$_3$, pH 8.3, containing 0.5 M NaCl. Store at room temperature (RT).
2. Collagen: Lyophilized acid-soluble collagen (100 mg) is dissolved in 30 mL of ice-cold coupling buffer and dialyzed against coupling buffer for 2 d with four changes of dialysis buffer in cold a room (*see* **Note 4**). Other adhesive proteins, such as fibronectin, laminin, fibrinogen, or von Willebrand factor, can also be bound to CNBr-activated Sepharose in a similar manner.
3. Bovine serum albumin (BSA, fatty-acid-free; Sigma): 5 mg/mL diluted in coupling buffer.
4. Dialysis tubing (Pierce, Rockford, IL).
5. CNBr-activated Sepharose 4B (Pharmacia Biotech, Uppsala, Sweden, cat. No 17-0430-01). Note that CNBr-Sepharose has a limited shelf life and should be used soon after purchase.
6. Blocking buffer: 1% ethanolamine or 1 M glycine dissolved in coupling buffer.
7. Washing buffer: 0.1 M sodium acetate at pH 4.0, with 0.5 M NaCl.
8. 10X stock solution of phosphate-buffered saline (PBS): 0.01 M sodium phosphate buffer at pH 7.4, 0.15 M NaCl.
9. Rotating platform (*see* **Note 5**).

2.3. Adhesion Assay and Microadhesion Column

1. T-junction, plastic tubes, syringes.
2. Microadhesion column—see sketch in **Fig. 2**. The column consists of three parts: an upper 30-mm-long microcolumn drilled to 1 or 2 mm diameter containing the adhesion beads, a lower microcolumn 30 mm long and drilled to 0.5 mm diameter, and a nylon mesh filter (25–μm pore size) that is placed between columns. A screw-thread union joint connects the upper and lower parts to provide tight sealing between the filter and columns. All parts are made of machinable clear plastic/resin material.
3. Multiple syringe pump from the Harvard Apparatus Co. (Natick, MA) or another similar pump.
4. Resistive-particle counter for platelet counting, such as that manufactured by Coulter (Hialeah, FL) with sensing apertures of 50 μm or similar diameter.
5. Counting vials: 20 mL, polystyrene, disposable.
6. Repeater pipet (manual or automated) for 10-mL delivery of diluent (0.15 M NaCl).

3. Methods
3.1. Isolation of Washed Human Platelets

1. Venous blood is drawn from healthy donors who have not taken aspirin or other antiplatelet drugs for 7 days. Blood is mixed with ACD (10 vol blood plus 1 vol ACD).
2. The anticoagulated blood is then distributed in 10- or 15-mL polypropylene tubes, which are centrifuged at 350g for 3, 3, and 5 min, respectively, with the platelet-rich plasma (PRP) collected at each step.
3. The resulting PRP is separated and centrifuged at 620g for 20 min in the presence of inhibitors of platelet aggregation and secretion, such as indomethacin, apyrase, and PGI$_2$.
4. The platelet pellet is then gently resuspended in ACD containing BSA, and apyrase.
5. After centrifugation at 620g for 20 min, the platelet pellet is resuspended in a modified HEPES-Tyrode's buffer containing 2 mM Mg^{2+} and 0.3% (w/v) BSA at concentration 4–6×10^8 platelets/mL.

These procedures are described in detail in earlier publications *(17,18)*.

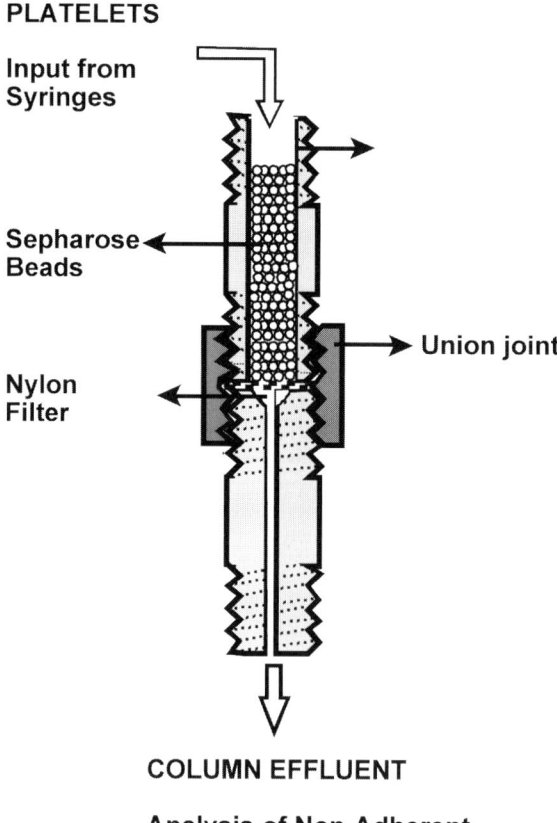

PLATELETS

Input from Syringes

Sepharose Beads

Union joint

Nylon Filter

COLUMN EFFLUENT

Analysis of Non-Adherent Platelets

Fig. 2. Adhesion column/chamber design. The assembly is composed of three parts: an initial cylinder, typically 3 cm long and drilled to 1 or 2 mm internal diameter for containing the adhesion beads (~100 μm diameter); a standard, screw-thread union joint to enable tight sealing of a nylon mesh filter (typically 20- to 30-μm holes); and last, an endpiece with internal diameter of 0.5 mm. All parts are made of machinable plastic/resin material. The syringes and assembly are typically connected via 0.8-mm internal diameter Teflon tubing. Adhesion or contact times can be as short as 0.1 s to 3 s or longer with shear rates from 3000 down to 500 s^{-1}, or close to arterial. The amount of beads in the column and pumping speed define the adhesion time. Other shear rates are simply a matter of selecting the appropriate pumping speeds.

3.2. Preparation of Collagen-Coated Sepharose 4B Beads

1. Dissolve purified lyophilized collagen (or another matrix protein) in ice-cold coupling buffer at 6.7 mg/mL and dialyze against 2 L coupling buffer for 2 d in a cold room with four changes of dialysis (coupling) buffer. If the collagen does not dissolve in the cou-

pling buffer, add 500 m*M* acetic acid and leave the collagen solution overnight, and then dialyze against coupling buffer.

2. Centrifuge the collagen solution for 30 min at 10,000*g* and retain a small quantity of the supernatant for subsequent analysis of collagen concentration, if required.

3. Weigh enough CNBr-activated Sepharose 4B to produce 15 mL of swollen gel (see manufacturer's directions) and add this to a 500-mL flask containing 350 mL of 1 m*M* HCl. Gently swirl the contents of the flask periodically over a 20-min period to swell the gel.

4. Collect the CNBr-activated Sepharose on a small scintered-glass funnel under gentle vacuum. Drain off most of the 1 m*M* HCl (do not allow to dry out).

5. Wash the sepharose with 150 mL coupling buffer and drain under gentle vacuum until the sepharose is firm (do not allow to dry out).

6. Using a metal spatula, scoop the Sepharose out of the funnel and place in a 50-mL centrifuge tube. Add 30 mL of the collagen solution to the tube and mix gently. A few extra mL of buffer may be required to ensure the mixture is fluid.

7. Close the tube and allow the coupling reaction between the collagen and CNBr-activated Sepharose to proceed at 4°C overnight while rocking the tube gently on its side.

8. Centrifuge the contents of the tube at low speed (~350*g*) for 10 min and remove the supernatant using a plastic pipet. Save the supernatant in case the collagen does not bind to the CNBr-activated Sepharose. This can be checked by analyzing the proline content in the supernatant.

9. Wash the contents of the tube in 100 mL of coupling buffer and centrifuge at low speed (350*g*) for 5 min. Discard the supernatant.

10. Add 60 mL of blocking buffer to mask any excess activated groups that were not utilized for coupling, and rock the tube gently overnight at 4°C.

11. Wash the collagen-Sepharose beads with three sequential cycles of low- and high-pH washes using washing and coupling buffer to remove any adsorbed but noncovalently bound collagen (*see* **Note 6**).

12. Wash the gel beads twice with PBS, pH 7.4.

13. Finally, suspend the washed beads in PBS, pH 7.4, containing 0.02% (w/v) sodium azide for long-term storage at 4°C. Since azide is a strong platelet inhibitor, thoroughly prewash the beads prior to subsequent use for adhesion assay.

3.3. Adhesion Assay and Microadhesion Column

3.3.1. Performance of the Adhesion Assay

The general design of the microadhesion assay under flow conditions is based on the combination of quenched-flow and continuous-flow systems with affinity chromatography *(15,16)*. PRP, washed platelets, or reconstituted or whole blood can be pumped through narrow-bore tubing (0.2 to 0.3 mm i.d.) in the presence of inducing agents or inhibitors of platelet function. The original design has now been modified such that the microadhesion column (10–50 µL capacity) containing collagen (or another matrix protein) bound to CNBr activated-Sepharose 4B beads **(Fig. 2)** is inserted in place of the reaction tube of the quenched-flow apparatus **(Fig. 1)**. Blood, washed platelets, or PRP are pumped through the collagen-Sepharose beads in the microcolumn.

To assess the extent of adhesion, platelets are counted in the effluent emerging from the column, typically using a resistive-particle counter *(19)*. Aliquots of the original platelet suspension not exposed to the bead surface are counted to serve as static controls. The percent of platelets that adhere to the beads is equal to

$$[1 - (P_{eff}/P_{Con})] \times 100\%$$

where P_{eff} and P_{Con} are, respectively, the numbers of single platelets in column effluent and in static control.

The extent of adhesion depends on the contact time t_c, defined as the time during which platelets flow through the column and interact with the collagen surface. The contact time can be calculated from the formula

$$t_c = V_f/Q \tag{1}$$

where V_f represents the free volume in the column (volume accessible to platelet flow among the beads) and Q is a variable pumping speed. The ratio of the free volume to the total volume of the adhesion column filled by beads is called *porosity*. The theoretical maximum packing density of identical beads (in which the beads form a face-centered cubic lattice) has porosity of 0.26; for random packing, the porosity is 0.36. In practice, not all the beads have exactly the same radius and the actual porosity of the system should be measured experimentally. For example, for 12.5 µL of packed beads (25 µL of bead suspension) we found the free volume to be 3.8 µL and calculated contact times at pumping speeds of 6.7, 3.3, and 2 µL/s to be 0.56, 1.15, and 1.9 s, respectively.

3.3.2. Calculation of Shear Rates

As far as we know, the exact distribution of shear rates in the system of beads has not been determined analytically or numerically in the literature. An approximate measure of the shear rates at the surface of the beads can be obtained by considering the adhesion column as a porous medium. In this model, the "free volume" is represented by a system of pores in which the shear rate is given by the formula:

$$\gamma = 4 \, Q/(\pi N_p r_p^3) = 4 \, Q/(\pi \, \varepsilon \, R_t^2 \, r_p) \tag{2}$$

where Q is the flow-rate through the column, N_p is the number of pores, r_p the radius of a pore, R_t the radius of the column, and ε the porosity of the system of beads in the column (the ratio of the free volume to the total volume). For example, assuming random packing of a column with internal radius of 1 mm filled with beads 100 µm in diameter, and a flow rate $Q = 6.7$ µL/s, the formula above gives a shear rate of about 3300/s for a pore radius r_p approx 0.2 times the radius of the beads (*see* **Notes 7,8**).

3.3.3. Column Preparation

1. Prepare the microadhesion assembly using one adhesion column unit coupled to a narrow-bore effluent column (1 mm i.d.) unit **(Fig. 2)**, linking them with a screw-thread union joint with a nylon filter placed between the bottom of the upper column unit and the top of the lower column. Tighten with pliers.
2. Load the adhesion column with 50 µL (or appropriate volume) of prewashed Sepharose beads **(Fig. 2)**. Gently rinse the loaded beads twice with 1 mL of PBS buffer, pH 7.4, using

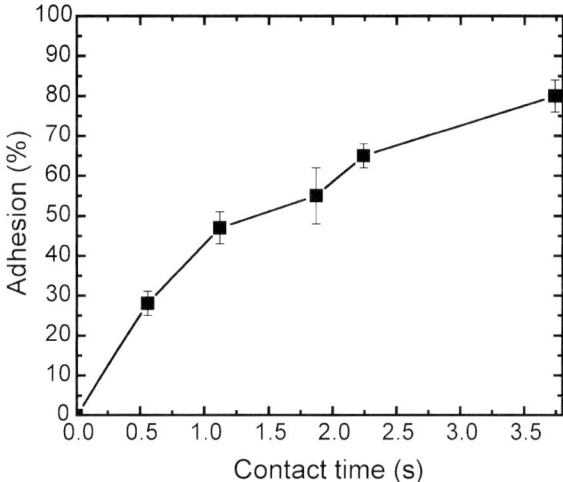

Fig. 3. A typical profile of platelet adhesion to collagen under arterial flow conditions. The different contact times were obtained by using 12.5 and 25 µL of packed collagen-coated sepharose beads and three different pumping speeds. The results are presented as mean ± SE from three experiments for one donor.

a 1-mL syringe. Place the loaded column assembly vertically in the continuous-flow system and keep the whole system at 37°C **(Fig. 1)**.

3. Fill the "cell" and "buffer" syringes with platelets or appropriate buffer or agonist solutions and then prime the line only until the beginning of the column.

4. Start pumping the solutions at 6.7 µL/s (or appropriate flow rate) and collect the nonbound effluent platelets (about 70 µL or three to four drops) in a plastic Eppendorf tube. The present design allows pumping platelets and mixing agonists or inhibitors before the adhesion column. Therefore, the roles of plasma proteins, platelet surface receptors, and modulators of platelet adhesion can be studied.

5. To evaluate the kinetics of platelet adhesion, the amount of the beads in the column and the pumping speed are varied to provide the appropriate contact (adhesion) time within the column. Using the microadhesion column, we have established that adhesion to type I collagen is extremely rapid, being essentially complete within several seconds **(Fig. 3)** as determined by the disappearance of single platelets from the effluent *(16)*. The potential contribution of platelet aggregation under the conditions of disturbed flow through the beads (shear stress between 15 and 50 dyn/cm^2, assuming porous medium) is an important question. Since particles counted by a resistive-particle counter can include not only singlets but also very small aggregates (up to four platelets), there is a possibility that small aggregates counted as single platelets could overestimate adhesion determined from counting single platelets in the column effluent. Determination of adhesion by following the loss in radioactivity of [^{51}Cr]-labeled platelets in the effluent confirms that particle counting of single platelets provides similar results. In addition, the presence of the RDG peptides that block GPIIb/IIIa-dependent aggregation do not significantly change adhesion values.

6. When preparing material for immunoblotting or immunoprecipitation (IP) of proteins in adherent platelets, about 300 μL of platelet suspension at 6×10^8/mL are pumped through the beads, the pump is then stopped and the column rapidly disassembled. Platelets bound to the beads are solubilized with 100 μL of ice-cold lysis buffer for IP or 2X SDS-PAGE sample buffer in preparation for SDS-PAGE and Western blotting. The amount of platelet protein is estimated from the percentage of platelets bound to collagen-coated beads compared with static platelet controls.

3.3.4. Analysis of Data

Controls should be run in which BSA-coated Sepharose beads are used in place of collagen-coated beads. This baseline (control) nonspecific adhesion to BSA-coated sepharose is typically less than 5–7% of that seen for collagen. All data should be corrected for this background or nonspecific adhesion. The data are usually expressed as the percentage of platelets attached to collagen-coated beads. The extent of adhesion is essentially a linear function of platelet concentration and does not depend on shear rate in the range of applied pumping speed from 1 to 7 μL/s. The adhesion is not due to trapping platelet aggregates that cannot pass through the column, since platelet treatments with aggregation inhibitors such as the GRGDSP peptide have no effect on platelet adhesion as mentioned above. In addition, scanning electron microscopy (SEM) reveals that aggregation does not occur initially, as only single platelets are seen attached to collagen-coated beads *(20)* and their discoid shape is only minimally altered.

3.3.5. Critique of the Method

Some characteristics of this in vitro test system need to be highlighted: (1) The use of Mg^{2+} in the suspending buffer, (2) incompletely defined flow conditions in a porous medium, and (3) ill-defined polymeric state of collagen. Despite these apparent limitations, the microadhesion assay to collagen under flow conditions has proved to be a valuable tool for understanding fundamental aspects of initial platelet-collagen interactions. The test is rapid, nonradioactive, highly reproducible, convenient, and relatively inexpensive. It enables detailed study of adhesive kinetics at very rapid (<1 s) times, and under flow conditions similar to arterial flow. In addition, it provides an opportunity to compare signal transduction events occurring in adherent cells versus nonadherent platelets.

4. Notes

1. Both human platelets and blood are considered biohazards. All procedures must be performed in compliance with appropriate institutional protocols and regulations for such potentially hazardous material.
2. Apyrases—enzymes extracted from potatoes that degrade ATP to ADP, and any ADP to AMP—are included in our suspending media to hydrolyze any ADP lost from the platelets during the course of experiments (often a number of hours), which otherwise accumulates and may cause the platelets to become refractory to stimulation. Prostacyclin (PGI_2), which can cause a transient increase in platelet cAMP, is a strong adhesion inhibitor and must be washed away. Platelets isolated in the presence of PGI_2 should be used for experimental purposes only after waiting 30 min following washing.

3. To avoid platelet aggregation, fibrinogen is omitted from the resuspension buffer. Because platelet adhesion to collagen in washed platelets mediated primarily via the $\alpha_2\beta_1$ integrin receptor is strongly blocked by the presence of external Ca^{2+} in the mM concentration range, calcium is also omitted from the final resuspension buffer. In the absence of Ca^{2+}, arachidonate-dependent pathways in suspended platelets may be activated, leading to the release of platelet granule contents. Therefore, aspirin or indomethacin should be added to inhibit this secondary activation by blocking the TXA_2 formation. To avoid potential effects of released ADP on platelet adhesion, apyrase should also be included in the resuspending buffer.

4. Collagens type I–VII can be obtained commercially from several companies (e.g., collagens types I, III, IV, and V [Sigma]; type VII [Chemicon Int., Temacula, CA]). Before commercially available collagens are used, they should be checked for integrity and cross-contamination with other major collagen types (types I, III, IV, and V), proteoglycans, or plasma proteins. Collagen preparation can be assayed by ELISA, inhibition-ELISA, and Western blotting.

5. All incubations during bead preparation should be done with mild agitation on a rotating platform.

6. The amount of collagen bound to Sepharose can be determined from the hydroxyproline content of a known weight of collagen-sepharose following hydrolysis under vaccum in 6 N HCl.

7. Formula (1) assumes that the flow is laminar (it can be shown that the Reynolds number for the porous medium model is less than 1). It also treats the platelet suspension as a Newtonian fluid. An alternative calculation of shear rates in the porous medium based on the Kozeny-Carman equation yields similar results to formula (1).

8. The porous-medium model does not take into account the fact that individual pores are not isolated "tubes" with uniform radius, but rather cross-linked "zigzags" having a complex geometry with a changing cross-section area. Shear rates at the walls of the pores are not uniform along the length of the pore, but depend on the position—they are highest in the narrowest parts, and lowest in the widest parts of the pore. Calculating these effects and evaluating the average shear rate at the surface of the beads are beyond the scope of the porous-medium approximation. Despite these limitations, we feel that the porous-medium model provides us with a useful approximation of the flow parameters.

Acknowledgments

The methods described in this chapter were developed with the support of the Carman Trust and the NIH (DK59004 NIH/DK), ARLG; and by the American Heart Association Mid-Atlantic Affiliate (Beginning Grant-in-Aid 0160500U to RPG).

References

1. Baumgartner, H. R. (1973) The role of blood flow in platelet adhesion, fibrin deposition, and formation of mural thrombi. *Microvasc. Res.* **5,** 167–179.
2. Baumgartner, H. R. (1977). Platelet interaction with collagen fibrils in flowing blood. I. Reaction of human platelets with alpha chymotrypsin-digested subendothelium. *Thromb. Haemost.* **37,** 1–16.
3. Ruckenstein, E., Marmur, A., and Rakower, S. R. (1976) Sedimentation and adhesion of platelets onto a horizontal glass surface. *Thromb. Haemost.* **36,** 334–342.
4. Baumgartner, H. R., Stemerman, M. B., and Spaet, T. H. (1971) Adhesion of blood platelets to subendothelial surface: distinct from adhesion to collagen. *Experientia* **27,** 283–285.

5. Turitto, V. T. and Baumgartner, H. R. (1975) Platelet interaction with subendothelium in a perfusion system: physical role of red blood cells. *Microvasc. Res.* **9,** 335–344.

6. Badimon, L., Turitto, V., Rosemark, J. A., Badimon, J. J., and Fuster, V. (1987) Characterization of a tubular flow chamber for studying platelet interaction with biologic and prosthetic materials: deposition of indium 111-labeled platelets on collagen, subendothelium, and expanded polytetrafluoroethylene. *J. Lab. Clin. Med.* **110,** 706–718.

7. Sakariassen, K. S., Aarts, P. A., de Groot, P. G., Houdijk, W. P., and Sixma, J. J. (1983) A perfusion chamber developed to investigate platelet interaction in flowing blood with human vessel wall cells, their extracellular matrix, and purified components. *J. Lab. Clin. Med.* **102,** 522–535.

8. Sakariassen, K. S., Muggli, R., and Baumgartner, H. R. (1989) Measurements of platelet interaction with components of the vessel wall in flowing blood. *Methods Enzymol.* **169,** 37–70.

9. Hellem, A. J. (1970) Platelet adhesiveness in von Willebrand's disease. A study with a new modification of the glass bead filter method. *Scand. J. Haematol.* **7,** 374–382.

10. Lindon, J. N., Rodvien, R., Brier, D., Greenberg, R., Merrill, E., and Salzman, E. W. (1978) In vitro assessment of interaction of blood with model surfaces. *J. Lab. Clin. Med.* **92,** 904–915.

11. Lindon, J. N., Kushner, L., and Salzman, E. W. (1989) Platelet interaction with artificial surfaces: in vitro evaluation. *Methods Enzymol.* **169,** 104–117.

12. Santoro, S. A. and Cunningham, L. W. (1982) Platelet-collagen adhesion. *Methods Enzymol.* **82,** 509–513.

13. Brass, L. F., Faile, D., and Bensusan, H. B. (1976) Direct measurement of the platelet collagen interaction by affinity chromatography on collagen/sepharose. *J. Lab. Clin. Med.* **87,** 525–534.

14. Cowan, D. H., Robertson, A. L., Shook, P., and Giroski, P. (1981) Platelet adherence to collagen: role of plasma, ADP, and divalent cations. *Br. J. Haematol.* **47,** 257–267.

15. Gear, A. R. (1982) Rapid reactions of platelets studied by a quenched-flow approach: aggregation kinetics. *J. Lab. Clin. Med.* **100,** 866–886.

16. Polanowska Grabowska, R. and Gear, A. R. (1992) High-speed platelet adhesion under conditions of rapid flow. *Proc. Natl. Acad. Sci. USA* **89,** 5754–5758.

17. Haver, V. M. and Gear, A. R. (1981) Functional fractionation of platelets. *J. Lab. Clin. Med.* **97,** 187–204.

18. Gear, A. R. (1984) Rapid platelet morphological changes visualized by scanning-electron microscopy: kinetics derived from a quenched-flow approach. *Br. J. Haematol.* **56,** 387–398.

19. Gear, A. R. (1976) Continuous-flow, resistive-particle counting. *Anal. Biochem.* **72,** 332–345.

20. Polanowska Grabowska, R., Geanacopoulos, M., and Gear, A. R. (1993) Platelet adhesion to collagen via the alpha 2 beta 1 integrin under arterial flow conditions causes rapid tyrosine phosphorylation of pp125FAK. *Biochem. J.* **296,** 543–547.

21. Geanacopoulos, M. and Gear, A. R. (1988) Application of spray-freezing to the study of rapid platelet reactions by a quenched-flow approach. *Thromb. Res.* **52,** 599–607.

22. Frojmovic, M. M., Milton, J. G., and Gear, A. L. (1989) Platelet aggregation measured in vitro by microscopic and electronic particle counting. *Methods Enzymol.* **169,** 134–149.

23. Jones, G. D. and Gear, A. R. (1990) Rapid blood platelet activation: continuous- and quenched-flow versus stopped-flow approaches [letter]. *Biochem. J.* **265,** 305–307.

24. Gear, A. R. and Raha, S. (1993) Calcium signalling and phosphoinositide metabolism in platelets: subsecond events revealed by quenched-flow techniques. *Adv. Exp. Med. Biol.* **344,** 57–67.

25. Raha, S., Jones, G. D., and Gear, A. R. (1993) Sub-second oscillations of inositol 1,4,5-trisphosphate and inositol 1,3,4,5-tetrakisphosphate during platelet activation by ADP and thrombin: lack of correlation with calcium kinetics. *Biochem J.* **292,** 643–646.
26. Polanowska Grabowska, R. and Gear, A. R. (1994) Role of cyclic nucleotides in rapid platelet adhesion to collagen. *Blood* **83,** 2508–2515.
27. Gear, A. R., Simon, C. G., and Polanowska Grabowska, R. (1997) Platelet adhesion to collagen activates a phosphoprotein complex of heat-shock proteins and protein phosphatase 1. *J. Neural. Transm.* **104,** 1037–1047.
28. Polanowska Grabowska, R., Simon, C. G., Jr., Falchetto, R., Shabanowitz, J., Hunt, D. F., and Gear, A. R. (1997) Platelet adhesion to collagen under flow causes dissociation of a phosphoprotein complex of heat-shock proteins and protein phosphatase 1. *Blood* **90,** 1516–1526.
29. Polanowska Grabowska, R. and Gear, A. R. (1999) Activation of protein kinase C is required for the stable attachment of adherent platelets to collagen but is not needed for the initial rapid adhesion under flow conditions. *Arterioscler. Thromb. Vasc. Biol.* **19,** 3044–3054.

15

Techniques to Examine Platelet Adhesive Interactions Under Flow

Suhasini Kulkarni, Warwick S. Nesbitt, Sacha M. Dopheide, Sascha C. Hughan, Ian S. Harper, and Shaun P. Jackson

1. Introduction

Platelet adhesion and aggregation at sites of vessel-wall injury are critical for the arrest of bleeding and for the development of vaso-occlusive thrombi at sites of athero-sclerotic-plaque rupture. These adhesive interactions are critically dependent on multiple receptors on the platelet surface (GPIb/V/IX, GPVI, integrins $\alpha_{IIb}\beta_3$ and $\alpha_2\beta_1$) and their specific ligands in the subendothelium (von Willebrand Factor, collagen) and plasma (von Willebrand Factor, fibrinogen) *(1,2)*. In vivo, these receptor-ligand interactions are exposed to a broad range of shear stresses generated by blood flow, ranging from 20–200/s in veins to 800–10,000/s in arteries *(3)*. In stenotic vessels, shear rates can approach 40,000/s. The development of in vitro methodologies mimicking physiological and pathophysiological flow conditions has significantly improved our understanding of the role of shear in regulating platelet functional responses. In general, the effects of shear stress have been studied with platelets in suspension using rotational devices such as the Couette or cone-plate viscometer. Alternatively, the effects of shear on platelets have been evaluated in a laminar-flow device such as the tubular, annular, or parallel-plate flow chamber. Rotational viscometers are ideal for the examination of shear effects on platelet adhesive interactions in the absence of platelet-surface interactions (i.e., platelets in suspension). Such studies are important in determining the mechanisms of platelet activation occurring in areas of vascular stenosis where shear rates are elevated well above physiological levels. Thrombus formation, however, does not generally occur with platelets in suspension but rather involves the progressive accrual of platelets onto vascular subendothelium and subsequently onto immobilized platelets. As such, the in vitro investigation of platelet function under conditions of physiological and pathological shear has been greatly facilitated by laminar flow devices.

From: *Methods in Molecular Biology, vol. 272:*
Platelets and Megakaryocytes, Vol. 1: Functional Assays
Edited by: J. M. Gibbins and M. P. Mahaut-Smith © Humana Press Inc., Totowa, NJ

Until recently, the morphometric and quantitative assessment of platelet adhesion and thrombus formation under high magnification has been limited to fixed samples. However, the advent of high-resolution microscopy techniques now enables the direct visualization of platelet adhesion processes down to a single-cell level in real time. Over the last five years, laminar-flow-based assays are increasingly being combined with confocal microscopy, allowing even higher resolution imaging and more accurate quantitation of platelet adhesion and aggregation events in three dimensions *(1,4–7)*. This chapter describes in detail the basic methodologies, evaluation procedures, and important troubleshooting information involved in a laminar-flow-based platelet assay developed in our laboratory. This technique allows very high-resolution imaging of the dynamics of platelet adhesion and thrombus growth under both physiological and patho-logical shear conditions in real time. Moreover, parameters defining various aspects of platelet function can be accurately quantitated using the methods described below.

2. Materials

The complete perfusion assembly established in our laboratory is photographically depicted in **Fig. 1**. On a per-flow basis, the following consumables and pieces of equipment are required.

2.1. Consumables

1. *Rectangular microcapillary tubes (microslides):* Microslides are flat rectangular glass capillary tubes **(Fig. 2A)** typically made from borosilicate. They are available with various internal dimensions (i.d.) and can be purchased from Vitro Dynamics Inc. (New Jersey) or can be custom-made by most scientific glassware suppliers. If custom-made, the microslide I.D. must be maintained at a constant value between production batches or batch-to-batch variation in shear rates will result. Furthermore, the outer diameter (o.d.) must be of a size that affords optimal optics for microscopy but is sufficiently thick to ensure that the microslides are not too fragile. Prior to use, all microslides are immersed in nitric acid (50% v/v in distilled water) overnight, washed thoroughly in distilled water to remove any traces of acid, dried at 37°C, and stored under dust-free conditions until required.

    In our laboratory, three sizes of microcapillary tubes are used depending on the range of shear rates required during perfusion **(Table 1)**. The flow rate is calculated using the formula:

    $$Q = \frac{wh^2t}{6\mu}$$

    where Q is the flow rate (mL/s), w is the microslide lumen width (cm), h is the microslide lumen height (cm), t is the desired shear stress (Pa), and μ is the final viscosity of the solution (whole or reconstituted blood) (Pa/s). Shear rate is inversely proportional to shear stress. To ensure that platelets do not settle out during perfusion at low shear rates (≤150/s) and to avoid the intake of air through weaker points in the perfusion apparatus at high shear rates (≥1800/s) flow rates are generally maintained between 0.1 mL/min and 2.0 mL/min.

    There are significant advantages to using microslides for perfusion studies over tradi-tional parallel-plate flow chamber apparatus:

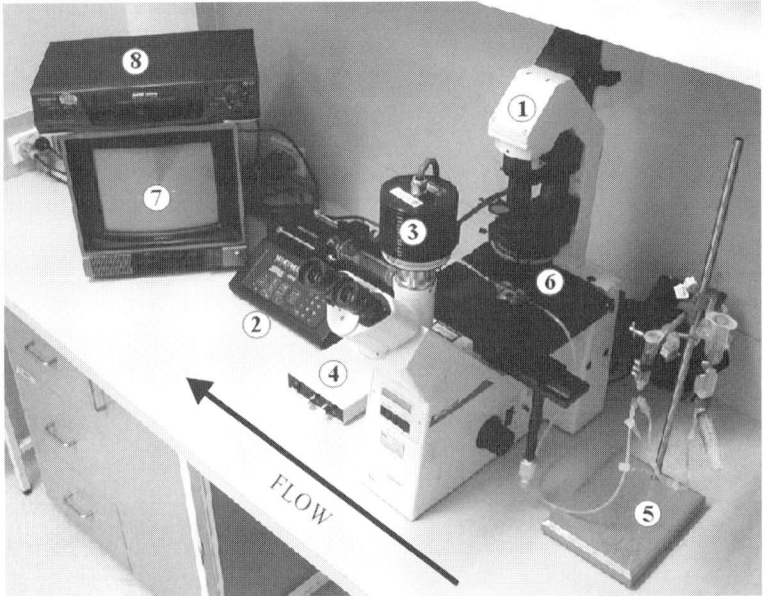

Fig. 1. Laminar flow perfusion assembly. (1) Leica DMIRBE inverted microscope with optical components enabling DIC microscopy and epifluorescence microscopy. This microscope can also be connected to a Leica TCS-SP confocal microscope. (2) Harvard PHD2000 Infusion/Withdraw Series pump with 2-syringe attachment. (3) DAGE-MTI RC300 CCD video camera connected to (4) Adjustable dials for light gain and offset functions. (5) Clamp stand with clamps holding blood and buffer reservoirs. The tubing attached to the reservoirs is connected to the tubing attached to the glass syringe on the Harvard pump via a glass microcapillary tube. (6) Custom-made metal stage plate for accommodating microslides during perfusion. (7) The video camera is connected to the TV monitor that in turn is connected to (8) A Panasonic VHS video recorder. *Note:* For better visualization of the perfusion assembly, the microscope-heating unit and Perspex hood have been omitted from this photograph. *Note:* Arrow represents direction of flow.

    a. Smaller volumes of blood are required, particularly for higher shear perfusions. This is beneficial when working with small rodents (e.g., transgenic mice) where only small volumes of blood can be obtained.

    b. The flat rectangular shape of microslides enables high-resolution imaging of platelet adhesion processes in real time, even in the presence of red blood cells (RBCs).

    c. Microslides are very easy to assemble. Due to their smaller size, more than one can be assembled at a time, enabling up to eight replicate experiments to be performed concurrently.

  2. *Tubing:* To connect the microslides to the inlet and outlet aspects of the perfusion system depicted in **Fig. 1, part 1**, Watson Marlow silicone tubing (ProScience, Melbourne, Australia) is used. This tubing is strong, durable, and easy to clean and does not support the

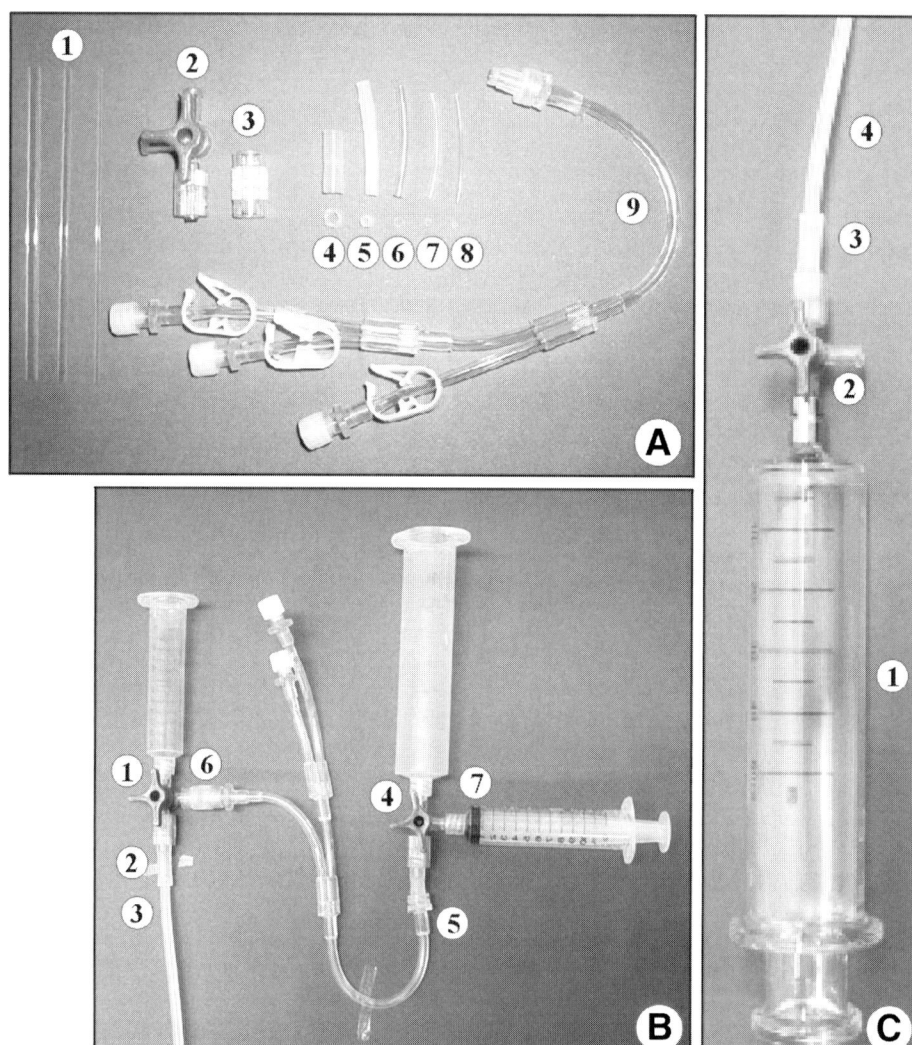

Fig. 2. Tubing Assembly Required for Perfusion. (**A**) Tubing Components Required for Flow—(1–3) The three sizes of flat, rectangular glass microcapillary tubes used for perfusion studies. Microslide dimensions are provided in **Table 1**. (4–9) represent the various types and sizes of tubing required for perfusion system assembly. Tubing dimensions are provided in **Table 2**. (**B**) Preparation of Blood/Buffer Reservoirs for Perfusion—(1) Polycarbonate syringes with luer-lock nozzles are divested of plungers and connected to a three-way tap. (2) The tap is then connected to a short length of tubing (No. 4.) (3) Tubing (No. 4) is in turn attached to a long length of tubing (No. 5). These syringes are used as blood reservoirs and are connected to microslides as shown in **Fig. 1**. (4) The syringes for buffer reservoirs are also connected to a three-way tap and a short length of tubing (No. 4). (5) This is then attached to the single opening of tubing (No. 9). (6) The other end of tubing (No. 9) (which has three openings) is connected to the three-way taps of blood and buffer reservoir(s) using a male-to-male

Table 1
Dimensions of Glass Microcapillary Tubes (Microslides) Used During Perfusion

Microslide size	Internal dimension (mm) [height × width]	Length (mm)	Shear range (s^{-1})	Flow rate range (mL/min)
Large	0.3 × 3.0	100	100–600	0.25–1.52
Intermediate	0.2 × 2.0	100	600–2000	0.4–1.33
Small	0.1 × 1.0	100	>2000	>0.17

Table 2
Dimensions of Watson-Marlow Silicone Tubing Required for Perfusion System Assembly

Tubing No.[a]	Internal diameter (mm)	Wall thickness (mm)	Lengths required (cm)
4	3.2	1.2	2
5	0.8	1.8	75
6	1.8	0.5	2
7	1.2	0.5	2
8	1.0	0.3	2

[a]Refer to **Fig. 2**.

nonspecific adhesion of platelets in a whole or reconstituted blood. **Figure 2A** photographically depicts the various sizes of tubing required for flow. For ease of reference, the different types of tubing will be referred to numerically (*see* **Note 1**).

3. *Plastic syringes:* Plastic syringes (divested of plungers) are used to hold buffer or platelet suspensions during perfusion. Although the size of the syringe used is up to the experimenters' discretion, it is advised that "luer-lock" syringes be used, as they attach more securely to three-way taps during flow.
4. *Double-sided tape:* This tape (0.6 cm wide) is available upon request from manufacturers of 3M products.

2.2. Buffers and Reagents

1. 15 mM trisodium citrate.
2. 200U/mL hirudin (α-thrombin inhibitor).
3. Acid-citrate-dextrose (ACD): 90 mM sodium citrate, 7 mM citric acid, 140 mM dextrose, pH 4.6.

Fig. 2. *(continued)* plastic adapter. (7) The second, smaller syringe attached to the three-way tap on the buffer reservoir is used to flush tubing or microcapillary tubes prior to or at the end of a perfusion. **(C)** Preparation of Harvard Syringes for Perfusion—(1) The plunger of the Harvard glass syringe is lightly greased to ensure smooth movement during flow. (2) The nozzle of the syringe is attached to a three-way tap. (3) This is in turn is connected to a short length of tubing (No. 4). (4) A longer length of tubing (No. 5) is then attached to this assembly.

4. Platelet washing buffer (PWB): 4.3 mM Na$_2$HPO$_4$, 24.3 mM NaH$_2$PO$_4$, pH 6.5, 113 mM NaCl, 5.5 mM glucose, 0.5% (w/v) bovine serum albumin (BSA), and 10 mM theophylline.
5. Red blood cell (RBC) washing buffer: 140 mM NaCl, 10 mM HEPES, pH 7.4, 5 mM glucose.
6. Modified Tyrode's buffer: 10 mM HEPES, pH 7.5, 12 mM NaHCO$_3$, 137 mM NaCl, 2.7 M KCl, 5 mM glucose, 1 mM CaCl$_2$, 1 mM MgCl$_2$.
7. Tris-buffered saline with protease inhibitor: 20 mM Tris-HCl, pH 7.2, 150 mM NaCl, 1 mM EDTA, 10 mM benzamidine.
8. Sepharose CL-6B size-exclusion chromatography column.
9. Buffer A (for purification of fibrinogen (**Subheading 3.6.2.**): 20 mM Tris-HCl, pH 7.4, 150 mM NaCl, 25 µg/mL PMSF, 1 mM benzamidine, 10 mM ε-amino-n-caproic acid.
10. Buffer B (for purification of fibrinogen (**Subheading 3.6.2.**): 20 mM Tris-HCl, pH 7.4, 150 mM NaCl.
11. 6 M β-alanine.
12. 3.7% Formaldehyde.

2.3. Equipment

1. *Harvard syringe pump:* The PHD2000 Infusion/Withdraw Series Pump can be purchased from Harvard Apparatus (Holliston, MA) and usually allows a maximum of two syringes to be run concurrently. A four-syringe adaptor kit (Model no. 2400–275) can also be purchased from the manufacturer; however, for experiments in which more than four runs need to be performed, customized pump attachments need to be made. In our laboratory, a maximum of eight syringes can be run simultaneously with ease (**Fig. 3A**).
2. *Inverted light microscope:* The details of the components of the light microscope below are largely available from the relevant company (e.g., Leica, Olympus, Zeiss). However, some components, such as the microslide stage plate, heating unit, and Perspex heating box, need to be custom-made.
3. Three-plate mechanical stage.
4. Microslide stage plate (**Fig. 3C**): Custom-designed stage plate assembly built to accommodate rectangular microcapillary tubes.
5. Side- or top-port: for connection to a video camera.
6. Tube lens (1.0X or 1.5X).
7. Condenser with a 23-mm working-distance cap and all necessary polarized light accessories and interference contrast prisms that are switched into the optical path as required.

Fig. 3. *(see facing page)* Peripheral components required for perfusion. (**A**) The Harvard PHD2000 infusion/withdraw series pump—This photo depicts the custom-made eight-syringe holder adapted to the Harvard pump. Two- and four-syringe holders can be purchased direct from Harvard Inc. (**B**) Microscope-heating unit—This custom-made microscope-heating unit has adjustable temperature settings and delivers heat to the Perspex hood surrounding the microscope via an insulated piece of tubing (black tube on left). The heating unit also has a precision temperature probe (arrow) to maintain a constant physiological temperature during flow. (**C**) Custom-made microscope stage plate—The stage plate can be custom-made by most metal workshops. The two raised metal strips are covered with double-sided tape to hold microslides flat during perfusion. These strips are approx 4 mm higher than the rest of the plate surface.

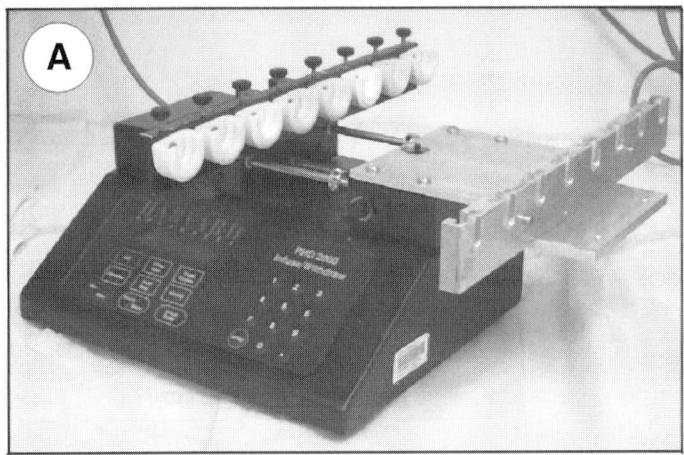

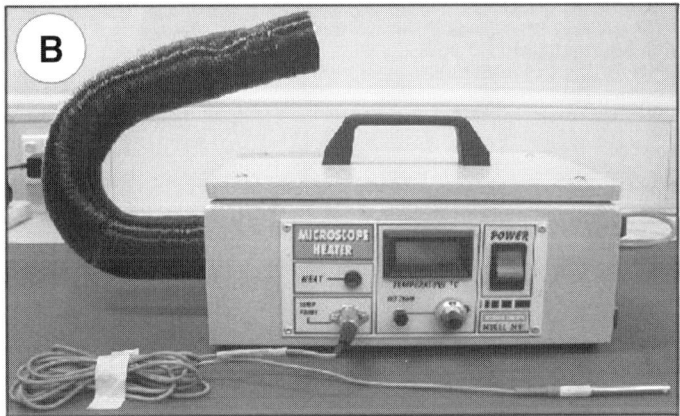

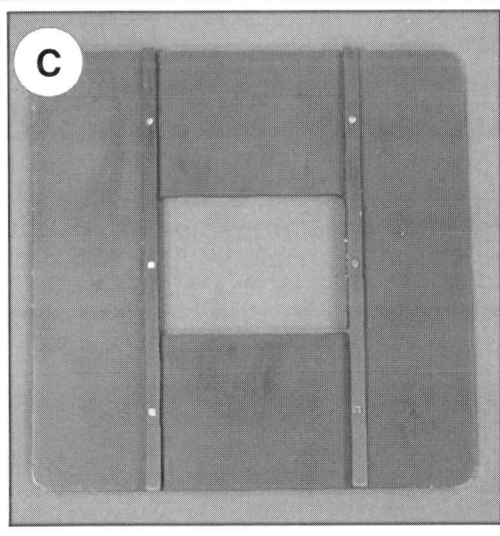

8. Optical components enabling techniques including phase-contrast, differential-interference-contrast (DIC), and fluorescence microscopy.
9. Objectives:
   a. Dry—40X and 63X. The 40X is a long-working-distance (1.9–3.3 mm) objective enabling visualization of cells at the lower internal surface of the microcapillary tube. Due to their small size, platelets are best visualized using objectives yielding ×40 or greater magnification.
   b. Immersion—Plan Apo 63X/1.20 water, 0.22-mm free working distance with a coverslip correction collar of 0.14–0.18 mm.
10. Components for fluorescence microscopy including a 50W or 100W high-pressure mercury burner acting as a light source, the higher wattage burner being more stable and furthermore, better suited to light microscopy.
11. *Fluorescence filter systems:* For visualization of cells labeled with single dyes, the excitation characteristics of dyes should be matched with those of the filters—for example, for fluorescein-type dyes (FITC, calcein, Fluo3, GFP) use a blue excitation filter system (BP 480/40, DM 505, BP 527/30 or LP512.5); for rhodamine (TRITC, CY3, DiI) a broad-band green excitation filter system (BP 515-560, DM 580, LP 590) is recommended (*see* **Note 2**).
12. *Video camera:* Although most microscope cameras are acceptable, in our experience, we have found the DAGE-MTI RC300 CCD camera (DAGE-MTI, Inc., IN) to be optimal for real-time image capture. The adjustable gain and offset functions are particularly advantageous, as they allow the contrast between background and fluorescent platelets to be enhanced while imaging in real time.
13. *Inverted confocal microscope:* Optical microscopes used for confocal microscopy are generally identical to those in general use, but are additionally fitted with a 100% beam splitter to ensure that laser excitation cannot inadvertently be directed through the eyepieces and hence cause eye injury. Other safety features include shutters to close the laser-beam path when not scanning and acquiring images. The choice of laser is usually made on the basis of fluorescence excitation required, and generally includes an argon-ion laser (488 nm) with additional green (543 nm) and red (633 nm) helium-neon lasers. Alternatively, and becoming less popular, is the single mixed-gas argon-krypton laser, providing 488-, 568-, and 647-nm laser lines. Options of UV and pulsed lasers may also be incorporated into the excitation system. When working in confocal mode, the microscope filter blocks are not used and all beam splitting and filtering of excitation and emission is done in the confocal scanhead. Full software control of these filters, scanning speeds, image capture, and focus allow automated imaging when in confocal mode. For these studies we have selected the TCS-SP confocal microscope, which can be coupled to either upright or inverted microscopes.
14. *Clamps and clamp stands:* These are readily available from most labware suppliers. As depicted in **Fig. 1**, the clamps are used to hold buffer and blood reservoirs during perfusion.
15. *Microscope heating hood and heating unit:* To ensure that experiments are performed at a physiological temperature, we use a custom-built microscope heater produced by Scientific Concepts (Victoria, Australia) **(Fig. 3B)**. A custom-made clear perspex hood is also fitted around the microscope, allowing efficient heating of the flow chamber while causing minimal hindrance during experimentation. The Perspex box requires several open ports, enabling easy access to the mechanical stage, the stage plate, the heating unit, and silicone tubing used for perfusion. An additional open port is also necessary for an unobstructed light path to ensure optimal optics during platelet visualization. The air temperature inside

the Perspex chamber is regulated by a precision temperature probe placed inside the chamber at a point distant to the heated air inlet.

16. *Video recorder/player and TV monitor:* The brand of video recorder and monitor used to record images of platelet adhesion is up to the experimenter's discretion. In our laboratory, we use the Panasonic VHS recorder (model no. AG7355) and a Sony Trinitron (14-inch) monitor.

3. Methods

3.1. Collection of Whole Blood

1. Blood is collected via venisection of the antecubital vein of consenting healthy volunteers who have not ingested any antiplatelet medication (e.g., aspirin or ibuprofen) in the two weeks preceding the procedure. Use of butterfly needles smaller than 19-*g* is not recommended, as high shear forces are generated when drawing through smaller-sized needles. For whole blood studies, blood is collected directly into polycarbonate syringes containing either 15 mM trisodium citrate or 200 U/mL of the α-thrombin inhibitor hirudin. Blood is withdrawn at a reasonably slow and steady rate, taking care to avoid frothing, and is immediately mixed by gentle inversions of the syringe.
2. To avoid the effects of trace amounts of thrombin generated during venipuncture, the first 2–5 mL of blood are discarded.
3. Anticoagulated blood is maintained at room temperature (~22°C) without agitation and used within 4 h postcollection.

3.2. Preparation of Washed Platelets

1. When isolating platelets, blood is anticoagulated at a 1:6 ratio (v/v) ACD containing 70 mM theophylline.
2. Platelet-rich plasma (PRP) is obtained by centrifugation of whole blood at 200g for 30 min.
3. The supernatant is aspirated and centrifuged at 2000g for 10 min to obtain a platelet pellet, which is subsequently resuspended at one-tenth the original volume in platelet-washing buffer (PWB).
4. Platelets in PWB are maintained in a 37°C water bath without agitation until required (*see* **Note 3**).

3.3. Preparation of Washed Red Blood Cells

1. The autologous RBC pellet resulting from the preparation of PRP (**Subheading 3.2., step 2**) is washed three times with an equal volume of RBC washing buffer via consecutive resuspension and centrifugation (2000g for 10 min).
2. Following the final wash, the RBC pellet is maintained as a packed-cell suspension until required (*see* **Note 4**).

3.4. Preparation of Reconstituted Blood

The environment experienced by platelets in whole blood is a complex milieu of plasma proteins (fibrinogen, vWF, albumin), nascent agonists (ADP, thrombin, adrenaline), and blood cells (leukocytes, erythrocytes), all of which can, and do, have an impact on platelet function and activation under flow conditions. In order to examine the impact of different blood components on platelet activation under flow, reconstituted blood is often utilized.

1. In reconstitution experiments, platelets are resuspended in modified Tyrode's buffer at a final concentration of 150×10^9/L.
2. The resulting suspension is then mixed gently with an equal volume of packed RBCs (50% hematocrit) (*see* **Note 5**).
3. Observation of reconstituted blood under physiological flow conditions has demonstrated that platelets under these conditions can efficiently tether and form adhesion contacts with immobilized matrix proteins, but are limited in their ability to form stable platelet aggregates due to the lack of soluble adhesive proteins such as fibrinogen and vWF. Therefore, when examining thrombus growth using reconstituted blood, the suspension buffer (Tyrode's) should be supplemented with purified vWF (10–20 µg/mL) and/or fibrinogen (1–2 mg/mL) prior to perfusion. Alternatively, platelets can be reconstituted with cell-free platelet-poor plasma (PPP), derived by centrifugation of fresh citrate- or hirudin-anticoagulated whole blood at 2000g for 10 min.
4. Reconstituted blood suspensions should be allowed to equilibrate for 10 min at 37°C prior to use in perfusion studies.

3.5. Preparation of Human Serum

1. Nonanticoagulated whole blood is collected into glass tubes and allowed to form a fibrin clot at 37°C for 2–3 h.
2. The clot is then manually compressed with a wooden taper and removed.
3. The resulting serum is clarified of remnant cells and debris by centrifugation at 2000g for 10 min, heat-inactivated (56°C for 30 min) to denature enzymes, cooled, and then stored at –20°C.
4. Matrices are blocked with 2% serum in Tyrode's buffer supplemented with 50 µg/mL of PMSF to inhibit residual thrombin activity. In our experience, blocking glass with <2% heat-inactivated serum leads to significant levels of nonspecific platelet adhesion to glass surfaces.

3.6. Preparation of Adhesive Proteins From Human Plasma

Although purified vWF and fibrinogen are available from commercial sources, in-house purification is less expensive over the long term and, in our experience, yields protein of higher quality and stability.

3.6.1. Preparation of Human vWF

von Willebrand factor is purified according to a modified method of Montgomery and Zimmerman *(10)* from cryoprecipitate derived from 20 L of pooled human PPP.

1. Initially, the pooled plasma is frozen at –70°C and then allowed to thaw at 4°C over a period of 2–3 d.
2. The resulting 4°C-insoluble cryoprecipitate is centrifuged at 15,000g for 60 min at 4°C and resuspended in Tris-saline buffer containing protease inhibitors (*see* **Subheading 2.2., item 7**) at one tenth of the original volume.
3. The cryoprecipitate is then clarified of lipoproteins by first adding 25% (w/v) sucrose, then centrifuging the dense suspension at 100,000g for 60 min at room temperature.
4. Following careful removal of the lipoprotein-containing upper tenth fraction of the supernatant, the remaining solution is loaded onto a sepharose CL-6B size exclusion column pre-equilibrated with Tris-saline buffer.

5. Fractions, eluted with Tris-saline buffer, are analysed for vWF activity and the presence of vWF antigen by ristocetin-induced platelet aggregation and SDS-PAGE (Chapter 9, vol. 2) analysis, respectively.
6. The purest fractions exhibiting the greatest vWF activity are pooled and concentrated using a YM-30 membrane at room temperature.
7. vWF preparations are usually concentrated to 100–500 µg/mL and stored in small aliquots (~1 mL) in polycarbonate tubes for up to one year at –20°C (*see* **Note 6**).

3.6.2. Purification of Fibrinogen

Fibrinogen is purified from human PPP as described by Jakobsen and Kierulf *(13)*.

1. Initially, 250 mL of 6 *M* β-alanine is added dropwise to 1 L of PPP while stirring continually.
2. The PPP is stirred for a further 60 min at room temperature; the resulting precipitate is pelleted by centrifugation at 2000*g* for 30 min.
3. The pellet, containing vWF and fibronectin, is discarded.
4. A further 375 mL of 6 *M* β-alanine is stirred into the supernatant for 30 min and the solution then centrifuged at 5000*g* for 30 min.
5. The supernatant is discarded and the fibrinogen-enriched pellet is resuspended in 250 mL of Buffer A (*see* **Subheading 2.2., step 9**).
6. The fibrinogen is then reprecipitated by adding 750 mL of 6 *M* β-alanine and stirred overnight at 4°C.
7. After centrifugation at 5000*g* for 30 min, the fibrinogen-containing pellet is resuspended in 250 mL Buffer A containing 2 m*M* EDTA to prevent any cation-dependent fibrinogen degradation. This solution can be stored for up to 2 yr at –20°C.
8. Prior to use, the fibrinogen preparation is dialysed against Buffer B (20 m*M* Tris-HCl, pH 7.4, 150 m*M* NaCl) for 24 h at 4°C.
9. It is important to assess the purified fibrinogen using SDS-PAGE to ensure the presence of all three subunits (Aα, Bβ, and γ). The activity of each fibrinogen preparation should also be routinely analyzed using functional assays (e.g., clotting, platelet-adhesion, and spreading assays).

3.6.3. Preparation of Purified Type I Collagen

Type I fibrillar collagen is prepared according to a modified method of Cazenave et al. *(14)*.

1. 2.5 mg/mL (w/v) type I fibrillar collagen derived from bovine tendon (Sigma Chemical Co., St. Louis, MO) is reconstituted in 3% acetic acid (v/v) and rehydrated overnight at 4°C with stirring.
2. The suspension is then homogenized with a medium-sized tissue homogenizer equipped with a fine cutting blade fitting (ProScience). Homogenization is performed on ice until >95% of particulate matter has been solubilized. This typically takes 6–8 h; it is recommended that the homogenization be performed in 30-min slots interceded by 15-min recovery periods to allow the homogenizer to cool down. In our experience, prolonged homogenisation without breaks usually leads to the collagen suspension overheating.
3. The homogenate is then centrifuged at 3000*g* at room temperature to remove nonsolubilized material.

4. The supernatant is stored at 4°C until further use and, in our experience, is stable over a period of 2 yr.

3.7. Coating of Microcapillary Tubes With Adhesive Proteins

1. Microslides are coated by drawing up solutions of vWF, fibrinogen (50–100 µg/mL in Tyrode's buffer) or collagen (2.5 mg/mL in 3% acetic acid) through capillary action.
2. Microslides are placed flat in humidified chambers for at least 2 h at room temperature or overnight at 4°C in order to achieve maximal and uniform coating.
3. Prior to perfusion, the microslides are gently flushed with cell-free Tyrode's buffer to remove unbound protein (*see* **Note 7**).

3.8. Blocking Matrix-Coated Microslides With Human Serum

For whole blood studies, microslides are left unblocked, as it has previously been shown that platelets in whole blood do not adhere to glass under flow *(1)*. However, when using platelets reconstituted with RBCs in the absence of plasma, microslides are blocked as follows:

1. First, unbound protein in microslides is removed by placing the microcapillary tubes in Tyrode's buffer, drawing up approx 500 µL of the solution by holding an absorbent tissue at the opposite end of the glass capillary tube.
2. To block exposed glass, 2% human serum in Tyrode's buffer is drawn into the microslides by capillary action.
3. Microslides are placed flat in a humidified chamber for 30 min at room temperature. At the end of this blocking period, the human serum must be exchanged for Tyrode's buffer, as prolonged exposure to human serum leads to a decrease in the capacity of the matrix to support efficient platelet adhesion and thrombus growth.

3.9. Fluorescent Labeling of Platelets

Although platelet adhesion to matrix proteins in the presence of RBCs can be easily visualised using DIC optics, formation of platelet aggregates and real-time quantitation of thrombus growth by confocal microscopy requires fluorescent labeling of platelets. To date, numerous dyes have been used to visualize platelets in real time, including mepacrine *(1,6)* and calcein *(15)*. However, using our perfusion system, we have found that prolonged exposure of such dye-labeled platelets to the excitation beam leads to photoactivation and artifactual platelet adhesion to matrix proteins under flow. As an alternative, we use the lipophilic carbocyanine dye, $DiOC_6$, which does not cause platelet activation, even with excitation times of 40 s or more. An additional advantage of this dye is that only platelets and leukocytes appear labeled in the presence of RBCs, as the hemoglobin in RBCs acts as a fluorescence quencher. Platelet loading with $DiOC_6$ is relatively straightforward and involves incubation of whole or reconstituted blood at room temperature with 1 µM $DiOC_6$ for 10 min prior to perfusion.

3.10. Basic Flow Assay

3.10.1. Perfusion System Assembly

The setup of the clamp stand and clamps is as shown in **Fig. 1**. The various connections involved in preparing the blood and buffer reservoirs are depicted in **Fig. 2B**.

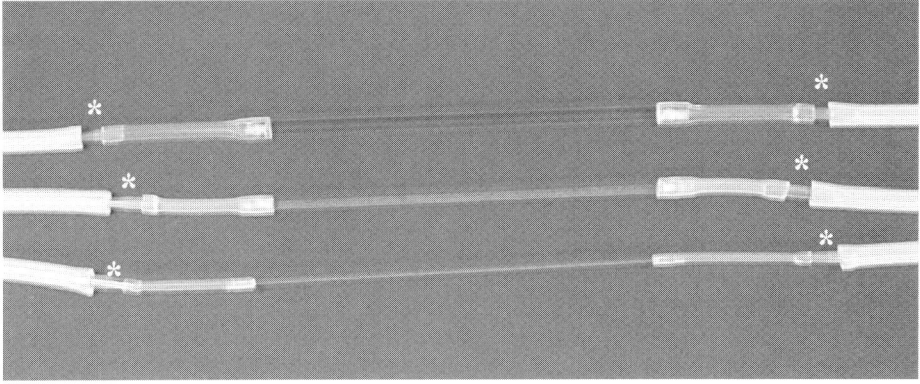

Fig. 4. Glass microcapillary tubes assembled for perfusion. In order to assemble the microcapillary tubes, the outer surfaces of either end of the tube are wrapped in short lengths (1.5 cm) of double-sided tape and gently inserted into the appropriate tubing (No. 6, 7, or 8, depending on the size of the microslide). The open ends of this tubing are then connected to tubing (No. 5) via a truncated-portion micropipettor tip (asterisks). On one end of the microslide, tubing (No. 5) should be connected to blood/buffer reservoirs, and the other end should be connected to glass syringes assembled in the Harvard pump.

1. The polycarbonate "luer-lock" syringes (to hold platelet preparations during perfusion) are attached to three-way taps that in turn are connected to a short length of tubing (No. 4) and a longer length of tubing (No. 5).
2. The third port of the three-way tap is connected to the three-port aspect of tubing (No. 9) using a male-to-male plastic adaptor (*see* **Fig. 2A**).
3. The single-port aspect of tubing (No. 9) is connected to the buffer reservoir syringe using another short length of tubing (No. 4). The three-way taps allow the experimenter to switch directly from cell suspensions to cell-free buffer during flow.
4. All tubing needs to be primed with buffer prior to the perfusion of blood, ensuring that there are no air bubbles present throughout the system.
5. Set up the Harvard syringe assembly as shown in **Fig. 2C**.
6. To ensure smooth movement of the glass syringe during perfusion, lightly grease the plunger assembly with petroleum jelly.
7. Assemble the glass syringe and prime by filling with deionized H_2O, leaving approx 5–10 mL in the syringe.
8. Attach the syringe to the three-way tap assembly that is in turn connected to a short length (~1 cm) of tubing (No. 4) and a long length (~75 cm) of tubing (No. 5).
9. Microcapillary tubes are assembled into the flow system as depicted in **Fig. 1** as follows: First, each end of the microcapillary tube is wrapped with a small length of double-sided tape. These ends are then gently pushed into a short length (~2 cm) of tubing (No. 6, 7, or 8, depending on the size of the microslide).
10. Each open end of this tubing is then connected to long lengths of tubing (No. 5) using a truncated portion of a micropipettor tip. Tubing (No. 5) at each end should already be connected to a glass syringe at one end and a platelet suspension reservoir at the other. The assembled microcapillary tubes should appear as shown in **Fig. 4**.

11. All microslides are then manually flushed with buffer ensuring the absence of any air bubbles throughout the closed-flow system (*see* **Note 8**).

3.10.2. Perfusion of Platelets in Whole or Reconstituted Blood

1. Prior to a perfusion experiment, establish the required rheological parameters for a given experiment. These parameters include:
   a. The desired wall shear rate (γ) and corresponding flow rate *(Q)*.
   b. The total volume *(V)* and period of blood perfusion (Δt) (*see* **Note 9**).
2. Once the desired rheological parameters have been established, whole or reconstituted blood is prepared as described in **Subheading 3.4.** and carefully transferred to the buffer reservoir of the perfusion assembly.
3. Flow is initiated by starting the refill function on the syringe pump and switching the three-way taps to the buffer reservoir(s) and subsequently to blood reservoir(s). When performing multiple flows simultaneously, it is advisable to draw buffer through the microslides for 1–2 min prior to blood perfusion to ensure that all samples start drawing simultaneously.
4. The perfusion experiment is terminated by continuous buffer perfusion to remove all non-adherent cells along with RBCs. Depending on the flow rate, the majority of nonadherent cells should be flushed from the microcapillary tubes within 1–5 min of buffer perfusion.
5. The adherent platelets can then be fixed with formaldehyde and stored at 4°C for visualization at a later date.

3.11. Monitoring Thrombus Formation Under Flow

The above sections have covered in detail the assembly and use of the standard flow rig utilized in our laboratory to examine platelet-adhesion dynamics at the surface of various immobilized matrices. The limitation of conventional light or epifluorescence microscopy in this context is that the investigator is limited to imaging in a single plane of view. Platelet thrombus development, on the other hand, involves both initial platelet-matrix adhesive interactions in one plane and subsequent platelet-platelet aggregation in three dimensions. This section will detail the method we have developed using confocal microscopy to examine platelet thrombus growth in three dimensions.

3.11.1. Visualization of Thrombus Growth by Confocal Microscopy

The thrombus growth assay developed in our laboratory is based around the standard Leica TCS-SP confocal system and is a direct adaptation of the flow system detailed in previous sections (*see* **Note 10**).

1. Blood platelets in whole or reconstituted blood are labeled with 1 μM of the lipophilic fluorophore, $DiOC_6$, for 10 min at 37°C prior to perfusion through matrix-coated microcapillary tubes, per the standard flow method. $DiOC_6$ fluorescence is excited at 488 nm using the argon laser source of the Leica TCS-SP confocal system, with fluorescence emission at 450–510 nm.
2. The rapidity of platelet adhesion and thrombus growth requires the use of a confocal system capable of relatively high rates of data acquisition. To optimize image capture for a large field of view and rapid sampling without compromising image quality, we advise setting image acquisition parameters to fast scan rates ($\leq$1 frame per 0.568 s), bidirectional scan and a lower resolution (256×256 pixels). The early and rapid onset of platelet aggregation at the initiation of platelet perfusion necessitates data acquisition at the earliest time

points of the perfusion process. For this reason the experimenter is limited to viewing a single microcapillary tube at a time with thrombus imaging restricted to a single randomly chosen field.

3. The time course studied in our laboratory typically ranges from 30 s to 5 min, with image capture occurring at 30–60-s time intervals. The "0" time point in these assays represents the point at which platelet-surface interactions are initiated.

4. Following 30 s of blood perfusion, the confocal scan is initiated at the adhesive surface (Z_0) and a predefined volume of 13–15 µm is sampled at 1-µm intervals using confocal sectioning techniques. The number of sections captured at each time point is dictated by the size of the growing thrombi and can thus be adjusted during the course of data acquisition.

5. Two additional requirements are to set the fluorescence detector gain so no pixels in the image are saturated (this prevents overestimation of thrombus size) and to acquire an average of two scans per section, which results in flowing platelets having reduced intensities and thus being easily eliminated though segmentation during thrombus 3-D reconstruction and analysis.

3.11.2. Analysis of Rate and Extent of Thrombus Growth in Real Time

A large number of software packages are available for confocal image analysis; the choice of which to use is dependent on the individual requirements of the investigator. In this section we describe the analysis protocol established in our laboratory to yield data on the height, surface area, and volume of developing thrombi **(Fig. 5)**:

1. Using a version of NIH Image for Macintosh (NIH, Bethesda, MD) modified by Scion Corp. for Windows, the acquired stack of confocal sections at each time point is converted to gray-scale and binarized.

2. The binarized image is imported into Image Tool (UTHSCA, TX) and the number of black (representing the background) and white (the fluorescent platelets) pixels calculated for each section in a stack.

3. The number of white pixels in the first stack (where platelet-matrix interactions occur) represents the total surface area (SA) in the field. Summation of the number of pixels representing fluorescent platelets from each consecutive stack then yields the total thrombus volume (in pixels) in the field of interest.

4. Absolute thrombus dimensions can be determined by calculating the volume for each section (pixels per slice × pixel size × section thickness), and then summing the successive section volumes. Pixel sizes are obtained from the calibrated dimensions read off the confocal software. The section thickness is the depth of field of the lens, in the case of the 63X water-immersion lens with 1.22 NA, this is about 1 µm (both calculated and measured) (*see* **Note 11**).

3.11.3. 3-D Reconstruction of Platelet Thrombi

Platelet thrombi can be reconstructed in 3-D using Vox Blast (VayTek, Fairfield, IA) volume-rendering software to better illustrate thrombus dimensions.

3.12. Monitoring the Dynamics of Platelet-Surface Interactions Under Flow

Although assessing the total thrombus volume using confocal microscopy provides important information regarding the overall rate and extent of thrombus formation, it does not allow investigation of the real-time dynamics of individual platelet adhesions

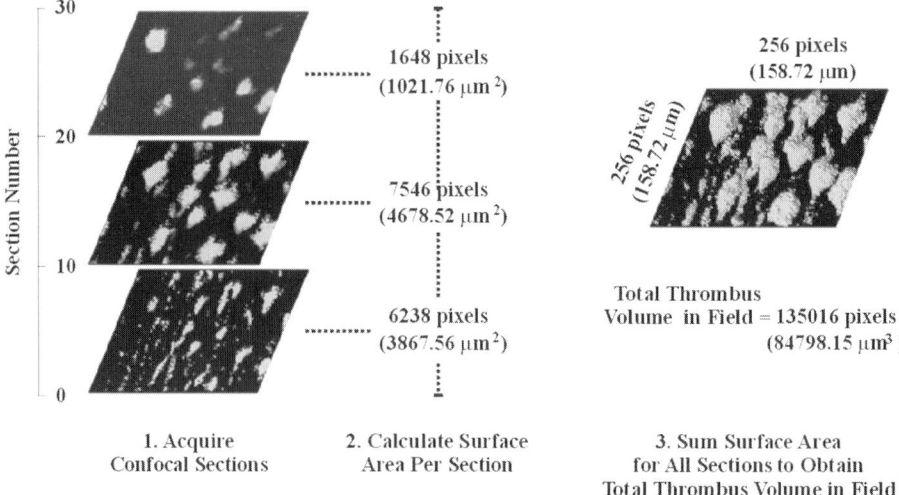

Fig. 5. Calculation of thrombus volume from confocal sections. This schematic exemplifies the steps involved in calculating thrombus volume from confocal sections. In the particular experiment shown, $DiOC_6$-labeled whole blood was perfused over a type I collagen matrix at 1800/s. After 5 min of perfusion, approx 25 optical sections (1 μm thick) were acquired using a 63X water-immersion objective. Images were captured at a resolution of 256 × 256 pixels (0.62 × 0.62 μm) and a frame rate of ≤1 frame/0.568 s. Confocal scans are initiated at the matrix surface (Section 0), progressing upward through the thrombi until fluorescent platelets are no longer observed. Once acquired, images are converted to gray-scale table and binarized, such that black pixels represent background and white pixels represent fluorescent platelets. Using Image Tool software, the number of white pixels in each consecutive section (i.e., the surface area coverage in each section) is analyzed. Summation of the surface area from each section then yields the total thrombus volume in the field of interest.

on purified matrices. It is now well established that upon tethering to an adhesive matrix such as vWF, platelets translocate before forming stationary adhesion contacts *(4)*. Furthermore, the proportions of tethering platelets translocating, detaching, or forming stationary adhesion contacts are important factors that determine the rate and extent of thrombus growth. Platelet tethering, translocation, detachment, and stationary adhesion behaviors are rapidly occurring and dynamic events; therefore, accurate assessment of these parameters requires visualisation of the earliest stages of platelet-matrix interactions.

3.12.1. Visualization of Platelet Adhesion Events in Real Time

1. The blood flow apparatus utilized for the analysis of early platelet-matrix interactions is identical to that described in **Subheading 3.10.1.** However, these experiments are

performed using a conventional light microscope fitted with DIC optics, connected to a DAGE CCD camera, allowing for real-time (25 frames/s) data acquisition.

2. Platelets in whole or reconstituted blood are perfused through matrix-coated microcapillary tubes at a predetermined shear rate (as described in **Subheading 3.10.2.**) and the early stages of platelet-surface interactions visualized by DIC microscopy (63X water objective).

3. Video recordings are made for at least 90 s and subsequently analyzed off-line. To exclusively analyze platelet-matrix interactions, a platelet density of 5×10^9/L is routinely utilized in our laboratory to eliminate the complicating effects of platelet-platelet interactions.

3.12.2. Analysis of the Dynamics of Platelet-Surface Interactions Under Flow

Analysis of platelet adhesion dynamics is typically conducted frame-by-frame ($50\frac{1}{2}$-frames/s). Based on extensive characterization studies in our laboratory *(7,17)*, we have developed the following definitions for scoring platelet behavior under flow:

1. *Platelet detachment:* A platelet is scored as detached when the cell body is no longer in contact with the adhesive surface and does not reattach downstream in the field being analyzed. This phenomenon occurs infrequently on purified matrices that present the platelet with a relatively continuous adhesive surface. However, platelet detachment does occur at relatively high frequency at the surface of preformed platelet monolayers and thrombi in vitro *(7)*.

2. *Tethered platelet* is defined as a platelet forming an adhesion contact with the matrix surface for more than 40 ms. Platelet-tethering analysis is usually calculated only over the first 5–10 s of flow (250–500 1/2-frames) as the occurrence of platelet-platelet interactions increase beyond this time point. This is particularly relevant at physiological platelet concentrations (150×10^9/L) perfused at relatively high shear rates.

3. *Translocating platelet* is defined as platelet movement >1 cell diameter from the point of initial attachment. Unlike leukocyte rolling under flow, platelet translocation occurs in a stop-start manner at the surface of vWF *(4,18)* wherein platelets remain stationary for extended periods of time (2–10 s) and then subsequently resume translocation. Therefore, it is important to ensure that platelets are not scored as translocating simply based on displacement from the point of initial contact, but rather scored based on a history of multiple adhesive contacts. **Figure 6A** shows representative data derived from this type of translocation analysis. Translocation velocities can be determined from this form of analysis by marking the centroid of a translocating cell and subsequently calculating the displacement per unit time. For accurate displacement measurements the TV monitor in use can be calibrated using a 0.01-mm stage micrometer (Olympus), enabling rolling velocities to be expressed in µm/s.

4. *Stationary adhesion:* Based on studies in our laboratory, if a tethered platelet is not displaced over a 10-s time period, then it is scored as having formed a stationary adhesion contact. Given the stop-start nature of platelet translocation, it is important to analyze tethering platelets for at least 10 s. It is also important to consider that platelet tether formation *(19)* may increase the "stop" phase of platelet translocation and may thus lead to the scoring of false positives during stationary adhesion analysis. **Figure 6B** shows the proportion of tethering platelets forming stationary adhesion contacts with a vWF matrix at increasing shear rates and at various time points during whole blood perfusion. Stationary adhesion of platelets with vWF requires ligand binding to active integrin $\alpha_{IIb}\beta_3$ *(1)* and the level of stable adhesion in a given field is thus a good indicator of the activation status of this receptor *(17)*.

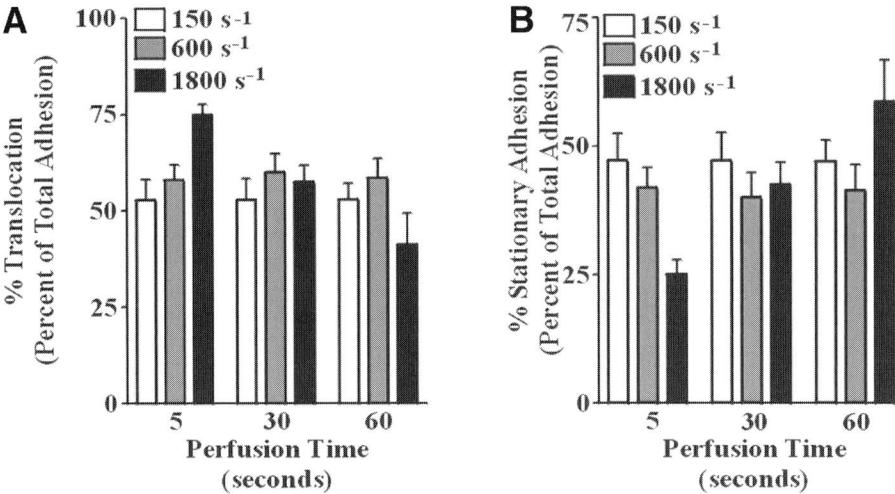

Fig. 6. Dynamics of platelet adhesion to a vWF matrix in whole blood under flow. Nonlabeled citrated whole blood was perfused over a vWf matrix at increasing shear rates for 90 s. Platelet-surface interactions were visualized by DIC microscopy using a 63X water-immersion objective. **(A)** The percentage of adherent platelets translocating over the vWF surface was quantitated at the indicated time points during perfusion. **(B)** The proportion of tethering platelets forming stationary adhesion contacts (no cell movement for >10 s) at the indicated times was also assessed. These results are an average of data from more than 10 independent experiments performed with blood obtained from different donors.

3.13. Monitoring the Dynamics of Platelet Aggregation Under Flow

While the assay described in **Subheading 3.12.** is well-suited to the evaluation of the dynamics of platelet-surface interactions, the assessment of less frequently occurring platelet-platelet interactions under flow can prove more problematic. Analysis of early platelet aggregation events under flow is further complicated by the highly dynamic and labile nature of these interactions. To more effectively monitor aspects of platelet-platelet tethering and adhesion, our laboratory has developed a flow-based platelet aggregation assay *(7)*. Briefly, this assay involves the perfusion of $DiOC_6$-labeled platelets in whole blood over spread platelet monolayers preformed in glass microcapillary tubes. The spread platelet monolayer presents platelets in free-flowing blood with a relatively continuous (in comparison to thrombi) and reproducible adhesive surface that can be used to model the complex adhesive surface found at the growing face of a developing thrombus.

3.13.1. Preparation of Confluent Spread Platelet Monolayers

Confluent monolayers are formed by drawing platelets, resuspended in Tyrode's buffer, into uncoated glass microslides via capillary action and allowing platelet adhesion and spreading to proceed for 30–60 min at 37°C. The platelet concentrations required to achieve a confluent spread platelet monolayer (i.e., >90% surface coverage) differ with respect to the size of the microslides as follows: large microslides (0.3 × 3.0 mm)—2×10^8/mL; intermediate microslides (0.2 × 2.0 mm)—5×10^8/mL; small microslides—1×10^9/mL (*see* **Note 12**).

3.13.2. Perfusion Over Spread Platelet Monolayers

1. The microcapillary tubes containing monolayers are assembled into the perfusion system as described in **Subheading 3.10.1.** and gently flushed with Tyrode's buffer to remove nonadherent cells. It is important to avoid the flushing of bubbles over the monolayers at any stage during assembly or perfusion, as air causes cell lysis.
2. Prior to whole blood perfusion, it is advisable to examine the quality of the monolayers by phase-contrast microscopy and discard monolayers exhibiting <90% confluency. Perfusion of $DiOC_6$-labeled platelets in whole blood over monolayers is identical to that described for thrombus-formation assays (**Subheading 3.11.**).

3.13.3. Visualization of Platelet–Platelet Interactions in Real Time

1. Platelet–platelet interactions are visualized using a 40X dry objective and an FITC-specific blue excitation filter system (488 nm), and video-recorded using the DAGE CCD camera. To avoid excessive photobleaching and to limit photo-damage of the platelet monolayer, visualization of platelet-platelet interactions using the fluorescence filter is restricted to 40-s periods interspersed by 15-s recovery periods.
2. The analysis of the dynamics of platelet–platelet interactions is identical to that described for platelet–matrix interactions (**Subheading 3.14.2.**).

3.16. Concluding Remarks

The flow-based assays detailed in this chapter enable the accurate and reliable assessment of the dynamics of platelet adhesive behavior in real time under both physiological and pathological shear conditions. Unlike traditional aggregation and cone-plate methodologies, flow-based systems enable detailed examination of platelet morphological change, platelet–matrix interactions, and platelet–platelet interactions within a shear environment. Furthermore, unlike the "closed" environment of traditional suspension-based systems, the recreation of the "open" flow environment using this apparatus more closely models the in vivo situation. The application of flow-based technology has greatly increased our understanding of platelet functional responses and associated signaling mechanisms at both the single-cell and population levels. Recent advances in confocal technology and the advent of more sophisticated probes of cellular function have paved the way for detailed investigations of the real-time signaling events driving platelet adhesion and thrombus development.

4. Notes

1. At the end of an experiment, all lengths of tubing should be flushed with copious volumes of hot water in the absence of detergent and air-dried. Depending on the level of use, most tubing should be replaced every 3–4 mo.

2. Long-pass (LP) emission filters are usually suitable to use if one is doing single-dye imaging only. Narrow-band filters are generally necessary when imaging two or more dyes simultaneously, to prevent bleedthrough.

3. Care should be taken to resuspend platelet pellets with minimal agitation to avoid mechanical activation of the cells.

4. RBC preparation, like platelet isolation, needs to be performed with minimal mechanical agitation of the cells to minimize the release of endogenous ADP. As an added measure, the packed RBC suspension is supplemented with 0.025 U/mL apyrase and 1 U/mL hirudin, to scavenge trace amounts of ADP, and α-thrombin generated during isolation. Both ADP and thrombin generated during the blood-fractionation procedure may have a significant impact on the level of platelet activation and therefore adhesion during flow experiments. RBC preparations where hemolysis has occurred are discarded.

5. RBCs are routinely included in reconstitution experiments because their presence increases the local platelet density at the matrix surface by effectively excluding platelets from the center of the bulk flow *(8,9)*. In our experience, hematocrits <50% lead to inefficient platelet tethering to physiological matrices, particularly under high-shear conditions, and should thus be avoided.

6. vWF prepared using this method contains higher-molecular-weight multimers than commercially available preparations. High-molecular-weight vWF multimers have been demonstrated to exhibit significantly greater functional activity than vWF consisting of lower-molecular-weight multimers *(11,12)* and give rise to superior platelet adhesion and thrombus growth under flow. The multimeric composition of different purified vWF preparations should be periodically assessed by native SDS-agarose gel electrophoresis to exclude any differences between preparations.

7. Titration studies in our laboratory have demonstrated that these coating concentrations are required for maximal platelet adhesion and thrombus growth under all shear conditions. Although lower coating concentrations may be used, the effect of decreased matrix density on platelet adhesive behavior needs to be considered.

8. The steps to set up the perfusion system with the inverted microscope for the purposes of light microscopy or confocal microscopy are essentially identical.

9. Strict attention should be paid to the volume of blood/buffer perfused, as this must not exceed the maximum capacity of the syringe, ensuring continuous perfusion throughout the observation period. This is particularly important when utilizing vWF as an adhesive substrate, where a drop in shear rate has been observed to result in platelet detachment (unpublished observations).

10. A number of key points need to be considered by the investigator when performing real-time thrombus-imaging studies, dependent on the adhesive matrix under study:

   a. In order to achieve optimal thrombus generation on a vWF or collagen matrix, whole blood needs to be perfused for at least 1–3 min, regardless of shear rate.

   b. Given the unique biomechanical properties of the vWF-GPIb/V/IX interaction, platelet adhesion to this adhesive surface can occur at shear rates exceeding 10,000/s *(4)*. Thrombus formation on fibrinogen however, due to the slow ligand-binding kinetics of the fibrinogen receptor (integrin $\alpha_{IIb}\beta_3$), can occur only at relatively low shear rates (<200/s).

   c. At low shear rates, initial platelet adhesion to a collagen matrix occurs primarily through platelet collagen receptors. However at higher shear rates, platelet adhesion to this matrix occurs through an indirect interaction between platelet receptor GPIb/V/IX and plasma vWF adsorbed to the collagen surface *(1,16)*. As a result, in the presence of plasma vWF, collagen is capable of supporting adhesion and thrombus growth over a broad range of shear rates.

11. Generally, for large objects, the volume calculation is performed by considering the optical section to have negligible volume (i.e., it is an infinitely thin slice) and using the focus step size between consecutive sections as the depth parameter. In this case the calculations are different, and this is what most volume-rendering software would use to calculate volumes. If this approach is undertaken, then the sampling of the thrombus could be different, but for simplicity and rapid imaging, we have used the setup described above, where optical step and section thickness are the same, and the calculations are similar. It is important to also ensure that platelets are sampled in at least two planes, which is generally true with 1-μm focus steps.

12. Uncoated glass is used in preference to adhesive matrices because empirically we have found that the different adhesive matrices produce poorly dispersed monolayers with inadequate surface coverage. Additionally, it has previously been demonstrated that platelets in whole blood do not interact with glass, therefore avoiding the occurrence of platelet adhesion events with surfaces other than the spread platelet monolayer.

References

1. Savage, B., Almus-Jacobs, F., and Ruggeri, Z. M. (1998) Specific synergy of multiple substrate-receptor interactions in platelet thrombus formation under flow. *Cell* **94,** 657–666.
2. Dopheide, S. M., Yap, C. L., and Jackson, S. P. (2001) Dynamic aspects of platelet adhesion under flow. *J. Exp. Pharm. Phys.* **28,** 355–363.
3. Kroll, M. H., Hellums, D., McIntire, L. V., Schafer, A. I., and Moake, J. L. (1996) Platelets and shear stress. *Blood* **88,** 1525–1541.
4. Savage, B., Saldivar, E., and Ruggeri, Z. M. (1996) Initiation of platelet adhesion by arrest onto fibrinogen or translocation on von Willebrand factor. *Cell* **84,** 289–297.
5. Alevriadou, B. R., Moake, J. L., Turner, N. A., Ruggeri, Z. M., Folie, B. J., Phillips, M. D., et al. (1993) Real-time analysis of shear-dependent thrombus formation and its blockade by inhibitors of von Willebrand factor binding to platelets. *Blood* **81,** 1263–1276.
6. Ruggeri, Z. M., Dent, J. A., and Saldivar, E. (1999) Contribution of distinct adhesive interactions to platelet aggregation in flowing blood. *Blood* **94,** 172–178.
7. Kulkarni, S., Dopheide, S. M., Yap, C. L., Heel, K. A., Harper, I. S., and Jackson, S. P. (2000) A revised model of platelet aggregation. *J. Clin. Invest.* **105,** 783–791.
8. Baumgartner, H. R., Stemerman, M. B., and Spaet, T. H. (1971) Adhesion of blood platelets to subendothelial surface: distinct from adhesion to collagen. *Experientia* **27,** 283–285.
9. Baumgartner, H. R. and Haudenschild, C. (1972) Adhesion of platelets to subendothelium. *Ann NY Acad. Sci.* **201,** 22–36.
10. Montgomery, R. R. and Zimmerman, T. S. (1978) von Willebrand's disease antigen II. A new plasma antigen deficient in severe von Willebrand's disease. *J. Clin. Invest.* **61,** 1498–1507.
11. Moake, J. L., Turner, N. A., Stathopoulos, N. A., Nolasco, L. H., and Hellums, J. D. (1986) Involvement of large plasma von Willebrand factor (vWF) multimers and unusually large vWF forms derived from endothelial cells in shear stress-induced platelet aggregation. *J. Clin. Invest.* **78,** 1456–1461.
12. Moake, J. L., Turner, N. A., Stathopoulos, N. A., Nolasco, L. H., and Hellums, J. D. (1988) Shear-induced platelet aggregation can be mediated by vWF released from platelets, as well

as by exogenous large or unusually large vWF multimers, requires adenosine diphosphate, and is resistant to aspirin. *Blood* **71,** 1366–1374.

13. Jakobsen, E. and Kierulf, P. (1970) A modified β-alanine precipitation procedure to prepare fibrinogen free of anti-thrombin III and plasminogen. *Thromb. Res.* **3,** 145–149.

14. Cazanave, J. P., Hemmendinger, S., Beretz, A., Sutter-Bay, A., and Launay, J. (1983) L'agrégation plaquettaire: outil d'investigation clinique et d'étude pharmacologique méthodologie. *Ann. Biol. Clin.* **41,** 167–179.

15. Denis, C., Methia, N., Frenette, P. S., Rayburn, H., Ullmann-Cullere, M., Hynes, R. O., et al. (1998) A mouse model of severe von Willebrand disease: defects in haemostasis and thrombosis. *Proc. Natl. Acad. Sci. USA* **95,** 9524–9529.

16. Baumgartner, H. R., Tschopp, T. B., and Weiss, H. J. (1977) Platelet interaction with collagen fibrils in flowing blood. II. Impaired adhesion-aggregation in bleeding disorders. A comparison with subendothelium. *Thromb Haemost.* **37,** 17–28.

17. Yap, C. L., Hughan, S. C., Cranmer, S. L., Nesbitt, W. S., Rooney, M. M., Giuliano, S., et al. (2000) Synergistic adhesive interactions and signaling mechanisms operating between platelet glycoprotein Ib/IX and integrin $\alpha_{IIb}\beta_3$. Studies in human platelets and transfected chinese hamster ovary cells. *J. Biol. Chem.* **275,** 41,377–41,388.

18. Nesbitt, W. S., Kulkarni, S., Giuliano, S., Goncalves, I., Nesbitt, W. S., Kulkarni, S., et al. (2002) Distinct glycoprotein Ib/V/IX and integrin $\alpha_{IIb}\beta_3$-dependent calcium signals cooperatively regulate platelet adhesion under flow. *J. Biol. Chem.* **277,** 2965–2972.

19. Dopheide, S. M., Maxwell, M. J., and Jackson, S. P. (2002) Shear-dependent tether formation during platelet translocation on von Willebrand factor. *Blood* **99,** 159–167.

16

In Vivo Models of Platelet Function and Thrombosis

Study of Real-Time Thrombus Formation

Shahrokh Falati, Peter L. Gross, Glenn Merrill-Skoloff, Derek Sim, Robert Flaumenhaft, Alessandro Celi, Barbara C. Furie, and Bruce Furie

1. Introduction

Our understanding of hemorrhagic and thrombotic diseases has expanded with use of models aimed at studying the vasculature using a variety of different animals. Unlike in vitro experiments, these animal models enable the study of the broad continuum of biological consequences induced by alterations made to a single variable. This chapter briefly reviews animal models used in the study of thrombosis research, focusing primarily on the use of intravital fluorescence microscopy.

Almost two centuries ago, the importance of vascular integrity in hemostasis was reported by Thackrah (*1*). He designed experiments with the aim of addressing "factors favourable to the concretion of blood" and concluded that the "fluidity" of blood is dependent principally on the "vitality" of the vessels containing it. Many years later, Donne provided the first description of platelets (*2*) and later still, in 1856, Virchow proposed his triad of factors responsible for thrombotic episodes—namely, alterations to the vessel wall, negation of blood flow, and coagulability of the blood (*3*).

Our understanding of hemostasis and thrombosis has advanced greatly since these early hypotheses. The incidence of thrombosis in the arterial or venous system, we now know, is associated with clinical outcomes common to industrialized countries, including myocardial infarction, cerebral infarction, transient ischemic attack, or deep-vein thrombosis. In the last several decades, experimental models of thrombosis have been developed that not only increased our knowledge of the pathogenesis of thrombus formation and dissolution, but also provided a tool for in vivo evaluation of potential antithrombotics and fibrinolytics.

A wide array of stimuli can activate platelets and/or the coagulation system leading to platelet activation and intravascular fibrin clot formation. The intravascular formation of a thrombus is mimicked in several animal models, including stasis/hypercoagulable

From: *Methods in Molecular Biology, vol. 272:*
Platelets and Megakaryocytes, Vol. 1: Functional Assays
Edited by: J. M. Gibbins and M. P. Mahaut-Smith © Humana Press Inc., Totowa, NJ

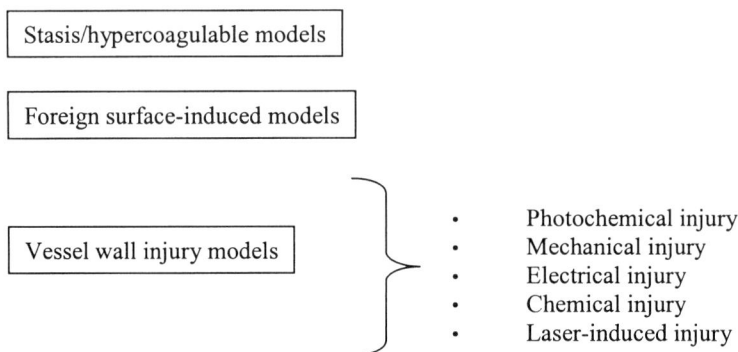

Fig. 1. Animal models of thrombosis. Numerous different models of thrombosis have been used for both arterial and venous thrombosis depending on the mechanism of induction (boxed text). Injury to the vessel wall can further be made by several mechanisms.

models, foreign surface-induced models and vessel wall injury models **(Fig. 1)**. The antithrombotic action of endothelial cells is well documented *(4)*. Upon injury or damage to the endothelium, the combined effect of the loss of the protective role of endothelial cells and the possible resultant exposure of prothrombotic subendothelial components, including tissue factor and collagen, are strong stimuli for thrombus formation. A number of experimental approaches have been taken to treat endothelial disruption in rodent thrombosis models. In this chapter, we describe several different vessel wall injury models with emphasis on the laser injury/intravital microscopy model we have been using.

1.1. Photochemical Injury

This reaction involves the irradiation of vessels with a high-intensity light in the presence of an intraluminal fluorescent dye, which is commonly either rose Bengal or sodium fluorescein *(5)*. Thrombus formation is monitored in real time using an intravital microscope-analog video system. It is believed that free-radical or molecular oxygen generation may be responsible for endothelial damage in this example. This system can be used in microvessels that are not suitable for mechanical or electrical injury, with the severity of the injury being controlled by adjusting light intensity and/or fluorescent dye concentration. Rats are the main animals used with this model. However, dogs, rabbits, and guinea pigs have also been reported. The major disadvantage one should consider here is whether endothelial injury is the sole cause of thrombus formation.

1.2. Mechanical Injury

Pinching arteries with needle forceps, denuding the endothelium via balloon catheters, or infusing a portion of a vessel with air or saline are all different mechanical models developed to induce endothelial injury. These models require large diameter vessels and have been used in clamping the coronary arteries of dogs, for example.

Cyclic flow variations or reductions can then be monitored as described first by Folts and colleagues. This Folts model has the advantage of enabling long-term studies and has been reported in conscious dogs *(6)*. This model has also been used in rats, and an adaptation of such a mechanical model has also been reported for use in mice *(7)*. A disadvantage of this model is the fact that it is less applicable for use in smaller vessels, and thus smaller animals such as mice, in which it is difficult to induce and monitor dynamic thrombus formation.

1.3. Electrical Injury

Application of an electrical current through the vessel wall using an electromicrocoagulator induces a thrombus composed of platelets and fibrin. This stimulus induces severe injury. However, the extent of the injury can be controlled to an extent by adjusting the current. Injury is induced in this model by first inserting an electrode into the lumen of the vessel in question so that it is in firm contact with the endothelium and then delivery of anodal direct current. The model has the advantage of being relatively easy to perform. Dogs, hamsters, and rats have been commonly used with this model.

1.4. Chemical Injury

This model has been documented for use in guinea pigs *(8)*, rats *(9)*, and mice *(10)*. In this model, the carotid artery is isolated, a flow probe attached distally to the thrombus induction site, baseline blood flow recordings obtained, and thrombus induced by placing a 2×2-mm piece of filter paper soaked in 10% ferric chloride on top of the vessel for three minutes. The parameter studied here is the time from removal of the stimulus to total occlusion, referred to as the TTO. The advantages of this model include its use without need for further surgery (e.g., intubation and mechanical ventilation of the animal) and thus short duration of each experiment. Disadvantages include extensive cell damage by oxidation and inflammation, which may not best ascribe to a physiological comparison. It should also be noted that ferric chloride can stimulate the vagal nerve which, by stimulating the vagal system, could interfere with blood flow itself.

1.5. Laser Injury

The model of endothelial injury we have been using involves laser-induced injury *(11)* followed by visualization of the injury and sequelae by bright-field and fluorescent intravital microscopy. It is possible with this system to monitor, quantitate, and analyze in real-time multiple components of a developing thrombus over a period of time, from its genesis to its dissolution. Our chosen vascular window is the microvasculature of the cremaster muscle in mice. However, laser-induced injury has previously been reported in other animals, including rats and guinea pigs. The advantage of this system is defined localized injury (typically, 1-µm diameter round of laser injury), study of multiple thrombi in the same animal and of different vessel types/sizes—for example, arteries vs veins—and investigation of multiple components of a developing thrombus in vivo in real time. Disadvantages of this system include potential access concerns of fluorescent antibodies to generated components within thrombi in vivo, concerns regarding injury

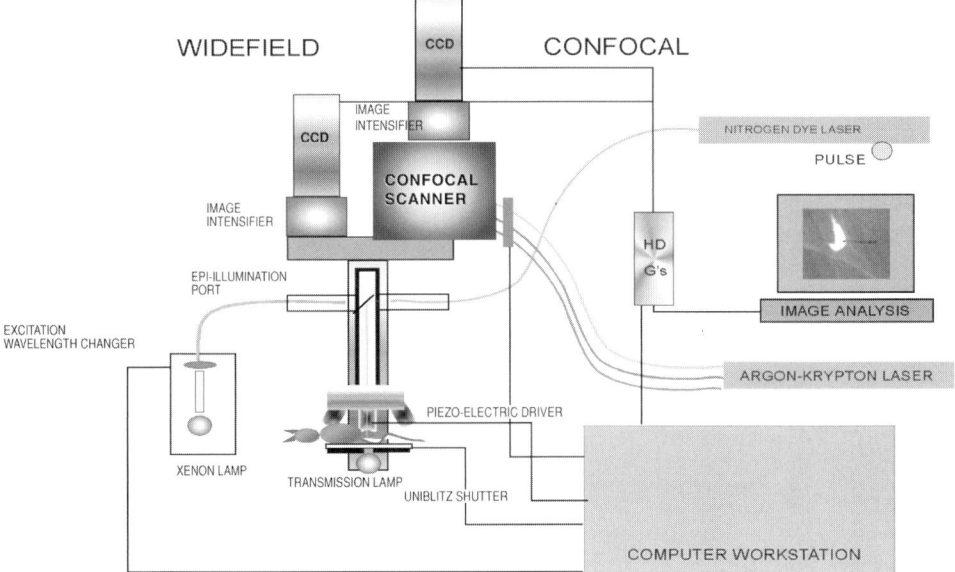

Fig. 2. Schematic representation of intravital setup for evaluation of real-time thrombus formation. Microvessel data can be obtained by intravital microscopy using a fluorescence microscope fitted with a water-immersion objective and long-distance condenser. The microscope's dual ports allow for both confocal and wide-field imaging systems. Images of the intravascular interactions are captured using a CCD camera and an image intensifier onto a computer workstation. (Reproduced from **ref. 12** with permission.) See color insert following p. 44.

reproducibility, and finally, initial and maintentance cost of the facility. The model of laser-induced injury with which we have been working is described here in detail.

2. Materials

2.1. Components of the Intravital System

It should first be noted that there are many options available for choosing different components. The system here described is by no means the only available means of conducting similar experiments. That said, the components are (*see* **Fig. 2**):

1. Olympus AX-70 fluorescence microscope with a special stage for physiological experiments, a long-distance condenser and triple ports for the binocular objectives, the confocal scanner, and the widefield port.
2. A full set of oil-immersion objectives and water-immersion objectives, including 100X, 60X, 40X, 20X, and 10X lenses.
3. Physiks International piezoelectric driver and its controller to allow computer-controlled changes in the focal plane as rapidly as every 20 ms and movements as small as 0.5 microns.

4. Yokogawa CSU-10 confocal scanner, a system based upon Nipkow disk technology. The scanner uses microlenses in the multiple pinholes on the disk and can collect up to 360 images per second.
5. Milles Griot argon-krypton three-line laser for excitation at λ_{ex} 488 nm, λ_{ex} 568 nm, and λ_{ex} 647 nm.
6. Sutter Lambda L-10 filter wheel on the excitation source.
7. Sutter Lambda DG-4 high-speed wavelength changer equipped with a high-intensity 175-watt xenon light source.
8. Single-wavelength excitation filters and triple-band pass emission filters.
9. Gen III Videoscope image intensifier.
10. Roper CoolSnap HQ CCD camera to capture high-resolution (1390 × 1024) images.
11. Cooke SensiCam high-speed camera (640 × 480).
12. Uniblitz shutter on the transmission light source.
13. Micropoint ablation laser.
14. Dell workstation used to control the components of the imaging system and to collect images. This workstation has dual 1-GHz processors, 1.5-GB of RAM, two SCSI hard drives (18 GB and 73 GB) and a high-end video card (*see* **Notes 1** and **2**).
15. 35/70 AIT drive for tape storage of data.
16. SlideBook, a custom-designed imaging software package from Intelligent Imaging Innovations (Bethesda, MD) that is able to control the above listed components and is used for image reconstruction and for all analysis of acquired data.

2.2. Buffers, Solutions, and Reagents

1. Perfusion buffer for use upon exteriorization of the mouse cremaster muscle consists of 135 mM NaCl, 4.7 mM KCl, 2.7 mM CaCl$_2$, 1 mM MgCl$_2$, and 18 mM NaHCO$_3$, pH 7.4.
2. Other reagents include mainly antibodies from commercial vendors and in most cases, dialyzing, concentrating, and subsequently labeling of antibodies with fluorescent dyes, including use of ALEXA dyes from Molecular Probes.

2.3. Anesthetics Used

Workers should obtain appropriate ethical approval, relevant training, and work within local and national guidelines for all animal studies.

1. Mice are pre-anesthetized with intraperitoneal injection of 125 mg/kg ketamine, 12.5 mg/kg xylazine, and 0.25 mg/kg atropine sulfate.
2. Anesthesia is maintained with 5 mg/mL Nembutal as required through the cannulated jugular vein.

2.4. Surgery-Related Items

A number of instruments and some hardware are necessary for the preparation of mice for the surgical procedures outlined below and also for others, including lymph node exteriorization, femoral vein cannulation, tail vein injections, and mouse ear preparation.

1. Dissection microscope with light source.
2. CO$_2$ gas supply.
3. Water bath with connected heat blanket.

4. Tray for cremaster setup.
5. Blunt and sharp-end surgical forceps, small and large surgical scissors, normal small scissors.
6. Braided silk sutures.
7. Polyethylene tubing for cannulation (specifications outlined below).
8. 1-mL insulin syringes with a 28.5-*g* needle.

3. Methods

3.1. Surgical Preparation of Mouse for Intravital Study

3.1.1. Tracheotomy

1. Mice are pre-anesthetised as described in **Subheading 2.3.** and surgically prepared in the following manner: The animal is immobilized by taping the front limbs down on a temperature-controlled blanket maintained at 37°C and a patch of skin approx 2 cm in diameter is removed from the neck. The trachea will be exposed and a small incision is made just proximal to the larynx.
2. A 4-cm-long piece of PE 90 tubing (inside diameter = 0.76 mm, outside diameter = 1.22 mm) is inserted into the trachea, penetrating to a depth of approx 1 cm.
3. The tubing is stabilized using 5-0 silk suture tied around the region of the trachea containing the tubing. This facilitates the animal's breathing for the remainder of the experiment.

3.1.2. Jugular and Carotid Cannulation

1. The jugular vein is exposed and cannulated using PE 10 tubing (i.d. = 0.28 mm, o.d. = 0.61 mm). This is also stabilized using 5-0 silk suture. Tying the distal end of the exposed region of the vessel prior to making an incision is a measure to control bleeding. This cannula is subsequently used to inject both maintenance anesthetic and experimental reagents.

   Monitoring blood pressure, as well as other methods, can be used to assess the degree to which the animal is anesthetised. The blood pressure can be monitored using a carotid-artery cannula whose free end has been connected to a pressure transducer. A steady rise in pressure of 5 mm Hg from baseline indicates lightening of anesthesia and the appropriate amount of maintenance anaesthetic can be administered.
2. For carotid cannulation, the vessel is exposed through the same incision used to establish the trachea tube and the jugular vein cannulated. The proximal end of the exposed vessel is clamped using a microvascular arterial clamp, while the distal portion of the vessel tied closed with 5-0 silk suture to prevent retrograde bleeding.
3. Heparinized PE 10 tubing is then inserted into the vessel through a small incision and stabilized with 5-0 silk suture. Removal of the clamp allows the blood pressure to register on the pressure transducer attached to the other end of the tubing.

3.1.3. Cremaster Muscle Exteriorization

1. Exposure of the mouse cremaster muscle allows for the visualization of blood flow. The testicle, epididymis, and associated structures are moved from the scrotum up into the abdomen by grasping the distal end of the scrotum with forceps and pushing the organs into the body.
2. Approximately 1.5 cm of the scrotum is then excised and the cremaster muscle exteriorized through this opening. There is little blood loss during this procedure.
3. Excess connective tissue is removed and an incision along the muscle made.

4. The muscle is then affixed over a glass slide, allowing illumination from below. A steady drip of perfusion buffer is maintained throughout the experiment to keep the exposed muscle moist.

5. Blood flow in the muscle will be visualized using the desired magnification water-immersion lens (e.g., 40X or 60X) and epi-illuminated with an appropriately filtered light source.

3.2. In Vivo Blood Velocity Determination

Centerline red blood cell (RBC) velocity can be determined in two ways:

1. The first is applicable to bright-field applications and utilizes the Microvessel Velocity OD-RT System from CircuSoft Instrumentation. This system uses a dual-slit photometric method by projecting the image of a blood vessel across two sequential photodiodes positioned in close proximity. As a RBC passes between the light source and the first photodiode, a change in light intensity is registered. A corresponding change in second photodiode is next registered and velocity is calculated. This process occurs in real time during data acquisition.

2. The second method requires the use of small (1 μm or less), fluorescently labeled beads. These beads are injected intravenously and their movement captured by digital video. After measuring the interframe distance traveled along the centerline and by knowing the frame rate, a velocity can be calculated. Averaging tens of these events allows for a good approximation of RBC velocity. This determination is done after data acquisition.

3.3. Pre-Alignment of Ablation Laser and Laser-Induced Endothelial Injury

It is important to align the ablation laser to a spot in the binocluar objectives in order to ensure accurate induction of injury to the desired site.

1. This is achieved by using the laser to uncoat a glass mirror that is coated with a thin layer of chromium.

2. Using this mirror, adjust the laser position to the cross-hairs seen in the binocular objectives.

Thrombosis can then be initiated by damaging the vessel wall with a laser pulse from a MicroPoint laser attached to the microscope. The pulse delivered causes damage in an area of approx 1 μm^2. Because of anesthesia and the tiny damage the laser pulse causes, the mouse has no sensation from the laser.

3.4. Real-Time Thrombus Formation I: Detecting Multiple Components Using Wide-Field Fluorescence Microscopy

1. Prepare buffers, pass 5% CO_2 gas through for buffering, and perfuse through tubing (37°C).

2. Turn on heat pad on which surgery will take place and leave for warming up; check CO_2 gas supply.

3. Turn on all equipment (*see* **Note 2**) including camera, microscope, intensifier, injury laser, DG-4 Sutter wide-field light source, or confocal laser and computer. Open software and check software connecting all components.

4. Align the cross-hairs of microscope to position of laser for injury (*see* **Subheading 3.3.**).

5. Weigh mouse and anesthetize accordingly.

6. Begin surgical procedure I: jugular cannulation and tracheotomy (*see* **Subheadings 3.1.1.** and **3.1.2.**).

7. Begin surgical procedure II: cremaster muscle exteriorization (*see* **Subheading 3.1.2.**).

8. Transfer the stage on which the mouse is positioned to the microscope stage.
9. Secure tray to stage (*see* **Note 3**).
10. Secure all tubing and immediately begin superfusion of exteriorized mouse cremaster muscle with prepared perfusion buffer (*see* **Subheading 2.2.**).
11. Move stage and using buffer meniscus, focus on the blood vessels of the cremaster muscle.
12. Arteries and veins may be distinguished at this stage in a wild-type mouse (i.e., should see rolling leukocytes in veins, but absent from arteries). The velocity of blood can be determined at this stage (*see* **Subheading 3.2.**).
13. In vitro labeling of desired antibodies (*see* **Note 4**).
14. Infuse antibodies through jugular cannula and wait 5–10 min (*see* **Note 5**). After infusion of each antibody, check cross-over to other channels.
15. Choose vessel type/size in question and focus on endothelial cell.
16. Set and digitally record the pre-injury state on computer using desired exposure times/ binning/high vs low resolution camera for each fluorescent channel.
17. Induce injury using the in-line laser (laser prepositioned to cross-hairs in eyepiece of microscope) (*see* **step 4** and **Subheading 3.3.**).
18. Immediately start recording fluorescence detected for each channel for the injured area (the Uniblitz shutter may be used to record a bright-field exposure for every round of fluorescent channels or as regularly as desired (**Fig. 2** and **3**).
19. Move upstream in vessel to induce laser injury and repeat another recording duration (recordings may be made continuously or at intervals if interested in long-time courses for thrombus composition/architecture).
20. At end of experiment, sacrifice mouse by anesthetic overdose.

3.5. Real-Time Thrombus Formation II: Detecting Embolization Events Using Wide-Field Fluorescence Microscopy

The method described in this section mirrors that of the last; however, of critical note here are the exposure time settings. The interest here is not in what is formed at the injured site, but the instability of the thrombus as measured by parts of it embolizing to flow downstream. Due to the rapid flow of blood in the vessels, the exposure settings have to be very short (i.e., <3 ms). It is also of note that in such studies, a combination of 8×8 binning (to reduce file sizes) and a single fluorescent antibody (e.g., anti-CD41 or its Fab fragments) provides the most effective method to detect fluorescent sections embolizing from the labeled thrombus. Using computer software (Slidebook), these embolization events can be recorded for subsequent analysis either as a fluorescent percentage value of the parent thrombus or as absolute integrated intensity values and plotted as spikes (since each embolized section is detectable

---

Fig. 3. *(see facing page)* Time course of thrombus formation in vivo and fluorescent labeling of venous thrombus components. Inititation and propagation of thrombus formation after laser ablation is here shown in four time points in bright field (**A**). Surgical preparation of mouse, laser ablation, and acquisition of data are detailed in text. White arrow at t = 0 s marks the site of laser ablation and for subsequent time points, arrows indicate thrombus progression (**A**). Platelets can be labeled with rat anti-mouse CD41

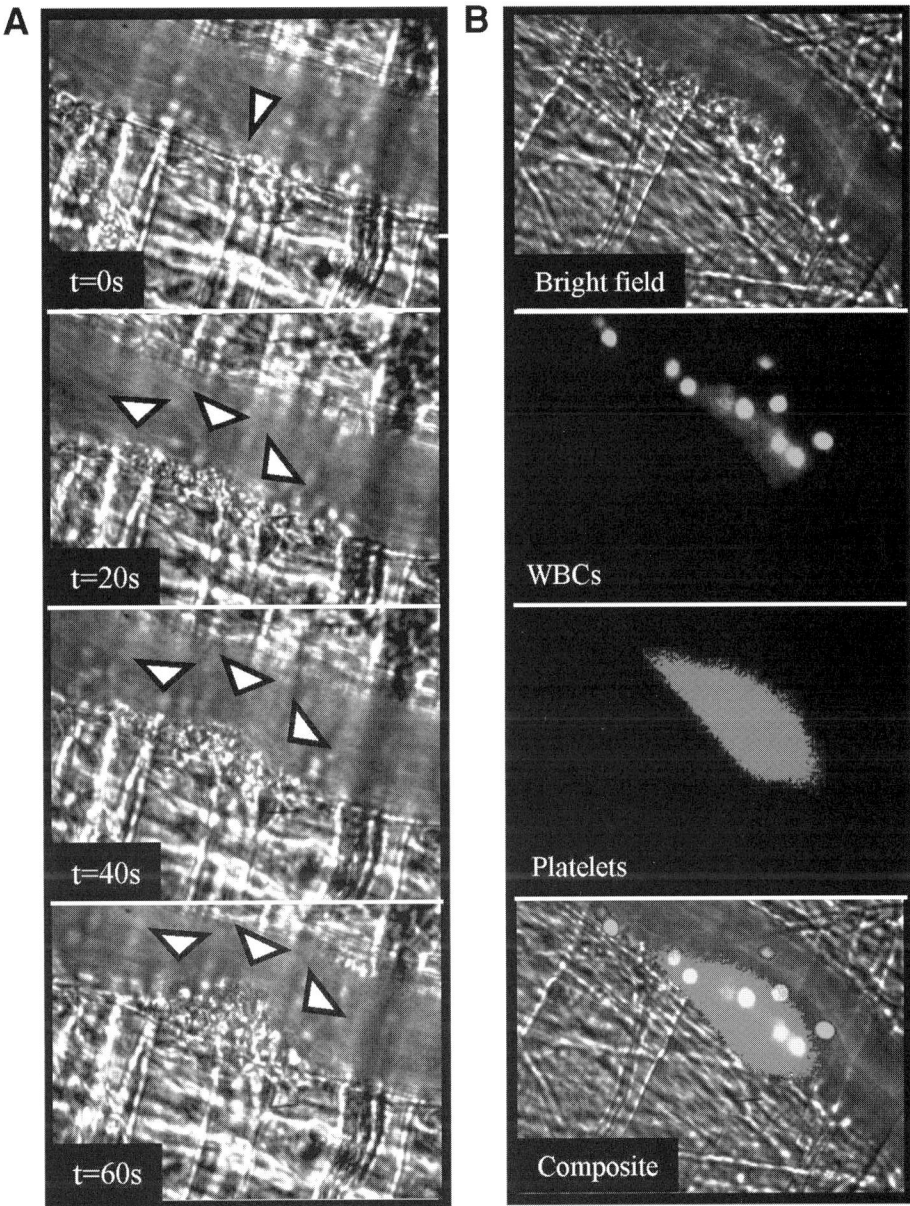

Fig. 3. *(continued)* antibody (0.1 mg/g body weight) and ALEXA 488-conjugated chicken anti-rat antibody (1 mg/g body weight). Circulating nucleated cells are labeled in vivo with SYTO 17 dye. Separation of fluorescent spectra allow for three-fluorescent-channel acquisition as well as bright-field; however, in this example, only two of the channels are used to label platelets as well as white blood cells. See color insert following p. 44.

for only a small number of frames) superimposed on the integrated intensity of a growing thrombus.

3.6. Determination of Thrombus Volume and Composition In Vivo Using High-Speed Scanning Confocal Microscopy

The volume and density of thrombi formed in vivo can be determined by confocal microscopy and image analysis. Confocal microscopy allows for the quantification of fluorescence in an optical plane. The imaging of many parallel narrow-spaced optical planes allows for three-dimensional depiction of a fluorescent object.

We employ a high-speed confocal imaging device, the Yokogawa CSU-10, which typically can image a plane in less than 30 ms. Fast acquisition is paramount to imaging thrombi in vivo. The combination of a piezoelectric objective focuser, which allows for fast control of planes in the Z-dimension and an argon-krypton laser with a filter wheel allowing excitation wavelength selection in 50 ms, achieves this aim. The computer software program coordinates the imaging of each plane at each excitation wavelength before moving on to the next plane. The Z-series can be repeated to allow imaging of a three-dimensional object over time.

The experimental setup and method are as described above for wide-field experiments. Follow the procedure in **Subheading 3.4.** through **step 15**. Continue as follows:

1. Focus on the center of the vessel.
2. Using the software, select the top and bottom planes such that the Z-series comfortably encompasses the vessel. Select a spacing between the planes—as low as 0.5 μm—but limited by speed of acquisition of the series.
3. Set the Z-plane to the center of the series.
4. Continue as in **Subheading 3.4., steps 16** through **20**.

For analysis of data, software can quantify the volume of each fluorochrome expressed either as spatial volume or intensity density. Software can also render multidimensional images using computer reconstruction of the Z-series and the combination of multi-wavelength images.

4. Notes

1. To date, many intravital microscopy studies have been done using either an analog CCD camera or a SIT camera with images being captured on videotape. It is possible to capture data in digital format with numerous advantages including quantitative analysis of pixel magnitude, subarray readouts from the camera at high frame rates without increased noise ratio, background subtraction capabilities, image reconstruction, color analysis, and obtaining a permanent data set that could retain original resolution. The disadvantage of digital capture is file size. It is not incomprehensible to acquire one data set from one thrombus which is one GB. As a result, although the software is able to capture long video rate images, the computer used must be adequate for such demands mainly with regard to having sufficiently high RAM, processing speed, and hard drive.
2. For turning on the equipment and in order for the software to recognize all components, all equipment should be turned on first (some take a few minutes, e.g., camera) followed by the computer and software.

3. The tray can be secured to the stage by fixing it to a movable aluminium plate secured to the stage. We are in the process of modifying this technique, however, to include a motorized stage with a custom-made stage for this application.

4. In vitro labeling of antibodies involves the initial conjugation and subsequent separation of unbound dye from protein/antibody. There are many fluorescent dyes to choose from. It is important for this application to choose dyes with minimal bleaching; thus, dyes such as the ALEXA family are preferred.

5. Antibodies are diluted in saline and injected slowly; upon completion, 5–10 min of equilibration time is allowed before the start of the experiment.

Acknowledgments

We thank Drs. Boris Tchernychev and Erik Vandendries for their comments and discussion on this chapter and during the developmental period of this intravital system.

References

1. Thackrah, C. T. (1820) An inquiry into the nature and properties of the blood, as existent in health and disease. *N. Engl. J Med. Surg.* **9,** 186–193.
2. Donne, M. A. (1842) De Forgine des globules du sang, de leur mode de formation et de leur fin. *C. R. Acad. Sci. (Paris)* **14,** 366–368.
3. Virchow, R. (1856) Uber die Verstopfung der Lungenarterie. *Gesammelte Abhandlungen zur wissenschaftlichen Medicin*, Frankfort, Meidinger Sohn, p. 221.
4. Gross, P. L. and Aird, W. C. (2000) The endothelium and thrombosis. *Sem. Thromb. Hem.* **26,** 463–478.
5. Rosenblum, W. I. and El-Sabban, F. (1977) Platelet aggregation in the cerebral micro-circulation: effect of aspirin and other agents. *Circ. Res.* **40,** 320–328.
6. Gallagher, K. P., Osakada, G., Kemper, W. S., and Ross., J. (1985) Cyclical coronary flow reductions in conscious dogs equipped with ameroid constrictors to produce severe coronary narrowing. *Basic Res. Cardiol.* **80,** 100–106.
7. Stockmans, F., Deckmyn, H., Gruwez, J., Vermylen, J., and Acland, R. (1991) Continuous quantitative monitoring of mural, platelet dependent, thrombus kinetics in the crushed rat femoral vein. *Thromb. Haemost.* **65,** 425–431.
8. Aoki, T., Cox, D., Senzaki, K., Seki, J., Tanaka., A., Takasugi, H., et al. (1998) Comparison of the antithrombotic effects of FK633, GPIIb-IIIa antagonist, and aspirin in a guinea pig thrombosis model. *Thromb. Res.* **89,** 129–136.
9. Kurz, K. D., Main, B. W., and Sandusky, G. E. (1990) Rat model of arterial thrombosis induced by ferric chloride. *Thromb. Res.* **60,** 269–280.
10. Fay, W. P., Parker, A. C., Ansari, M. N., Zheng, X., and Ginsburg, D. (1999) Vitronectin inhibits the thrombotic response to arterial injury in mice. *Blood* **93,** 1825–1830.
11. Rosen, E. D., Raymond, S., Zollman, A., Noria, F., Sandoval-Cooper, M., Shulman, A., et al. (2001) Laser-induced noninvasive vascular injury models in mice generate platelet- and coagulation-dependent thrombi. *Am. J. Pathol.* **158,** 1613–1622.
12. Falati, S., Gross, P., Merrill-Skoloff, G., Furie, B. C., and Furie, B. (2002) Real-time imaging of the assembly of platelets, tissue factor and fibrin during arterial thrombus formation in the mouse. *Nat. Med.* **8,** 1175–1181.

17

Adhesion Between Platelets and Leukocytes or Endothelial Cells

Gerard B. Nash

1. Introduction

Activated platelets expose P-selectin and thereby adhere to leukocytes of all main classes *(1–4)*. If neutrophils or monocytes are also activated, then adhesion can be stabilized by binding of their β2-integrins to fibrinogen and possibly other ligands on the platelet surface *(5–9)*. Experimentally, adhesion can be demonstrated when leukocytes are flowed over immobilized platelets *(3,4,6–8)*, or when suspensions of isolated leukocytes and platelets are mixed together *(1,5)*. Platelet-leukocyte aggregates can also be found in whole blood *(10,11)*. Mutually activating interactions can also occur between leukocytes and platelets through released substances, and these interactions are promoted by adhesion between the cells *(12)*. Platelet-leukocyte adhesion may thus be influential in the development of inflammation or of thrombi. Platelets are not thought to bind to intact endothelium normally, but increasing evidence suggests that adhesion can occur when endothelial cells are stimulated or exposed to pathogenic agents (e.g., *13–15*). Among other actions, platelets attached to endothelium might assist capture of flowing leukocytes *(16)*.

Methods for studying the adhesion of platelets to matrix proteins are described in Chapters 13–15, vol. 1. Here, detailed methods are described for studying the adhesion of flowing leukocytes to platelets already bound to a surface (e.g., modeling a situation that may occur in damaged blood vessels). Less-definitive descriptions are also given for assays of binding between these cells in mixed suspensions, or of binding of platelets to endothelial cell monolayers.

The main flow-based assay described subjects adhesive interactions to dynamic constraints similar to those present in vivo. Firm adhesion between leukocytes and platelets follows a stepwise process resembling that between leukocytes and activated endothelium. Unstable, selectin-mediated adhesion is followed by leukocyte activation, followed by firm integrin-mediated adhesion. Critical parameters influencing adhesion

From: *Methods in Molecular Biology, vol. 272:*
Platelets and Megakaryocytes, Vol. 1: Functional Assays
Edited by: J. M. Gibbins and M. P. Mahaut-Smith © Humana Press Inc., Totowa, NJ

are the wall-shear rate (which determines velocity of leukocytes before interaction with immobilized platelets) and wall-shear stress (which determines the force applied to leukocytes, and hence adhesive bonds, immediately after initial attachment). These parameters can be calculated and controlled for the flow geometries used (*see* **Subheading 3.3.1.**). It may be noted at this stage that the values up to which leukocyte adhesion to selectins can occur (maximum wall-shear rate ~300 s⁻¹) are much lower than those at which platelet capture to collagen can occur (>1000 s⁻¹). This disparity may arise partly because platelets are smaller. Thus, they travel slower when adjacent to an adhesive surface than do leukocytes for the same wall shear rate, and experience a lower force pulling them from the surface after they initially attach. Consequently, experiments at high shear rates may show platelet adhesion to a chosen substrate, but experiments to study leukocyte interaction with platelets will need to be carried out at lower wall-shear rates (typically ~150 s⁻¹).

The major procedures described here are those required to prepare isolated cells, to coat adhesive substrates, to connect substrates to a flow system and perfuse cells while making videomicroscopic recordings, and to analyze recorded events at the coated surface. Variants covered in **Subheadings 3.4.–3.6.** are the study of leukocyte-platelet aggregation in suspension, use of whole blood in assays, and adhesion of platelets to endothelial cells.

2. Materials
2.1. Blood Cell Isolation and Activation

1. Anticoagulants: K_2-EDTA (1.5 mg/mL) in 10-mL tubes (Sarstedt, Numbrecht, Germany). 50 µL of preservative-free Na-heparin (1000 U/mL CP Pharmaceuticals Ltd., Wrexham, UK) in 10-mL tube. 100 µL of concentrated K_2-EDTA/theophylline/prostacyclin (160 mg/mL 0.7 M 500 ng/mL respectively, all Sigma Chemical Co., Poole, UK) in a sterile 10-mL syringe. 1 mL of buffered citrate-phosphate-dextrose-adenine (CPDA; Sigma) in a sterile 10-mL tube.
2. Density gradient media: Histopaque 1077 (H1077) and Histopaque 1119 (H1119) (Sigma).
3. Washing/resuspending buffers: phosphate-buffered saline with or without 1 mM Ca^{2+} or 0.5 mM Mg^{2+} (PBS Gibco, Invitrogen Ltd., Paisley, UK), with 0.15% (w/v) bovine albumin (dilute from 7.5% culture-tested solution, Sigma) (PBSA).
4. Platelet agonist: Thrombin (100 U/mL stock dissolved in PBSA, stored at –20°C, Sigma).
5. Neutrophil agonist: *N*-formyl-methionyl-leucyl-phenylalanine (fMLP, 10 mM stock in ethanol stored at –20°C, diluted to 1 µM in PBSA for use, Sigma).
6. Fixatives: 2% formaldehyde or 2% glutaraldehyde (both BDH Laboratory Supplies, Poole, UK) in PBS.
7. Fluorescent dyes: Rhodamine 6G (Sigma) or calcein-AM (Molecular Probes, Eugene, OR), both 1 mg/mL stock solution in Ca^{2+}/Mg^{2+}-free PBS stored at –20°C.

2.2. Adhesive Substrates

1. Microslides: Glass capillaries with rectangular cross-section (0.3 mm × 3 mm) (Vitro Dynamics Inc., NJ).
2. Glass treatment: Aminopropyltriethoxysilane 4% (v/v) in acetone (Sigma) with molecular sieve (BDH Laboratory Supplies) added to ensure anhydrous APES.

2.3. Flow-Based Adhesion Assay

1. Flow system: Syringe pump with smooth flow (e.g., PHD2000 infusion/withdrawal, Harvard Apparatus, South Natick, MA). Electronic three-way microvalve with zero dead volume (LFYA1226032H Lee Products Ltd., Gerrards Cross, Buckinghamshire, UK) with 12-V DC power supply for valve. Silicon rubber tubing, ID/OD of 1/3 mm and 2/4 mm (Fisher Scientific, Loughborough, UK). Scotch double-sided adhesive tape, approx 1 cm wide (3M Ltd., Bracknell, Berkshire, UK). Three-way stopcocks (BOC Ohmeda AB, Helsinborg, Sweden). Sterile, disposable syringes (2, 5, 10 mL Becton Dickinson, Oxford, UK).

2. Videomicroscope: Microscope with stage enclosed in a temperature-controlled chamber at 37°C. Fluoresence capability desirable for some variants of assay. Video camera (e.g., Hitachi KP-110 b/w CCTV camera, or JVC TK-S350 for low light/fluorescence). Black-and-white monitor (e.g., Hitachi VM-1202X). Video recorder (e.g., time lapse, Panasonic AG-6730).

3. Image analysis: Computer with video capture card and specialist software for counting cells, measuring motion, etc. There are a range of commercial packages available, as well as image analysis software (NIH Image http://rsb.info.nih.gov/nih-image/) available free over the Internet. We currently use Image Pro software (DataCell Limited, Finchampstead, UK).

2.4. Culture of Endothelial Cells

1. Culture medium, Medium 199 (Earles Modification ICN Flow Laboratories Ltd., High Wycombe UK) supplemented with gentamycin sulfate (28 µg/mL Cidomicin Injectable, Roussel Laboratories Ltd., Uxbridge, UK), glutamine (4 mM, ICN Flow Laboratories Ltd.), human epidermal growth factor (1 ng/mL, Sigma E9644), and fetal calf serum (20% v/v heat-inactivated). Adding hydrocortisone (1 µg/mL, from 1 mg/mL stock in ethanol) improves growth if going beyond first passage.

2. 1% bovine skin gelatin (Sigma, culture-tested solution).

3. Collagenase (Sigma type IA) stored at –20°C at 10 mg/mL in phosphate-buffered saline (PBS); thawed and diluted to 1 mg/mL with M199 for use.

4. Autoclaved cannulae and plastic ties (electrical).

5. EDTA solution (0.02%, culture-tested, Sigma).

6. 70% (v/v) ethanol or industrial methylated spiritis.

3. Methods

3.1. Blood Cell Isolation and Activation

3.1.1. Blood Withdrawal

1. For preparation of leukocytes, draw from the antecubital vein of normal human volunteers with a minimum of stasis; dispense into K_2EDTA tubes.

2. For isolation of platelet-rich plasma (PRP), use preservative-free Na-heparin (5 U/mL final concentration).

3. For preparation of washed platelets in a minimally activated state, draw directly into a 10-mL syringe containing 100 µL K_2EDTA/theophylline/prostacyclin (final concentrations 1.6 mg/mL, 7 mM, and 5 ng/mL, respectively).

4. For blood to be used in whole blood adhesion assays, dispense 9:1 in CPDA and add 5 mM $MgCl_2$ (e.g., from 0.5 M sterile-filtered stock).

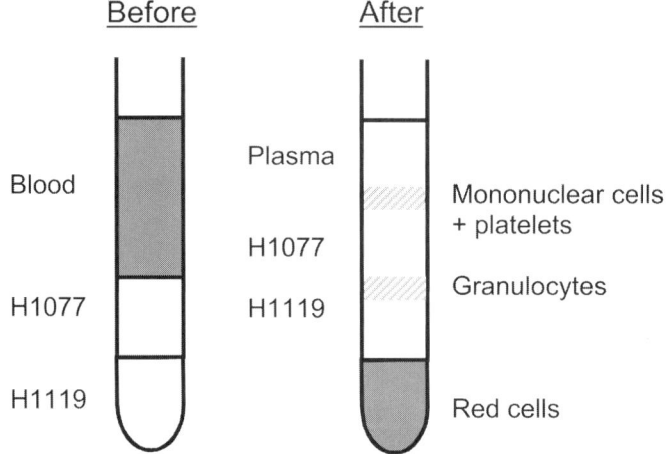

Fig. 1. Layering of liquids used for density gradient fractionation of blood. "Before" = 2.5 mL Histopaque 1077 (H1077) layered on 2.5 mL Histopaque 1119 (H1119), with 5 mL blood layered on top. "After" shows redistribution of cells and liquids after centrifugation at 800g for 25 min.

3.1.2. Preparation of Platelets

1. For PRP: centrifuge heparinized blood at 300g for 5 min and retrieve supernatant.
2. For "resting" platelets: centrifuge EDTA blood at 300g for 5 min, retrieve supernatant, wash once with PBS without Ca^{2+}/Mg^{2+} containing theophylline and prostacyclin (7 mM and 5 ng/mL, respectively), and resuspend in the same buffer.
3. Count platelets (e.g., with Coulter counter, Coulter Electronics, Luton, UK) and dilute to 2×10^8 platelets/mL.

3.1.3. Isolation of Leukocytes

1. Place 2.5 mL H1119 in 10-mL centrifuge tube and gently layer 2.5 mL H1077 on top. An interface should be visible between the layers.
2. Layer whole blood (5 mL) on top (**Fig. 1**).
3. Centrifuge at 800g for 25 min.
4. Retrieve the mononuclear cells from the top of the gradient, at the interface of plasma and H1077 (**Fig. 1**).
5. Discard the middle section of H1077.
6. Retrieve the granulocyte (mainly neutrophil) layer from the H1077-1119 interface.
7. Wash cells twice in PBSA with Ca^{2+}/Mg^{2+}.
8. To deplete mononuclear cells of monocytes, place in culture dish for 30 min at 37°C for monocytes to sediment and adhere. Gently wash off enriched lymphocytes.
9. Count leukocytes and dilute to 10^6 cells/mL in PBSA (*see* **Note 1**).

3.2. Adhesive Substrates

3.2.1. Pre-Treatment with APES

1. Immerse microslides in nitric acid (50% (v/v) in distilled water) for 24 h (e.g., in batch ~100–300).
2. Wash thoroughly in copious amounts of running tap water and rinse through once with deionized distilled water.
3. Dry at 37°C and store until required.
4. Place in polystyrene tubes and rinse twice with anhydrous acetone.
5. Immerse in a freshly prepared solution of APES (4% v/v in anhydrous acetone) for 1 min, ensuring that all capillaries are filled (*see* **Note 2**).
6. Remove microslides from the APES and blot out onto tissue, ensuring that all capillaries are emptied.
7. Re-insert into a fresh aliquot of the solution for another 1 min.
8. Remove APES by blotting and rinse the microslides once with anhydrous acetone, followed by three washes with deionized distilled water, and then dry at 37°C. Between each change, care must be taken to remove all the liquid from the microslides.
9. Autoclave the microslides at 121°C for 11 min and store aseptically, indefinitely.

3.2.2. Formation of Monolayer of Adherent Platelets

1. Attach short length of 2-mm i.d. silicon rubber tubing to APES-coated microslide and draw in heparinized PRP using pipettor. Microslides hold approx 50 µL, but if enough is available, approx 100 µL can be used to flush and fill. The tubing also assists in handling and avoidance of fingerprints on microslides.
2. Allow platelets to sediment and adhere to the inside of the microslide for 30 min.
3. To test quality of coating with new batches of microslides, rinse through with PBSA. Using heparinized PRP, a nearly confluent layer of mainly spread platelets should be visible under phase contrast microscopy. Using resting platelets, discrete, roughly discoidal platelets should form a carpet on the APES.

3.3. Flow-Based Assay of Adhesion of Leukocytes to Platelets

3.3.1. Setting Up the Flow Assay

1. Assemble the flow system shown in **Fig. 2** but without the microslide attached. The electronic valve has a common output, and two inputs, from "Wash reservoir" and "Sample reservoir," which can be selected by turning the electronic valve on and off.
2. Fill the wash reservoir with PBSA and rinse through all tubing, valves, and connectors with PBSA, ensuring that bubbles are displaced (e.g., using syringe attached to three-way tap for positive ejection). Fill sample reservoir with PBSA and rinse through valve, etc. PBSA can be degassed under vacuum to avoid formation of small bubbles as it is warmed. Prime downstream syringe and tubing with PBSA and load into syringe pump. All tubing must be liquid-filled.
3. Glue a coated microslide across the middle of a glass microscope slide using two spots of cyanoacrylate adhesive (Superglue Loctite UK, Welwyn Garden City, UK) applied to the edges of the slide. Discard tubing adaptor used for filling.

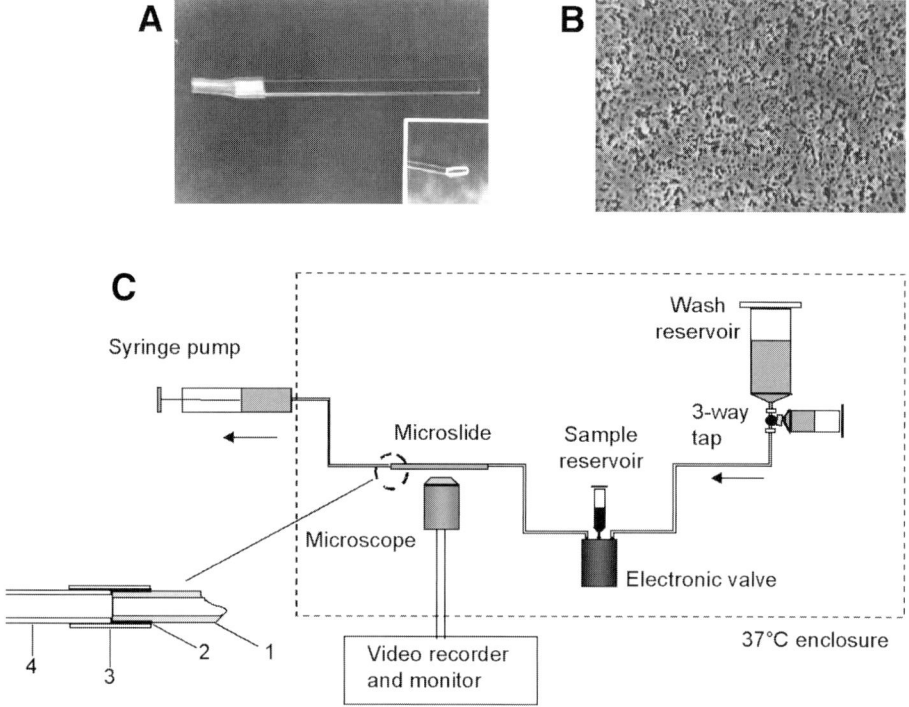

Fig. 2. Illustrations of (**A**) a microslide; (**B**) platelet monolayer deposited by settling PRP in an APES-coated microslide; (**C**) schematic of flow system. In expanded section of (**C**), 1 = microslide, 2 = double-sided tape, 3 = silicon rubber tubing with i.d./o.d. 2/4 mm, 4 = silicon rubber tubing with i.d./o.d. 1/2 mm.

4. Wrap double-sided adhesive tape around each end of the microslide, without obstructing lumen.
5. Connect microslide to silicon rubber tubing by pushing over each of the taped ends. Start at the upstream (sample) end to avoid injection of air. Squeeze the 2-mm i.d. silicon rubber tubing (**Fig. 2**) to flatten and ease over rectangular end of microslide, one corner first.
6. Place microslide onto microscope stage and start flow by turning on the syringe pump in withdrawal mode, with electronic valve and three-way tap in position to allow delivery of PBSA from wash reservoir (**Fig. 2**).
7. Wash out nonadherent platelets and observe surface using phase-contrast microscopy.
8. Adjust flow rate to that required for assay. The flow rate (Q) required to give a desired wall-shear rate (γ in s^{-1}) or wall-shear stress (τ in Pascal, Pa) is calculated from the internal width (w) and internal depth (h) of the microslide and the viscosity (n) of the flowing medium using the formulae:

$$\gamma = (6 \cdot Q)/(w \cdot h^2)$$
$$\tau = n \cdot \gamma$$

Since $w = 3$ mm, $h = 0.3$ mm, and $n = 0.7$ mPas for PBSA at 37°C, this can be manipulated to give

$$Q \text{ (mL/min)} = 0.0027\gamma \text{ (s}^{-1})$$

or

$$Q \text{ (mL/min)} = 3.8\tau \text{ (Pa)}$$

For instance, to obtain a wall-shear rate of 1000 s^{-1}, the flow rate is 2.7 mL/min, and to obtain a wall-shear stress of 0.1 Pa (wall-shear rate = 140 s^{-1}), the flow rate is 0.38 mL/min (*see* **Note 3**).

9. Perfusion of leukocytes is typically carried out at a flow rate ($Q = 0.38$ mL/min) equivalent to a wall-shear rate of 140 s^{-1} and wall-shear stress of 0.1 Pa (= 1 dyn/cm^2).

3.3.2. Perfusing Leukocytes and Activating Agents and Recording Behavior

1. Load isolated leukocytes into sample reservoir **(Fig. 2)** and allow to warm for 5 min.
2. Switch electronic valve so leukocyte suspension is drawn through microslide.
3. Deliver timed bolus (e.g., 4 min). Typically, flowing leukocytes will be visible after about 30 s, the time required to displace dead volume in valve and tubing.
4. Switch electronic valve so PBSA from wash reservour is perfused. Again, 30–60 s will be required before all leukocytes have been washed through the microslide.
5. Video recordings can be made as desired during inflow and washout of leukocytes. Typically, a series of fields should be recorded along the centerline of the microslide during inflow (e.g., 6 fields recorded for 10 s each during the last minute of the bolus), for off-line analysis of the behavior (e.g., rolling or stationary adhesion) of the leukocytes. Another series should be made after 1 min washout (when the bolus is complete) for analysis of the numbers of adherent cells. This may be extended if changes in leukocyte behavior are to be studied (e.g., if activatory agents are added).
6. If the surface of the microslide has been coated with minimally activated washed platelets, there will be relatively rare, short-lived interactions of flowing leukocytes. If the surface has been coated with platelets from PRP, there should be numerous, steady rolling adhesive interactions. Existence of stationary adhesion indicates spontaneous activation of leukocyte integrins.
7. To study effects of platelet activation, leukocytes can be perfused in the presence or absence of thrombin (0.2–1.0 U/mL), which will activate the platelets and not the leukocytes. Thus, changes in behavior will depend on up-regulation of P-selectin and/or on leukocyte-activating agents generated by the platelets upon stimulation. For neutrophils, platelet-generated agonist(s) tend to transform P-selectin-mediated rolling adhesion to integrin-mediated stationary adhesion *(17)*.
8. To directly study effects of leukocyte activation, at the end of washout of the bolus, the sample reservoir can be filled with agent (e.g., 1 μM fMLP) and this can be perfused over the leukocytes already rolling on the platelets. This will cause rapid activation of neutrophils, integrin-mediated immobilization, and subsequent migration *(7,18)*.
9. To study inhibitory antibodies, pretreat either leukocytes or platelet monolayers for 20 min before perfusion. If competitive inhibitors are to be used (e.g., RGD peptide), they need to present in media throughout; otherwise, they will be washed out.

3.3.3. Analysis of Leukocyte Behavior from Video Recordings

3.3.3.1. SIMPLE APPROACH WITHOUT COMPUTERIZED IMAGE ANALYSIS

1. Make video recordings of microscope stage micrometer (typically with 10-μm "ruler") oriented parallel and perpendicular to flow. Use this to calibrate the size of the video field observed on the monitor during playback.
2. Count cells present on a stop-frame, video field at the start of a sequence. Average the counts over sequences recorded. Convert this to count of adherent cells/mm².
3. Divide this by the numbers of leukocytes perfused (in units of 10⁶ cells) to obtain number adherent/mm²/10⁶ perfused. The number perfused is simply calculated by multiplying the concentration of the suspension (usually 10⁶/mL) by the flow rate (e.g., 0.395 mL/min) by the duration of the bolus (e.g., 4 min). This normalization allows correction for changes in conditions (bolus duration, cell concentration, flow rate) between experiments, and effectively calculates an efficiency of adhesion.
4. The count includes cells that are rolling or stationary. Both will be visible as bright circles on stop-frame recordings made using phase contrast microscopy, or if leukocytes have been fluorescently stained and viewed using fluorescence microscopy. Nonadherent cells will be visible only as blurred streaks.
5. To estimate the percentage of adherent cells rolling, mark cells in a stop-frame at the start of a sequence, play forward, and re-mark the cells. Those moving continually and displaced by greater than half a cell diameter in 10 s may be considered as rolling (*see* **Note 4**).

3.3.3.2. ANALYSIS USING COMPUTERIZED IMAGE ANALYSIS

1. Digitize a series of images at regular intervals from the start of a recording on a particular field; typically use 10 images, 0.5 or 1 s apart, depending on the rate of rolling.
2. Software may be able to locate and count the adherent leukocytes, as they are bright against a darker background. This is done by thresholding (choosing a level of intensity above which areas are deemed white, and below which they are deemed black). If small bright objects are present, they can be filtered out according to a separate size threshold. It may be easier simply to count cells manually.
3. Record the count for the first image.
4. Mark the leading edges of a series of cells to be followed and move to the second captured frame. Re-mark the leading edges and record the distance moved (calibration is achieved using the recording of the stage micrometer). Repeat through series. This will yield data for position versus time. Velocity for each cell can be averaged over the observation time, and estimates of variation in velocity made if desired. Alternatively, mark only the first and last frames to obtain average rolling velocity.
5. Repeat the analysis for the different recorded video fields and average the data. Convert counts to numbers adherent/mm²/10⁶ perfused, as above.
6. To obtain data for percentage of adherent cells rolling or stationary, there are two approaches. Either take the digitized sequence and play as a loop, observe cells in turn, and assign them to rolling or stationary depending on whether their position varies by >0.5 cell diameter, or measure changes in position for every cell (as above) and assign all cells below a certain velocity as stationary. We have used 0.4 μm/s as a cutoff (essentially, half a cell diameter in 10 s) *(19)*. For point-attached cells, flow may induce a movement of about half a cell diameter without requiring the breaking and making of bonds that underlie rolling adhesion. There is, however, no hard rule for this. For instance, at low

temperature, rolling may continue at a very low velocity *(20)* and it becomes difficult to separate rolling and stationary adherent cells.

7. In experiments where leukocytes have been activated and undertake migration on the surface, the above method can be adapted for measuring velocity and direction of migration. This requires prolonged recording of a single video field, usually during the washout phase, when, for instance, an activating agent has been added. A sequence of 5–10 images is captured 1 min apart. The positions of cells are recorded in each image and the distance moved between images calculated. The rate of migration (μm/min) can be determined and averaged. The direction of migration can be quanitifed as the net distance moved in a chosen direction (e.g., parallel with the flow axis) divided by the sum of the individual distances moved in the separate minutes. A value of 1 represents movement in a straight line along the chosen axis. A value of 0 means no net displacement in that direction (*see* **Note 4**).

3.4. Adhesion of Leukocytes to Immobilized Platelets in Whole Blood

Adhesion between leukocytes and platelets on surfaces has rarely been done using whole blood. No definitive methods can be given, only guidance for those interested in using more physiologically relevant models. In principle, leukocyte adhesion to deposited platelets can be observed in whole blood if fluorescent dyes are used *(26)*. The two types of cell can be distinguished by size. The different types of leukocytes are not so clearly different, although small, paler lymphocytes adherent to a surface can be distinguished from larger, brighter cells (mainly neutrophils).

There are two possible approaches:

1. Precoat microslides with platelets as in **Subheading 3.2.2.**, and perfuse blood instead of isolated leukocytes (essentially as in **Subheading 3.3.2.**). Fluorescent leukocytes will be visible attaching to the platelets and can be analyzed essentially as in **Subheading 3.3.3.** A complication is that platelets will adhere from the blood onto the precoated platelets, and these may not become activated as fully as those laid down originally.
2. Precoat microslides with collagen, e.g., as described in Chapter 12, vol. 1, and then perfuse blood through them at the chosen shear rate. Platelets will adhere to the collagen and leukocytes may bind to them as the surface gets coated (*see* **Note 5**). Studies in which blood has been perfused over collagen type 1 and washed out show that platelet aggregates can include adherent leukocytes *(27)*. For important variables for these approaches, refer to **Note 6**.

3.5. Adhesion Between Platelets and Leukocytes in Mixed Suspensions

Adhesion between leukocytes (mainly neutrophils or monocytes) and platelets has also been widely studied in mixed suspensions (e.g., *1,5,23,24*). This may be relevant to the formation of microaggregates in blood in vivo, and indeed, all leukocytes bind platelets to some degree in blood *(10,11)*. In general, aggregation requires expression of P-selectin on platelets for initiation and can be stabilized by activated β2-integrins on the leukocytes.

3.5.1. Method A—Based on Jungi et al. *(23)* and Spangenberg et al. *(5)*

1. Prepare resting platelets at 2×10^8/mL as in **Subheading 3.1.2.**
2. Incubate with 0.2 U/mL thrombin for 10 min at room temperature without stirring.
3. Fix by addition of an equal volume of 2% formaldehyde in PBS for 1 h.
4. Wash twice and resuspend at 1×10^8/mL in PBSA.

5. Isolate leukocytes and adjust concentration to 5×10^6/mL as in **Subheading 3.1.3.**
6. Mix suspensions of leukocytes and platelets 1:1 in a multiwell plate, e.g., in triplicate for each condition to be studied (final ratio 20 platelets per leukocyte).
7. Incubate under rocking conditions for 30 min at room temperature.
8. Fix aliquots at chosen times (e.g. 0, 10, 20, 30 min) by mixing 1:1 with 2% glutaraldehyde in PBS.
9. Place 10 µL on a microscope slide and cover with coverslip. Observe with interference contrast or phase-contrast microscopy.
10. Count 100 neutrophils, and assign them as having either (a) no platelets attached; (b) 2–4 platelets attached; (c) 5–6 platelets attached; (d) 7 or more platelets attached.
11. Express data as percentage of neutrophils with platelets (2 or more) adherent, and average number of platelets adherent to 100 neutrophils (assigning 3, 4, or 7 platelets to the three categories B–D).

3.5.2. Method B—Based on Maeda et al. (24)

1. Prepare heparinized PRP and adjust concentration to 4×10^8/mL as in **Subheading 3.1.2.**
2. Isolate leukocytes and adjust concentration to 10^7/mL as in **Subheading 3.1.3.**
3. Mix suspensions in a test tube in proportions of leukocytes, platelets, PBSA of:

1:1:0	(40 platelets per leukocyte)
1:0.5:0.5	(20 platelets per leukocyte)
1:0.25:0.75	(10 platelets per leukocyte)
1:0.125:0.875	(5 platelets per leukocyte)

4. Place tubes on roller mixer at approx 80 rpm.
5. Fix aliquots at chosen times (e.g., 0, 5, 10, 20 min) by mixing 1:1 with 2% glutaraldehyde.
6. Count the number of single leukocytes using a Coulter counter and/or count aggregates as particles with volume >1.8 × mean leukocyte volume (25).
7. The two parameters give related indices of platelet-induced aggregation (reduction in singlet neutrophils or formation of multicellular aggregates) as a function of time, compared to time zero (before mixing). At these low mixing shears, platelets act as cross-bridges in leukocyte aggregates.
8. In the absence of a Coulter counter, single neutrophils and aggregates can be counted manually using a hemocytometer and a microscope (*see* Chapter 3, vol. 1).
9. Aggregation is largely ablated, for instance, by addition of 5 m*M* EGTA.

3.6. Adhesion of Platelets to Endothelial Cells

Intact endothelial monolayers have generally been considered nonadhesive for platelets because of their ability to generate prostacyclin and nitric oxide. This is not strictly correct. A number of studies have shown that a variety of endothelial treatments increase adhesion, and activated platelets simply sedimented onto cultured endothelial cells adhere in small numbers (e.g., *see* **ref. 16** for commentary).

Assays of platelet adhesion to endothelial cells are variants of the assays of platelet adhesion described in Chapters 13 and 15, vol. 1, with a confluent monolayer of cultured endothelial cells used as a substrate instead of purified proteins such as collagen. The essential requirements are ability to culture a confluent monolayer on a convenient substrate and a means for distinguishing adhesion of platelets on a cellular background. There are various methods for culture of endothelial cells from different sources, and for the novice, it is probably best to start by buying cells and media from commercial suppliers. Our current method for isolating and culturing human umbilical-vein endothelial cells (HUVEC) is given below, adapted from Cooke et al. *(30)*.

3.6.1. Isolation and Primary Culture of HUVEC

1. Place the umbilical cord in a tray on paper toweling and spray liberally with 70% ethanol. Choose sections of about 6 inches that do not have any clamp damage. Each 6-in piece of cord equates to 1 flask of primary cells.
2. Add approx 2 mL gelatin to 25 cm^2 culture flasks.
3. Locate the two arteries and one vein at one end of the cord.
4. Cannulate the vein and secure the cannula with an electrical tie.
5. Carefully wash through the vein with PBS using a syringe and blow air through to remove the PBS.
6. Cannulate the opposite end of the vein and tie off.
7. Inject collagenase (~10 mL per 6 in) into vein until both cannulae bulbs have the mixture in them.
8. Place the cord into an incubator for 15 min at 37°C.
9. Remove from the incubator and tighten the ties. Massage the cord for approx 1 min.
10. Flush the cord through using a syringe and 10 mL PBS into a 50-mL centrifuge tube. Push air through to remove any PBS. Repeat this twice more (3 × 10 mL).
11. Centrifuge at 400g for 5 min. Discard supernatant.
12. Resuspend the cells in approx 1.5 mL of culture medium and mix well with pipet.
13. Make up to 4 mL in complete medium.
14. Remove gelatin from flask and add cell suspension.
15. Change medium after 2 h and again the next day. Cells should be confluent in about 3–4 d.

3.6.2. Seeding of Multiwell Plates for Static Assays

1. Rinse a single flask containing a confluent primary monolayer of HUVEC with 4 mL EDTA solution.
2. Add 2 mL of trypsin solution for 1–2 min at room temperature, until the cells became detached.
3. Add 8 mL of culture medium to the flask, remove the resulting suspension, and centrifuge at 400g for 5 min.
4. Remove supernatant and resuspend the cell pellet in 0.5 mL of culture medium and disperse by sucking them in and out of a pipet tip.
5. Make up to 12 mL with culture medium and add 0.5 mL to each well of a 24-well plate.
6. After 2 h, replace medium with 1 mL fresh culture medium. Culture for 24 h or until confluent.

3.6.3. Static Platelet-Endothelial Cell Adhesion Assay

1. Prepare resting platelets or PRP at 2×10^8/mL as in **Subheading 3.1.2.**
2. Add rhodamine 6G or calcein-AM at 1 µg/mL for 20 min.
3. Wash and resuspend at 1×10^8/mL in PBSA with Ca^{2+}/Mg^{2+}.
4. Add 100 µL to culture medium in each well coated with HUVEC in 24-well plate and allow platelets to settle for 30 min at 37°C.
5. Remove medium, and add PBSA gently. Swirl plate and remove PBSA. Repeat up to 4 washes. Fix by addition of an equal volume of 2% formaldehyde.

6. Observe using inverted fluoresence microscope and count adherent fluorescent platelets in field of known dimensions.

7. Convert count to number/mm^2, multiply by area of well, and divide by number of platelets added × 100% to obtain percent adherent.

8. Compare resting platelets with platelets activated with, e.g., 0.2 U/mL thrombin.

9. Compare resting HUVEC with HUVEC activated with, e.g., 0.2 U/mL thrombin for 15 min (washed out before addition of platelets).

3.6.4. Flow-Based Platelet-Endothelial Cell Adhesion Assay

HUVEC can be cultured inside microslides *(30)* or on coverslips that can be incorporated in flow chambers (e.g., *31*). In principle, platelets in suspension or in blood can be perfused over endothelial cells in microslides or in flow chambers. There have been few reports of use of this technology for studying adhesion of platelets to intact confluent monolayers of endothelial cells. We have perfused washed platelets over human microvascular endothelial cells (HMEC-1) in microslides and found negligible adhesion *(16)*. We have also perfused heparinized blood over HMEC and found sporadic attachment of platelets, usually in clumps (C. Kirton and G. Nash, unpublished observations). However, there is no well-defined or widely used method that can be recommended.

4. Notes

1. There are various methods described for isolating leukocytes from blood; **Subheading 3.1.3.** describes a simple one that we use regularly. The cells should appear spherical and form predominantly rolling attachments (~90% of adherent cells rolling) on platelets immobilized as described above, without addition of thrombin. If the cells have a distorted shape and/or become stationary adherent spontaneously, one must suspect unintentional activation, so that integrins have become engaged. It is advisable also to test viability of preparations (e.g., ~99% viable judged with trypan blue) and purity (e.g., 95% polymorphonuclear when isolating neutrophils judged with crystal violet), especially when first starting this type of work.

2. Successful coating with APES requires that the reagent be anhydrous. We buy small volumes adequate to coat a batch of microslides, use a fresh bottle for each batch, and discard any unused reagent. It is important to efficiently remove all liquid from each microslide between changes, and to ensure that all bubbles are displaced on refilling with agents. This requires patience.

3. Flow parameters: The formulae for shear rate and stress (**Subheading 3.3.1., step 8**) apply for fully developed, laminar flow in a parallel-plate geometry. It assumes the chamber is much wider than it is deep. The ratio in microslides is 10:1. One should make all recordings along the centerline for the predictions of shear rate and stress to be accurate, as both will fall off toward the side walls. Reynold's number in microslides under most conditions will be in the range 1–30, well below that predicting turbulence. If deviation from simple straight flow of particles is seen, there may be bubbles stuck in the microslide. Deposition of large particles, debris, or clots should not occur unless contamination has occurred or inadequate anticoagulant has been used.

4. The behavior of leukocytes on the immobilized platelets depends on how the platelets have been treated and deposited. There may be the following variations:

   a. Using heparinized PRP settled on APES, neutrophils roll continuously until they are activated with an agent such as fMLP, upon which they immobilize rapidly and then commence active migration *(7,18,19)*. If thrombin is added to the platelets with the neutrophils, then a proportion of the neutrophils becomes immobilized, indicating that the platelets have generated a neutrophil-activating agent *(17)*.

b. Using resting washed platelets on APES, perfused neutrophils make relatively few, short-lived attachments. If thrombin is added to the platelets with the neutrophils, then the level of adhesion increases dramatically and a proportion of the neutrophils becomes immobilized, indicating again that the platelets have generated a neutrophil-activating agent *(17)*.

c. Washed platelets settled on fibrinogen support rolling adhesion of neutrophils, which gradually transform into stationary adhesion *(21)*.

d. Washed platelets settle on fibronectin and then, stimulated with thrombin, support capture of flowing neutrophils, which rapidly become immobilized *(8)*.

e. Washed platelets settle on collagen type I-support rolling adhesion of flowing neutrophils, of which ~50% become immobilized over minutes *(22)*.

It is evident that the state of platelet activation determines the expression of P-selectin and also the presentation of neutrophil-activating agent(s). The two do not necessarily happen together, and P-selectin can be expressed before a state is reached where a leukocyte-activator is generated.

5. We are not aware of any published study using this method to study the dynamics of adhesion as it occurs. Our experience with this system is that leukocyte interactions with deposited platelets are short-lived and analysis has to be modified accordingly (e.g., by counting the number of adhesive interactions seen in a given area per minute rather than counting the number of cells adherent after a fixed bolus).

6. *Anticoagulant:* CPDA with added $MgCl_2$ (5 mM) is adequate, although there is some dilution of the blood. We have made up a 10X concentrated version to avoid this *(26)*. Heparin does not appear suitable because of formation of large clumps in the flowing blood and on the surface.

Storage: Adhesiveness of leukocytes appears to decrease quite rapidly in stored CPDA or heparinized blood *(26)*.

Fluorescent dye: Dyes may affect properties of leukocytes and/or platelets. We have found rhodamine 6G or calcein-AM (both at 1–5 µg/mL) have little effect on leukocyte adhesion. It is notable that when surfaces are illuminated with high-intensity mercury-arc lamps, adhesion of platelets increases on the illuminated area if rhodamine, calcein-AM, or quinacrine are used as dyes. Prolonged exposure to light in any spot must be avoided.

Conditions of flow: Blood is not Newtonian (its viscosity decreases with increasing shear rate), and the flow profile is not parabolic, but blunted (plug flow) (*see*, e.g., *28*). For a given volumetric flow rate, plug flow will cause the wall-shear rate and cell velocity near the wall to be greater than predicted. At the same time, exclusion of red cells from the layer closest to the wall, and the tendency of red cell aggregates to migrate toward the centerline, will cause the hematocrit near the vessel wall to be lower than the bulk average. This means that the effective viscosity near the wall, and hence the wall shear stress, cannot be predicted exactly. There is no exact solution to this problem. It is best either to calculate wall shear rate as in **Subheading 3.3.1.** and quote it as a value for "ideal" flow, or to apply a multiplicative correction of 2.1, based on measurement of actual platelet velocity profiles in plug flow in arterioles *(29)*.

References

1. Hamburger, S. A. and McEver, R. P. (1990) GMP-140 mediates adhesion of stimulated platelets to neutrophils. *Blood* **75,** 550–554.

2. Moore, K. L., Stults, N. L., Diaz, S., Smith, D. F., Cummings, R. D., Varki, A., et al. (1992) Identification of a specific glycoprotein ligand for P-selectin (CD62) on myeloid cells. *J. Cell Biol.* **118,** 445–456.

3. Lalor, P. and Nash, G. B. (1995) Adhesion of flowing leucocytes to immobilized platelets. *Br. J. Haematol.* **89,** 725–732.

4. Nash, G. B., Morland, C., Sheikh, S., Buttrum, S. M., and Lalor, P. (1996) Adhesion between leucocytes and platelets, rheology, mechanisms and consequences. *Prog. Appl. Microcirc.* **22,** 98–113.

5. Spangenberg, P., Redlich, H., Bergmann, I., Losche, W., Gotzrath, M., and Kehrel, B. (1993) The platelet glycoprotein IIb/IIIa complex is involved in the adhesion of activated platelets to leukocytes. *Thrombo. Haemost.* **70,** 514–521.

6. Diacovo, T. G., deFougerolles, A. R., Bainton, D. F., and Springer, T. A. (1994) A functional integrin ligand on the surface of platelets, intercellular adhesion molecule-2. *J. Clin. Invest.* **94,** 1243–1251.

7. Sheikh, S. and Nash, G. B. (1996) Continuous activation and deactivation of integrin CD11b/CD18 during de novo expression enables rolling neutrophils to immobilize on platelets. *Blood* **87,** 5040–5050.

8. Weber, C. and Springer, T. A. (1997) Neutrophil accumulation on activated, surface-adherent platelets in flow is mediated by interaction of Mac-1 with fibrinogen bound to $\alpha_{IIb}\beta_3$ and stimulated by platelet-activating factor. *J. Clin. Invest.* **100,** 2085–2093.

9. Kuijper, P. H. M., Torres, H. I. G., Lammers, J. W. J., Sixma, J. J., Koenderman, L., and Zwaginga, J. J. (1998) Platelet associated fibrinogen and ICAM-2 induce firm adhesion of neutrophils under flow. *Thromb. Haemost.* **80,** 443–448.

10. Rinder, C. S., Bonan, J. L., Rinder, H. M,, Ault, K. A., and Smith B. R. (1991) Dynamics of leukocyte-platelet adhesion in whole blood. *Blood* **78,** 1730–1737.

11. Rinder, C. S, Bonan, J. L., Rinder, H. M., Mathew, J., Hines, R., and Smith B. R. (1992) Cardiopulmonary bypass induces leukocyte-platelet adhesion. *Blood* **79,** 1201–1205.

12. Evangelista, V., Piccardoni, P., White, J. G., deGaetano, G., and Cerletti, C. (1993) Cathepsin G-dependent platlet stimulation by activated polymorphonuclear leukocytes and its inhibition by antiproteinases, role of P-selectin mediated cell-cell adhesion. *Blood* **70,** 2947–2957.

13. Rosenblum, W. I. (1997) Platelet adhesion and aggregation without endothelial denudation or exposure of basal lamina and/or collagen. *J. Vasc. Res.* **34,** 409–417.

14. Venturini, C. M., Weston, L. K., and Kaplan, J. E. (1992) Platelet cGMP but not cAMP inhibits thrombin-induced platelet adhesion to pulmonary endothelium. *Am. J. Physiol.* **263,** H606–H612.

15. Frenette, P. S., Johnson, R. C., Hynes, R. O., and Wagner, D. D. (1992) Platelets roll on stimulated endothelium in vivo, an interaction mediated by endothelial P-selectin. *Proc. Nat. Acad. Sci. USA* **92,** 7450–7454.

16. Kirton, C. and Nash, G. B. (2000) Activated platelets adherent to an intact endothelial cell monolayer bind flowing neutrophils and enable them to transfer to the endothelial surface. *J. Lab. Clin. Med.* **136,** 303–313.

17. Stone, P. C. W. and Nash, G. B. (1999) Conditions under which immobilised platelets activate as well as capture flowing neutrophils. *Br. J. Haematol.* **105,** 514–522.

18. Rainger, G. E., Buckley, C., Simmons, D., and Nash, G. B. (1997) Cross-talk between cell adhesion molecules regulates the migration velocity of neutrophils. *Curr. Biol.* **7,** 316–325.

19. Buttrum, S. M., Hatton, R., and Nash, G. B. (1993) Selectin-mediated rolling of neutrophils on immobilised platelets. *Blood* **82,** 1165–1174.

20. Nash, G. B., Abbitt, K. B., Tate, K., Jetha, K. A., and Egginton, S. (2001) Changes in the mechanical and adhesive behaviour of neutrophils on cooling in vitro. *Eur. J. Physiol.* **442,** 762–770.

21. Yeo, E. L., Sheppard, J. A. I., and Feuerstein, I. A. (1994) Role of P-selectin and leukocyte activation in polymorphonuclear cell adhesion to surface adherent activated platelets under physiologic shear conditions (an injury vessel wall model). *Blood* **83,** 2498–2507.

22. Ostrovsky, L., King, A. J., Bond, S., Mitchell, D., Lorant, D. E., Zimmerman, G. A., et al. (1998) A juxtacrine mechanism for neutrophil adhesion on platelets involves platelet-activating factor and a selectin-dependent activation process. *Blood* **91,** 3028–3036.

23. Jungi, T. W., Spycher, M. O., Nydegger, U. E., and Barandun, S. (1986) Platelet-leukocyte interactions, selective binding of thrombin stimulated platelets to human monocytes, polymorphonuclear leukocytes and related cell lines. *Blood* **67,** 629–636.

24. Maeda, T., Nash, G. B., Christopher, B., Pecsvarady, Z., and Dormandy, J. A. (1991) Platelet-induced granulocyte aggregation in vitro. *Blood Coag. Fibrinol.* **2,** 699–703.

25. Rhee, B.-G., Hall, E. R., and McIntire, L. V. (1986) Platelet modulation of polymorphonuclear leukocyte shear induced aggregation. *Blood* **67,** 240–246.

26. Abbitt, K. B. and Nash, G. B. (2001) Characteristics of leukocyte adhesion directly observed in flowing whole blood in vitro. *Br. J. Haematol.* **112,** 55–63.

27. Kirchhofer, D., Riederer, M. A., and Baumgartner, H. R. (1997) Specific accumulation of circulating monocytes and polymorphonuclear leukocytes on platelet thrombi in a vascular injury model. *Blood* **89,** 1270–1278.

28. Goldsmith, H. L. and Turitto, V. T. (1986) Rheological aspects of thrombosis and haemostasis, basic principles and applications. *Thrombos. Haemost.* **55,** 415–435.

29. Tangelder, G. J., Slaaf, D. W., Arts, T., and Reneman, R. S. (1988) Wall shear rate in arterioles in vivo, least estimates from platelet velocity profiles. *Am. J. Physiol.* **254,** H1059–H1064.

30. Cooke, B. M., Perry, I., Usami, S., and Nash, G. B. (1993) A simplified method for culture of endothelial cells and analysis of adhesion of blood cells under conditions of flow. *Microvasc. Res.* **45,** 33–45.

31. Kuijper, P. H. M., Torres, H. I. G., vanderLinden, J. A. M., Lammers, J. W. J., Sixma, J. J., Koenderman, L., et al. (1996) Platelet-dependent primary hemostasis promotes selectin- and integrin-mediated neutrophil adhesion to damaged endothelium under flow conditions. *Blood* **87,** 3271–3281.

18

In Vitro Measurement of High-Shear Platelet Adhesion and Aggregation by the PFA-100®

Paul Harrison

1. Introduction

1.1. Background

In recent years there has been considerable progress in the availability of tests to assess platelet function (*1*). The gold standard of platelet-function testing, "platelet aggregometry," was invented in the 1960s and has provided a vital research and diagnostic tool. However, because of the comparatively low shear conditions under which platelets are aggregated, the test does not accurately simulate in vivo platelet adhesion. In response to this problem a number of researchers have developed tests in an attempt to mimic or simulate in vivo platelet adhesion and aggregation. Many of these techniques remain as specialized research tools because of their inherent complexity; however, some tests have been developed into commercial instruments (*1*). In 1985 Kratzer and Born (*2*) developed a prototype instrument, the "Thrombostat-4000," which simulates high-shear platelet adhesion and aggregation. In the mid-1990s, Dade/Behring (Deerfield, IL) further developed the test into a commercially available instrument called the platelet function analyzer, or PFA-100® (*3,4*). Compared to most platelet function tests the PFA-100 is simple and rapid, and requires less training. However, as with other laboratory tests of platelet function, good PFA-100 practice guidelines and a number of quality control procedures are required to ensure optimal performance and data interpretation. This chapter will focus mainly on these issues and also on how to interpret PFA-100 data. Although general experience with the instrument is increasing, there is still a need to standardize platelet testing methodology with incorporation of the test into normal laboratory practice.

1.2. Principle of Test

The PFA-100 system measures primary hemostatic function in vitro. The instrument attempts to mimic the conditions to which platelets are exposed during blood-vessel

From: *Methods in Molecular Biology, vol. 272:*
Platelets and Megakaryocytes, Vol. 1: Functional Assays
Edited by: J. M. Gibbins and M. P. Mahaut-Smith © Humana Press Inc., Totowa, NJ

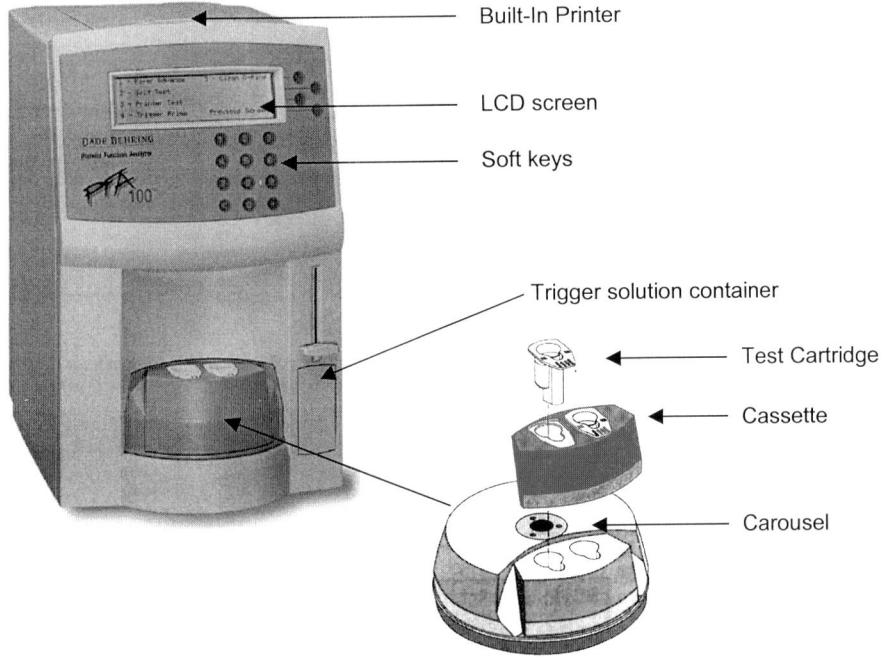

Built-In Printer

LCD screen

Soft keys

Trigger solution container

Test Cartridge

Cassette

Carousel

Fig. 1. The PFA-100 instrument (courtesy of Dade-Behring).

injury. The disposable test cartridges are composed of a sample reservoir, a capillary, and a membrane with a 150-μm central aperture. The membrane is coated with the platelet agonist collagen, in combination with either ADP or epinephrine (*see* **Figs. 1–3**).

A constant vacuum (40 mbar) is applied to aspirate the citrated whole blood from the reservoir through the capillary, onto the membrane, and through its central aperture. The platelets are subjected to high shear (5000–6000/s) within the capillary and become activated when they contact the membrane, resulting in adhesion, spreading, degranulation, and recruitment of other platelets to form aggregates (*see* **Fig. 2**). Eventually the platelets form a plug, which occludes the aperture (*see* **Fig. 3**). The instrument monitors the flow of blood through the aperture and determines the end of the test when blood flow stops. This parameter is recorded as the closure time (CT). Experimental parameters that may also be recorded include the total volume of blood used in the test and the initial flow rate (*see* **Fig. 4**).

2. Materials

1. PFA-100; available from Dade/Behring (Deerfield, IL). The instrument is a bench-top analyzer with integral printer, which is easily transportable if moved with care (*see* **Fig. 1**). Up to two test cartridges can be loaded into the cassette within the carousel. The software

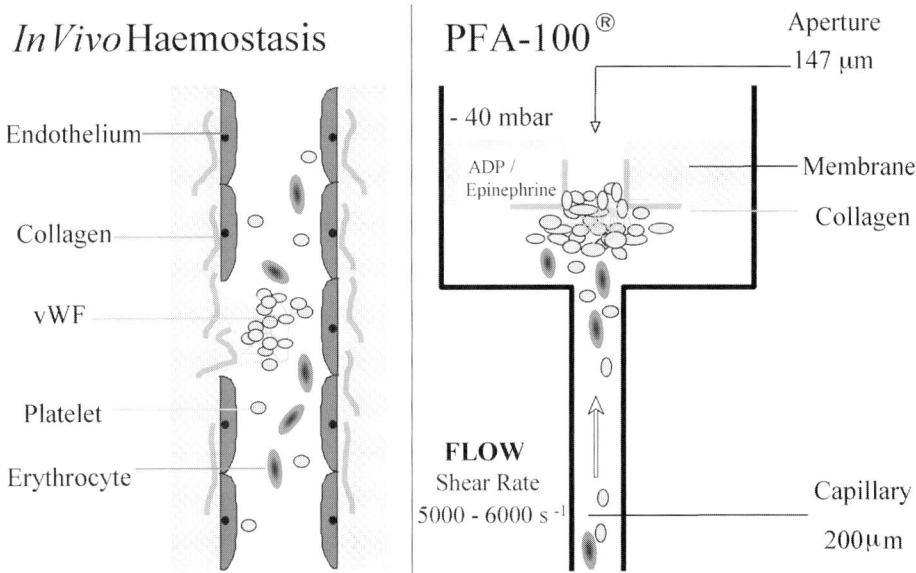

Fig. 2. Cross-section of cartridge (right-hand side) showing the principle of the PFA-100 test, which mimics high-shear-dependent platelet adhesion and aggregation (left-hand side) (courtesy of Dade-Behring). See color insert following p. 44.

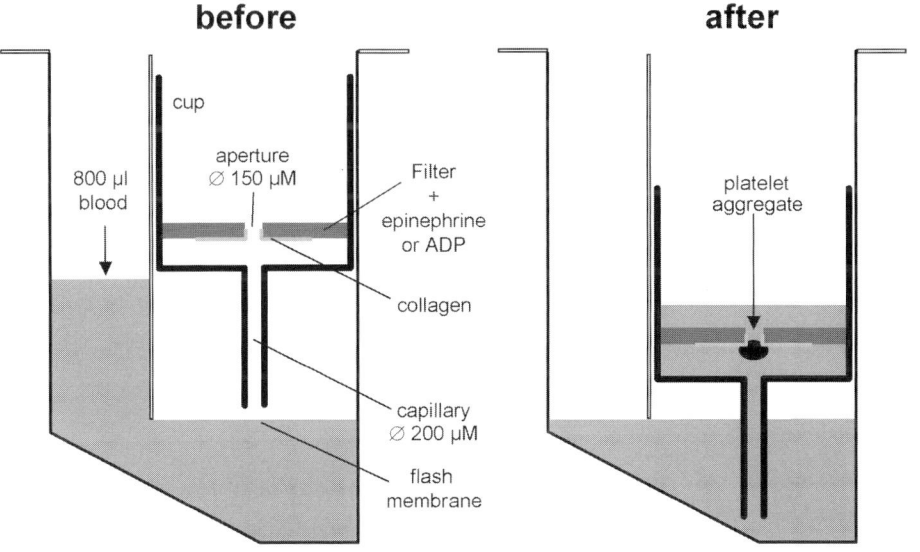

Fig. 3. Cross-section of a cartridge before and after performing the PFA-100 test (courtesy of Dade-Behring). See color insert following p. 44.

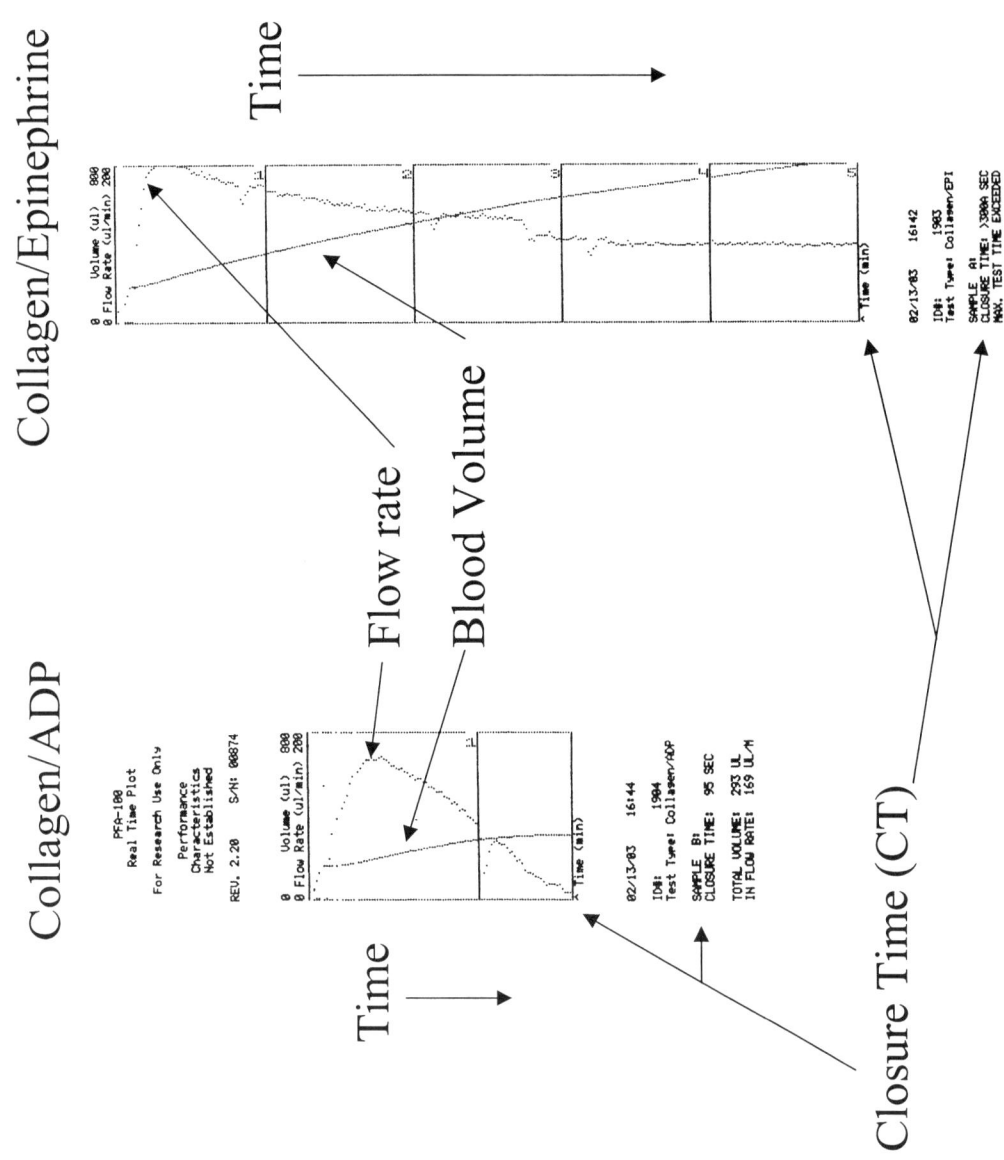

Collagen/Epinephrine

Time

Collagen/ADP

Time

Flow rate

Blood Volume

Closure Time (CT)

keys simplify operation by running built-in programs. The machine also has a bar-code reader port and external PC port.

2. Trigger solution, catalog number B4170-50–3 × 11 mL vials/box. Unopened vials are stable at room temperature until the expiration date. The solution is stable for 60 d once placed in the instrument. Vials should be inspected regularly and discarded if particulate matter is present.

3. Cartridges: Test cartridges within unopened pouches are stable at 40°C until the expiration date and at 4°C for 30 d after opening the pouch. Individual test cartridges are stable for 4 h at room temperature. Two types are available:
   a. Collagen/epinephrine: Catalog number B4170-20 (packs of 20)—a test cartridge unit containing a membrane coated with 2 µg of equine Type I collagen and 10 µg of epinephrine bitartrate.
   b. Collagen/ADP: Catalog number B4170-21 (packs of 20)—a test cartridge unit containing a membrane coated with 2 µg of equine Type I collagen and 50 µg of adenosine 5′-diphosphate.

4. Printer paper, catalog number B4170-71.

5. Printer ribbon, catalog number B4170-72.

6. Cassettes, catalog number B4170-70; pack of 5.

7. Priming cartridges, catalog number B4170-74; pack of 10.

8. Vacuum test cup, catalog number B4170-75; pack of 35. The cups are inserted into the priming cartridge to assemble the vacuum cartridge.

9. O-ring maintenance: cleaning pads (catalog number B4170-73); O-ring service tool (catalog number B4170-77); and O-rings (catalog number B4170-78).

10. 21-gauge needles and other consumables for blood taking (see other chapters in this book).

11. Siliconized evacuated tubes. Two different tube types are required: one containing EDTA and the other containing buffered trisodium citrate (*see* **Note 1**).

12. Isopropanol.

3. Methods

3.1. Maintenance and General Operation

1. After switching on, the PFA-100 performs a self-test and requires a warm-up period before tests can be conducted. If the instrument is in regular (i.e., daily or several times per week) use, it is recommended that it be left permanently switched on.

2. O-ring maintenance: Automatic O-ring cleaning is carried out as part of the daily quality control (QC) procedure (*see* **Subheading 3.2.**). However, it is also recommended that manual cleaning be carried out on a weekly basis (*see* **Note 2**). The O-ring should also be replaced on a yearly basis (*see* **Note 2**). In addition the O-ring should also be checked, cleaned, and replaced (if damaged or worn) when either the status messages "Vacuum Test Fail" or "Test terminated due to Air Leak" are displayed.

Fig. 4. *(see opposite page)* Examples of PFA-100 results from a sample taken from a subject 2 h post-aspirin ingestion (300 mg). The collagen/ADP cartridge gives a normal closure time (CT) and the collagen/epinephrine cartridge gives a maximal or >300 CT (courtesy of Dade-Behring).

3.2. Daily Self-Test of Instrument Components

A daily self-test should always be performed to check instrument performance. The test takes approx 7 min and verifies machine operation by checking various systems/ components. These include the vacuum chuck, the carousel drive, AIL (air in line) sensor, and the vacuum, trigger, and incubation systems. The instrument also cleans the O-ring during this procedure.

1. Select "Self-Test" from the maintenance menu.
2. The system will instruct the operator to load a vacuum test cartridge in position A and a priming cartridge in position B.
3. The carousel rotates and the user is instructed to place an O-ring cleaning pad within the instrument and then to place a few drops of 100% isopropanol onto the pad.
4. After the self-test, the operator will be prompted to remove the cleaning pad. Under no circumstances should this pad be left inside the instrument.
5. After completion of the self-test, the instrument records the date and time and prints any pass/fail results. If the machine fails any component, then testing cannot be performed until the fault is rectified or corrected. The most common fault is a vacuum failure, usually caused by a faulty, worn, or dirty vacuum seal. This seal can be checked and replaced according to the procedures in **Note 2**.

3.3. Blood Samples and Anticoagulant

1. Blood is drawn via a 21-gauge needle from an antecubital vein with minimal trauma and a standardized procedure. All samples are obtained and discarded following local ethical and safety guidelines. Control and test subjects are not generally rested before sampling for PFA-100 analysis.
2. Blood is drawn from an antecubital vein into two 4.5-mL evacuated tubes. The first 4.5 mL of blood is drawn into an EDTA tube and used for a full blood count. The second 4.5 mL of blood is drawn into buffered trisodium citrate (*see* **Note 1**) and analyzed in the PFA-100. 0.8 mL of citrated whole blood is required for each cartridge, so if both types of test cartridge are to be used, a minimum of 1.6 mL is needed.

3.4. Performing a Test

1. Remove the test cartridge(s) for a single run from their sealed foil container packs stored at 4°C and warm at room temperature for at least 15 min before analysis. Immediately return the resealed pack to the cold room or refrigerator.
2. Remove the foil seals of the cartridge and snap the appropriate cartridge(s) into positions A and B within the PFA-100 cassette. The user has the option to perform a single test using one cartridge (in either position A or B), a duplicate test on one type of cartridge, or a test on both types of cartridge (i.e., collagen/epinephrine and collagen/ADP) within the same run.
3. Mix the blood sample by gentle inversion three to four times and pipet 0.8 mL of blood into the front small opening (the sample reservoir) of each test cartridge (*see* **Fig. 1**). Pipetting is performed slowly and against one of the inside corners of the opening to prevent trapping of air bubbles below the blood in the sample reservoir.
4. Lower the cassette into position within the carousel and push down to ensure that the cartridges are even with the carousel surface. It is also important that the test be performed as soon as possible after the blood is pipetted into the cartridges to avoid sedimentation of the blood cells.

5. Press the "Run" softkey and the machine automatically performs the test.
6. After the test, remove and discard the cartridges.
7. A sample printout is shown in **Fig. 4**. Volume (μL) and flow rate (μL/min) are plotted against time. As shown, time is on the vertical axis and increases from top to bottom of the trace. Also printed are the sample identification number, the cartridge or test type, whether it is sample A or B, the closure time (seconds), total volume (μL), and the initial flow rate (μL/min). The maximum closure time that can be given is 300 s.

Note: Only closure time results are included on the standard printout. Volume, flow rate, and the plot against time are seen in an experimental mode and are not commercially available.

3.5. Status Messages

The instrument will flag various status codes, depending on the nature of a particular condition occurring during a test run (for a complete list see the PFA-100 operating manual). The most common of these that can occur during testing are listed below. The instrument will usually stop the test and flag a greater-than symbol (>) followed by the time of the result with appropriate status codes and messages as shown below:

A—Maximum test time exceeded; >300 s.
B—Test terminated due to air leak.
C—Test terminated due to flow obstruction.
D—Test terminated due to insufficient sample.
E —Test terminated due to maximum syringe travel being reached.

3.6. Controls

For the purposes of quality control testing, a control donor group within each laboratory setting should be established. These individuals should ideally exhibit closure times (CTs) within the middle of the established laboratory reference ranges, be free from any medication known to affect platelet function, and exhibit duplicate CTs less than or equal to 15% on the collagen/epinephrine cartridge. It is also recommended that one of these normal control donors be tested alongside test samples using the same batches of cartridges. If the CT falls outside of the reference range, a second test should be performed with another normal donor. If the second result is abnormal then the user should contact technical services. In a similar fashion, new cartridge lots should also be tested with duplicates of samples from the control donor group. Repeat testing should again be performed with another normal donor if the results fall outside the reference range. If the results are abnormal again, the new cartridge lots are suspected and the user should contact technical services.

3.7. Normal Ranges

Each laboratory should always establish its own reference ranges on both cartridge types utilizing normal volunteers from its institution. These individuals should have no previous personal or family history of bleeding or bruising, they should not be taking any drugs that may interfere with platelet function, and previous laboratory investigations into platelet function and von Willebrand factor parameters should all be normal. Normal ranges should be tested on blood samples taken into the identical citrate anticoagulant that is used within the user's institution, i.e., either 3.8% (0.129 *M*) or 3.2% (0.105 *M*) buffered trisodium citrate. Typical normal ranges obtained with 3.8% trisodium citrate are 58–151 s for collagen/ADP and 94–202 s for collagen/epinephrine. With 3.2% trisodium citrate, typical ranges are 55–112 s for collagen/ADP and 79–164 s for collagen/epinephrine (2002 reference range from the Oxford Haemophilia Centre).

3.8. Interpretation of Results

1. Results are reported as the closure time in seconds. Results should be used to aid in detection of platelet dysfunction and not directly for diagnosis. Users should be cautious in interpreting results. CTs above the normal ranges (*see* **Subheading 3.7.**) indicate platelet dysfunction and that possible further diagnostic workup is required. CTs below the normal ranges may indicate the presence of hyperfunctional platelets. When utilized in a diagnostic algorithm, the PFA-100 test should always be evaluated in conjunction with the full clinical and family history of the patient (including knowledge of all drugs/medication that the patient has been taking) and other laboratory tests of clotting and platelet function. Repeat tests a few weeks apart are often advisable to exclude possible transitory acquired defects (e.g., from diet or drugs).

2. The maximum closure time is 300 s. If the test goes beyond this point the instrument displays >300 s as the CT.

3. A full blood count should always be conducted in parallel with the test so that results can be interpreted with respect to potential thrombocytopenia and anemia. For further details on platelet counting, see Chapter 3. Platelet counts <100×10^9/L and hematocrits <30% may result in prolongation of the CTs.

4. Results within the normal ranges suggest that platelet aggregometry and vWF parameters will be normal. However a small number of platelet-function defects (e.g., storage pool disease, Type I VWD, Factor V Quebec, and platelet release defects), as assessed by other methods such as aggregometry, can sometimes give normal results on both cartridges. Conversely, prolonged CTs will sometimes occur in a small number of patients with normal platelet function as measured by aggregometry or other low-shear methods.

5. If the CT test results are very prolonged or beyond the maximum value (300 s) then this usually signifies a severe hemostatic defect (e.g., Glanzmann's thrombasthenia, Bernard Soulier syndrome (BSS), or von Willebrand's disease).

6. If the test results give a normal collagen/ADP CT and prolonged collagen/EPI CT (often >300 s) then this typically indicates a deficiency in thromboxane generation (e.g., caused by aspirin ingestion). However, patients with dense granular storage and/or release defects can also present with this pattern.

7. Some samples have been observed to give a normal collagen/EPI CT and a prolonged collagen/ADP CT. Little is known about the actual incidence of this, although ingestion of cocoa-containing substances has been reported to produce this pattern *(5)*.

8. For further interpretation of results and utility of the PFA-100 see the recent review articles by Jilma *(6)*, Favaloro *(7,8)*, and Francis *(9)*.

4. Notes

1. All PFA-100 samples should be taken into siliconized evacuated tubes containing buffered 0.105 *M* (3.2%) trisodium citrate. Alternatively, 0.129 *M* (3.8%) tubes can be used

providing that normal ranges have been established using the same anticoagulant. The use of unbuffered citrate tubes is not recommended, as the instrument will flag a much higher incidence of premature closure times when performing the test *(10)*.

2. O-ring cleaning and replacement procedure (N.B. wear gloves, as the O-ring is in contact with blood and can have dried blood residues): From the "System Ready" display, select "menus" option, followed by the "maintenance" option and "remove O-ring" option. The system will display "Load O-ring service tool, then press continue." Place the O-ring service tool into the incubation wells of the carousel and then press "continue." The instrument then removes the O-ring and deposits it within position A and rotates back after about 30 s, allowing removal of the O-ring by inversion of the tool. If the O-ring is not removed then the operation should be repeated, but if the instrument consistently fails to do this then contact the service department. Remove the O-ring and rinse under cold tap water. Inspect for debris and cracks and replace if necessary. Otherwise, shake off the excess water and soak in 70% isopropanol for 15 s. Shake off excess isopropanol and reinstall. When reinstalling, minimize debris or dirt contact with the O-ring by storing the tool within the plastic packaging and checking the cleanliness of position B before use. To install the O-ring, select "Install O-ring" on the "maintenance" menu. The system will then display "Load O-ring service tool, then press continue." Load the O-ring into position B of the service tool and place it into the incubation wells of the carousel holder. Press "continue" and the instrument will rotate the O-ring into position and install it. After 30 s the carousel rotates to allow removal of the tool and the O-ring will have been installed. To ensure that the O-ring is functional, perform a self-test as described in **Subheading 3.2.**

References

1. Harrison, P. (2000) Progress in the assessment of platelet function. *Br. J. Haematol.* **111,** 733–744.
2. Kratzer, M. A. A. and Born, G. V. R. (1985) Simulation of primary hemostasis in vitro. *Haemostasis* **5,** 357–362.
3. Kundu, S. K., Heilmann, E. J., Sio, R., Garcia, C., and Ostgaard, R. A. (1996) Characterization of an in vitro platelet function analyser, PFA-100®. *Clin. Appl. Thromb. Haemost.* **2(4),** 241–249.
4. Kundu, S. K., Heilmann, E. J., Sio, R., Garcia, C., Davidson, R. M., and Ostgaard, R. A. (1995) Description of an in vitro platelet function analyzer—PFA-100. *Semin. Thromb. Haemost.* **21(Suppl. 2),** 106–112.
5. Holt, R. R., Schramm, D. D., Keen, C. L., Lazarus, S. A., and Schmitz, H. H. (2002) Chocolate consumption and platelet function. *JAMA* **287,** 2212–2213.
6. Jilma, B. (2001) Platelet function analyzer (PFA-100®): a tool to quantify congenital or acquired platelet dysfunction. *J. Lab. Clin. Med.* **138,** 152–163.
7. Favaloro, E. J. (2001) Utility of the PFA-100R for assessing bleeding disorders and monitoring therapy: a review of analytical variables, benefits and limitations. *Haemophilia* **7(2),** 170–179.
8. Favaloro, E. J. (2002) Clinical application of the PFA-100. *Curr. Opin. Hematol.* **9(5),** 407–415.
9. Francis, J. L. (2002) Platelet Function Analyzer (PFA)-100. In: *Platelets*, Michelson, A., ed. Academic Press, pp. 325–335.
10. Heilmann, E., Kundu, S., Sio, R., Garcia, C., Gomez, R., and Christie, D. (1997) Comparison of four commercial citrate blood collection systems for platelet function analysis by the PFA-100®. *Thromb. Res.* **87,** 159–164.

19

Flow-Cytometric Analysis of Platelet-Membrane Glycoprotein Expression and Platelet Activation

Alison H. Goodall and Jackie Appleby

1. Introduction

Flow-cytometric measurement of platelet-surface glycoproteins in unfixed whole blood is a sensitive and quantitative approach that offers many advantages over other methods of platelet analysis for the following reasons:

- It enables simultaneous analysis of multiple aspects of platelet biology to be conducted on large numbers of single platelets in a short time.
- Analysis can be carried out in whole blood, making sample preparation rapid and relatively simple and reducing in vitro handling artifacts.
- It enables 100% of the platelet population to be studied, including giant platelets, platelet-derived microparticles, and platelet-leukocyte aggregates.
- Analysis of unfixed blood samples allows investigation of the platelet response to agonist stimulation.
- Whole blood analysis means that platelets are studied in autologous plasma and in the presence of the other blood cells, which can contribute to the overall platelet response through and the release of soluble mediators.

The use of flow cytometry in the study of platelets has been extensively reviewed (for example, *1–3*).

1.1. Flow Cytometry

Flow cytometry (for a practical handbook, *see* **ref. *4***) allows the rapid analysis of many thousands of individual cells per second as they pass through the focused beam of a laser light source (**Fig. 1**). Reflected or refracted light is detected by photodiodes or photomultiplier tubes and translated into an electronic signal, which represents a measure of the cells' size and granularity, respectively. This allows discrimination of different cell types with distinct morphological characteristics within a complex mixture such as whole blood, thus enabling analysis of the platelets without the need for separation from the

From: *Methods in Molecular Biology, vol. 272:*
Platelets and Megakaryocytes, Vol. 1: Functional Assays
Edited by: J. M. Gibbins and M. P. Mahaut-Smith © Humana Press Inc., Totowa, NJ

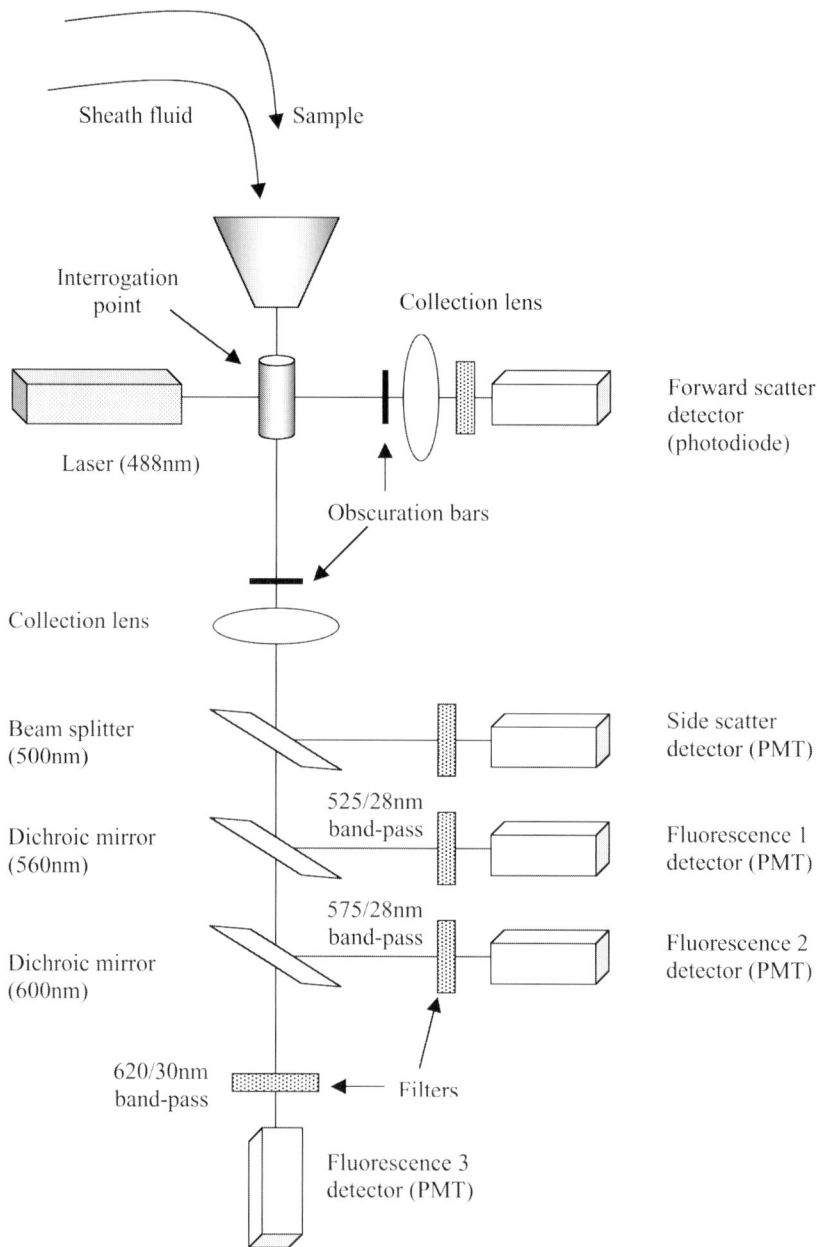

Fig. 1. Simplified schematic diagram of a flow cytometer. Sheath fluid is added with the sample to focus the fluid stream and ensure that the particles in the sample pass through the beam one at a time. The beam splitter reflects 10% of light to the side scatter detector and the remaining light to fluorescence channels. Beam splitters and dichroic mirrors reflect light below a specific wavelength, allowing light above that wavelength to pass through. Emission filters normally have bandwidth of 28–30 nm.

Table 1
Fluorochromes Commonly Used in Flow-Cytometric Analysis of Platelets

Fluorochrome	Peak excitation wavelength (nm)	Peak 3 emission wavelength (nm)
Fluorescein isothiocyanate (FITC)	495	520
Rhodamine-phycoerythrin (RPE)	495	576
Rhodamine-phycoerythrin-Cy5 (RPE-Cy5)	495	670

other blood cells. If the blood sample has been preincubated with fluorescently labeled antibodies that recognize antigens on the platelet surface, the fluorophore is excited as the platelets pass through the focused beam of the laser and emits fluorescence at a characteristic wavelength. This is detected in the flow cytometer by photomultiplier tubes and translated into an electronic signal that is directly proportional to the number of fluorescent antibody molecules on each cell, and thus to the number of antigens on each platelet. Modern flow cytometers normally have three or four such photomultiplier tubes, each set to detect fluorescence of different wavelengths by means of selective dichroic mirrors and filters. Thus, combinations of antibodies coupled to fluorophores with different emission spectra enable simultaneous analysis of a number of antigens on the same platelet, or selective gating of the cells of interest. The characteristics of the fluorochromes listed in this chapter are given in **Table 1**, but antibodies coupled to others are commercially available.

Directly conjugated reagents are preferred, as they provide a straightforward relationship between fluorescence and antigen density. Indirect methods can be used, in which antigens are identified with unlabeled primary monoclonal antibodies (MAbs), which are then identified with fluorescently labeled, isotype-specific secondary antibodies. This has the advantage of giving amplification of the fluorescence signal, but it may make precise quantification more complex. However, a well-standardized indirect technique can provide a very sensitive method for detecting antigens expressed at low density.

Fluorescence measurement can be expressed either as the percentage of positive cells above a threshold set with an appropriate negative control, or as the mean or median fluorescence intensity (MFI) of a population of cells; the median is the more appropriate measure for an antigen that shows a non-Gaussian, or heterogeneous, distribution on the platelet population. Percentage positive data are used primarily to measure increased expression of an antigen that is not normally present on the platelet surface (e.g., an activation antigen), or to discriminate between populations of cells, whereas MFI is used to quantify the level of expression of an antigen that is constitutively expressed. The MFI provides an arbitrary figure, but comparative studies have demonstrated a linear relationship between the binding of a fluorescently labeled antibody and conventional I^{125} binding assays *(5,6)*. This can be translated into a more precise measurement by incorporating calibrated fluorescent standards (e.g., Quantum, Sigma-Aldrich) and appropriate software to convert arbitrary fluorescent units into mean equivalent soluble fluorochrome (MESF). In addition, there are now commercially available kits that give an absolute number of antibody molecules bound to the

Table 2
Applications of Flow-Cytometric Analysis of Platelets

Diagnosis of congenital and acquired platelet defects:
- Glanzmann's thrombocytopenia (deficiency in GPIIb-IIIa)
- Bernard-Soulier syndrome (deficiency in GPIb-IX-V)
- Collagen response defects (deficiency in GPIa-IIa or GPVI)
- Gray platelet syndrome (deficiency in P-selectin)
- Heparin-induced thrombocytopenia

Platelet activation in vivo:
- Activation-dependent platelet antigens
- Platelet-platelet and platelet-leukocyte aggregates
- Procoagulant microparticles

Blood transfusion:
- Monitoring platelet concentrates
- Detection of platelet-associated Ig
- Immunophenotyping of platelet alloantigens (HPA)

Platelet turnover studies:
- Platelet counting
- Detection of reticulated platelets

platelets (e.g., Biocytex, Marseille, France; Quantum Simply Cellular Microbeads Kit, Sigma-Aldrich, St. Louis, MO). The limit of antigen detection is generally calculated to be ≥500 molecules per platelet.

There are increasing numbers of applications for flow-cytometric investigation of platelets (**Table 2**), but in this chapter we will deal with two basic aspects of platelet biology that can be studied using essentially the same methodology.

1.2. Expression of Platelet-Membrane Glycoproteins

Flow cytometry is an accurate method for detecting and enumerating constitutively expressed platelet membrane glycoproteins. The method can form part of a routine laboratory screening program for the diagnosis of patients with congenital platelet defects, such as Glanzmann's thrombasthenia (GT; deficiency in the GPIIb-IIIa complex) and Bernard-Soulier syndrome (BSS; deficiency in the GPIb-IX-V complex), to give a clear diagnosis of patients with severe, homozygous defects. Levels of receptors can also be measured in relation to gene polymorphisms and platelet function. For example, levels of the collagen adhesion receptor, GPIa-IIa *(7)*, and agonist receptor GPVI have each shown a gene-dose relationship with specific polymorphisms *(8)*. Any of the constitutively expressed platelet-adhesion or agonist receptors can be measured in this way, provided they are present at a high enough density to reach the level of detection by flow cytometry.

Measurement of glycoproteins on platelets can be carried out by single-color analysis (illustrated in **Fig. 2**) in which the platelets are identified solely on the basis of their forward scatter (FS, a measure of cell size) and side scatter (SS, a measure of cell

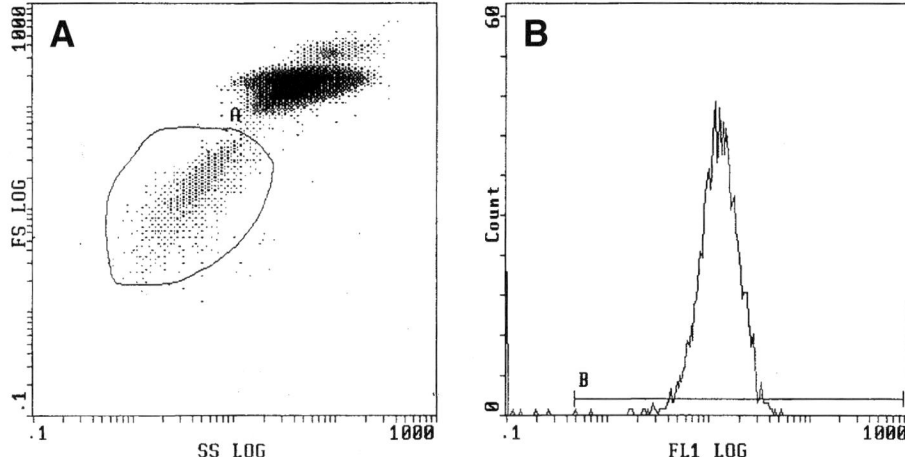

Fig. 2. Example of flow-cytometric analysis of the constitutive platelet-membrane glycoprotein GPIbα. (**A**) Whole blood samples incubated with FITC-conjugated anti-GPIbα antibody and analyzed by side scatter (SS; *x* axis) and forward scatter (FS; *y* axis). Platelets are identified in electronic gate "A." The large population of cells to the top right of the platelet population in histogram 1 are red cells and those with the highest FS signal are leukocytes. (**B**) Histogram of the fluorescence (FL1; 488 nm excitation, 520 emission) particles from gate A.

granularity), then analyzed for antigen expression. This approach has the advantage of simplicity and economy, and for many applications is the method of choice. However, to ensure that all platelets are identified, and more importantly, to ensure that any platelet-sized particles derived from other cells are eliminated from the analysis, a two-color approach can be used. In this case the sample is co-labeled with an antibody to a highly expressed, platelet-specific antigen and an antibody to the antigen being studied. The two antibodies are labeled with different fluorophores. The pan-platelet markers of choice are usually either the GPIIb-IIIa complex, or GPIbα or GPIX, the latter being theoretically preferred as it is neither cleaved by proteases such as thrombin, nor directly involved in ligand binding. Two-color analysis is particularly important if the platelets being investigated fall outside the normal platelet size range, for example, when analyzing samples from patients with giant platelet conditions such as BSS or some storage pool disorders, since the FS and SS characteristics of these platelets can take them into the red-cell region of the flow-cytometric profile. When a single-color method is used, the identity of events in the platelet gate should, in any case, be confirmed using a pan-platelet marker in a separately labeled sample.

1.3. Platelet Activation

Whole blood flow cytometry can also be used for the investigation of platelet activation through the expression of a variety of activation-dependent changes on the platelet

Table 3
Antigens on Platelets

Antigen			Antibodies	Refs
Platelet-membrane glycoproteins				
• GPIIb-IIIa	CD41/61		Y2/51	*57*
• GPIb-IX-V	CD42b/42a/42d		HIP1	*58*
			FMC 25	*59*
			V3	*60*
• GPIa-IIa	CD29/49b		AK-7	
			CLB-thromb/4	*61*
Platelet-activation antigens				
• Activation of GPIIb-IIIa:				
• Bound fibrinogen			rabbit α-fibrinogen	*19,20*
• Fibrinogen binding site			PAC-1	*22*
• RIBS			9F9	*1*
			2G5	*21*
			F26	*62*
• LIBS			LIBS1	*23*
			LIBS6	*63*
			PM1.1	*64*
• Degranulation:				
• P-selectin	α-granules	CD62P	AK-6	*65*
			CLB-thromb/6	*66*
• GP53	lysosomes/ dense granules	CD63	CLB-gran12	*25*
• LAMP-1	lysosomes	CD107a	H5G11	*67*
• LAMP-2	lysosomes	CD107b	H4B4	*68*
• CD40L			TRAP1	*69*

surface (**Table 3**) *(1,2)*. Flow cytometry is such a sensitive technique that even small changes in platelet activation status or responsiveness can be readily detected. This technique can be used to detect platelets that have been activated either in vivo (for example, in patients with thrombotic disease states *[9–11]*), ex vivo (for example, in stored platelet concentrates *[12,13]*), or within in vitro models of hemostasis *(14–16)*. In addition, the analysis of unfixed whole blood allows investigations of the responsiveness of platelets to agonists and antagonists in vitro and the study of antiplatelet drugs *(17,18)*.

1.3.1. Activation Markers on Single Platelets

Intracellular signals generated by physiological platelet agonists cause a conformational change in the platelet-membrane GPIIb-IIIa complex, opening up the receptor site for fibrinogen. This "final common pathway" of platelet activation, which results in platelet-platelet aggregation, can be considered an early marker of platelet activation, since it is induced by virtually all physiological platelet agonists. Activation of the GPIIb-IIIa receptor can be detected either by polyclonal antibodies that recognize fibrinogen (this chapter and *see* **refs.** *19,20*), or with MAbs to ligand-induced neo-epitopes on fibrinogen that are seen only when fibrinogen has bound to the GPIIb-IIIa receptor *(21)*. Activation of GPIIb-IIIa can also be detected with MAbs to neo-epitopes on the GPIIb-IIIa complex such as PAC-1 (Becton Dickinson 340507), which recognizes the fibrinogen-binding site and therefore binds only to activated platelets *(22)*, or with MABs to occupancy-dependent, ligand-induced binding sites (LIBS) *(23)* on GPIIb-IIIa.

Platelet activation can also result in degranulation, which leads to exposure of platelet granule membranes, and their associated antigens, to the outside of the cell **(Table 3)**. Of these the CD62P (P-selectin, GMP-140, PADGEM) antigen of the α-granule membrane has been studied the most, as well as being the most highly expressed *(24)*. Other markers of degranulated platelets that have been used to measure activation of single platelets are listed in **Table 3**. These include the CD63 (GP53) antigen of lysosome/dense-granule membranes *(25)* and changes in the absolute levels of GPIIb-IIIa (which increase by up to 50% as intracellular pools of the complex are revealed), or of the GPIb-V-IX complex, which can fall by 20–30% due to internalization of this receptor to intracellular membranes *(26)*.

1.3.2. Platelet-Leukocyte Aggregates

Expression of P-selectin on the platelet surface initiates interaction with its counter-receptor, PSGL-1, on leukocytes to form platelet-leukocyte aggregates *(27)*. This interaction occurs rapidly in vivo, resulting in loss of p-selectin positive platelets *(28)*. It is becoming widely appreciated that platelet-leukocyte aggregates are probably a better marker of platelet activation in vivo than P-selectin-positive platelets *(29)*. These conjugates can be detected by flow cytometry using a two-color analysis **(Fig. 3)** in which the leukocyte population is identified by means of their FS and SS characteristics. The major leukocyte subsets can be further discriminated with either a pan-leukocyte marker (usually CD45) or a specific marker to a particular leukocyte cell type (e.g., monocytes, identified with a CD14 MAb). Alternatively, leukocytes can be identified initially by positivity for a pan- or specific leukocyte marker and then further discriminated by their FS/SS characteristics *(11,29–31)*. Platelets bound to the leukocytes are identified with a pan-platelet marker to calculate the percentage of leukocytes with bound platelets, normally using MAbs to either GPIbα or GPIX. Antibodies to GPIIb-IIIa or P-selectin are best avoided, since these antigens participate in bridging the two cell types, potentially blocking access to the epitopes recognized by the MAbs. Measurement of platelet antigens on platelet-leukocyte aggregates is not recommended, as the number of individual platelets bound per leukocyte may vary.

1.3.3. Procoagulant Microparticles

Under some conditions, following stimulation with strong platelet agonists such as collagen and thrombin, the phospholipids of the platelet plasma membrane can undergo reorientation, leading to a translocation of negatively charged phospholipids (predominantly phosphatidylserine, PS) to the outer leaflet of the bilayer *(32)*. This movement (often termed "flip-flop") *(33)* is accompanied by budding of small, negatively charged

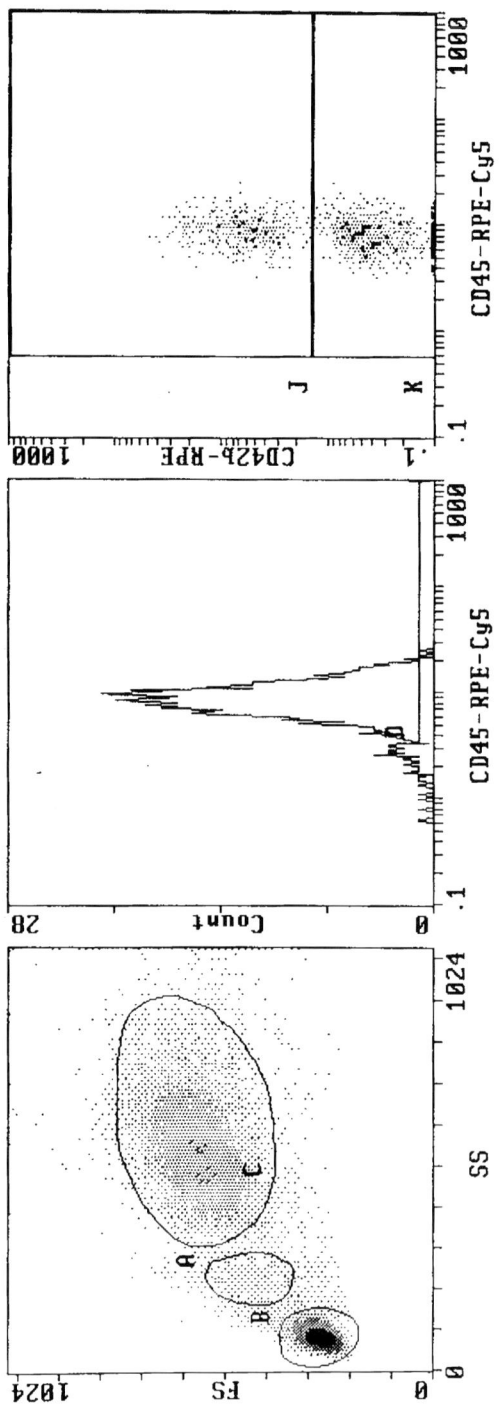

Fig. 3. Flow cytometric analysis of platelet-leukocyte aggregates. Whole blood has been incubated with RPE-Cy5-conjugated CD45 (anti-leukocyte) antibody and RPE-conjugated anti-GPIbα (CD42b) antibody. Leukocyte populations are identified by SS/FS characteristics (left-hand histogram). Cells in gate "A" are monocytes, those in gate "B" are lymphocytes, and those in gate "C" are granulocytes. Leukocyte populations (in this example, the monocytes) are then analyzed for expression of CD45 antigen by single-color (FL4) analysis (gate "D"), shown in the center histogram. In the right-hand histogram the CD45-positive monocytes are then put through a two-color analysis to separate the GPIbα-positive particles (seen in the top gate "J") from the GPIb-negative monocytes (gate "K"). The cells in gate "J" represent monocyte-platelet aggregates. Data can be represented as the percentage of monocytes with attached platelets. This sample is from blood in which the platelets have been partially activated.

membrane vesicles (microparticles). These changes can also be induced by elevating the level of intracellular calcium using A23187 or C5b (*33–35*). The negatively charged surface allows the tenase (FVIIIa.FIXa) and prothrombinase (FVa.FXa.) complexes to bind and results in the generation of thrombin at the platelet surface (*34*). These changes can be measured in the flow cytometer by the presence of the various coagulation proteins on the platelet surface (*35*) or by using fluorescently conjugated annexin V, which binds preferentially to negatively charged phospholipids (*36*). Annexin V binding, together with cell size (FS), can be used to identify and quantify the number of procoagulant microparticles in a whole blood sample. A two-color approach is recommended, in which platelets and platelet-derived microparticles are identified with a pan-platelet marker (e.g., GPIbα) and then subjected to a two-parameter analysis for annexin V fluorescence and forward scatter (size) as illustrated in **Fig. 4**. Methods based on discrimination by particle size alone are less satisfactory as there is no clear cut-off between platelets and microparticles, and under some conditions platelet-sized particles can express a procoagulant surface.

1.4. Platelet Responses to Agonist Stimulation

Agonist stimulation can be used to measure platelet responsiveness in samples from different individuals, to assess the effects of antiplatelet drugs in vivo and in vitro, or to study a wide range of aspects of platelet biology. Of the physiological agonists, ADP gives good activation of GPIIb-IIIa, but minimal degranulation (*37*). ADP induces significant degranulation only if the platelets are allowed to aggregate, leading to generation of thromboxane, which then acts through specific surface receptors to induce platelet degranulation. Since flow-cytometric methods are designed to avoid platelet-platelet aggregation, relatively little degranulation is observed in response to ADP. Strong agonists, such as thrombin and collagen, can induce platelet degranulation in the absence of aggregation. If thrombin is added to whole blood samples it will also cleave fibrinogen and other coagulation proteins, leading to cross-linked fibrin and, therefore, clotting. A synthetic peptide analog of the fibrin-fibrin recognition site, GPRP (glycine-proline-arginine-proline), should be included in the incubation mixture to prevent clotting (*38*). Alternatively, platelets can be activated by peptides that act directly on the PAR-1 (SFLLRN or TRAP) (*39*) or PAR-4 (GYPGKF) (*40*) thrombin receptors. These methods are described below. Examples of flow-cytometric images of maximum P-selectin expression in response to ADP and TRAP are shown in **Fig. 5A**, and typical concentration-response curves for ADP, thrombin, and TRAP are shown in **Fig. 5B**.

Other agonists can also be used. Fibrillar collagen presents problems for flow cytometry as it cross-links and therefore aggregates the platelets, but synthetic peptide analogs of the agonist-receptor binding site on collagen have been generated and used very successfully in flow-cytometric studies. These are not commercially available (although they can be synthesized using published sequences *[41]*) and their use will not be covered in this chapter. Platelets can be activated via the thromboxane pathway using either a synthetic thromboxane analog (e.g., U46619; Calbiochem 538944) or with arachidonic acid (Sigma; A8798). Epinephrine can also be used to stimulate the platelets. However, it should be noted that the concentrations of epinephrine that have

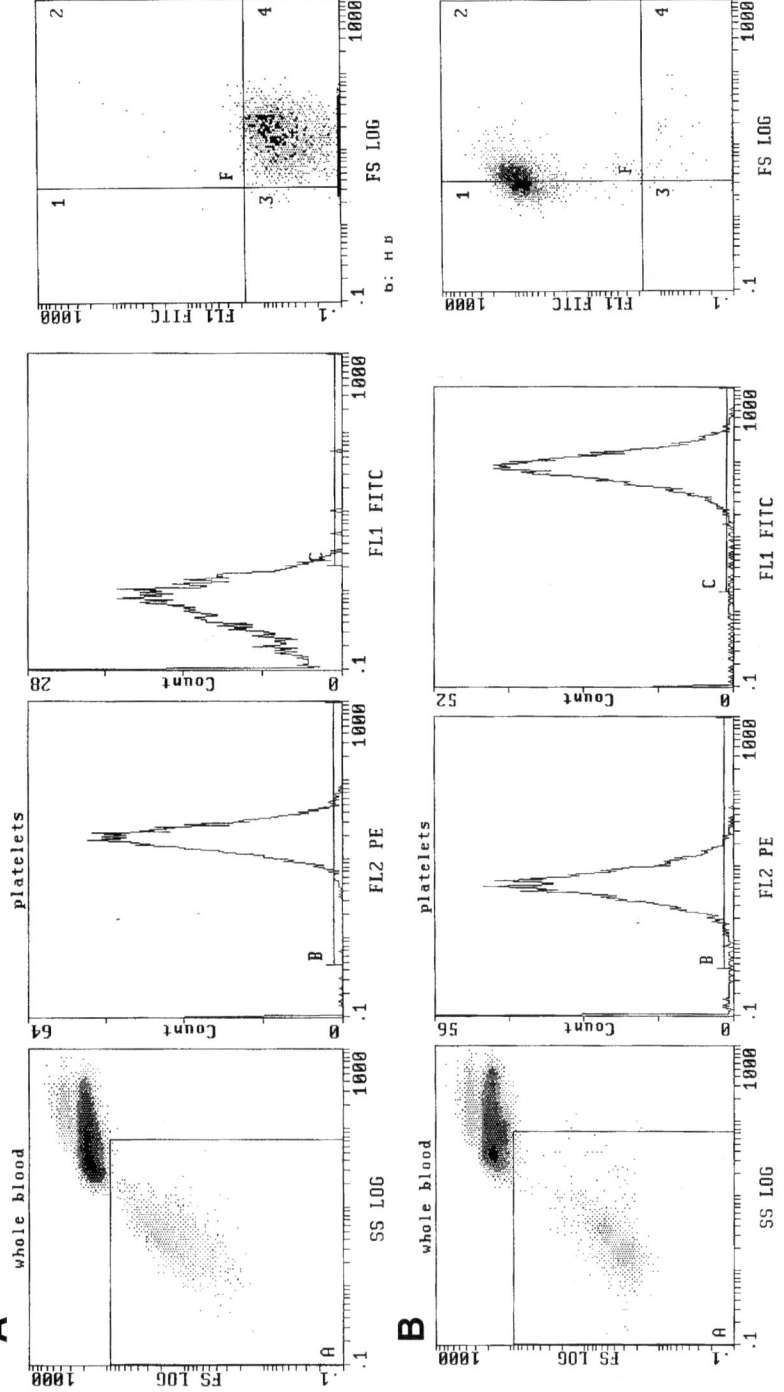

been traditionally used as a platelet agonist (i.e., in the μ*M* range) are not physiologically relevant. Levels of epinephrine do not normally rise above the n*M* range in vivo. At these concentrations epinephrine does not have a significant effect on platelets, but does potentiate the effects of other agonists *(42,43)*.

1.5. Disadvantages of Flow-Cytometric Analysis of Platelets

While whole blood flow cytometric analysis of platelets is a powerful research and diagnostic tool, there are some disadvantages. From a practical perspective, the need for rapid and careful sample preparation and the need for ready access to a flow cytometer make it a demanding technique. Fluorescently labeled antibodies are relatively costly, as is the purchase and maintenance of a flow cytometer. From a mechanistic viewpoint the technique is primarily limited to the analysis of single cells and thus to aggregation-independent (and thromboxane-independent) platelet activation *(44,45)*.

1.6. Sample Preparation

Although there are various standardized methods in the literature *(46–48)*, differences remain. Those given here are based on our experience over the past 15 yr. For all applications the same basic approach to sample preparation can be used, based on methods developed in the 1980s *(6,49–51)*. Simple dilution of the blood is followed by incubation with appropriate antibodies, followed by a final dilution/fixation step before analysis in the flow cytometer. Where appropriate, agonists or inhibitors can be included in the incubation mixture. **Figure 6** illustrates a generalized flow diagram for the basic methodology.

Although sample preparation is relatively simple, great care is needed, perhaps even more than with many other platelet methods, to ensure that the platelets do not become activated, aggregated, or in any way altered during sample processing. The key points are:

Fig. 4. *(see opposite page)* Dual-color flow-cytometric analysis of platelet-derived procoagulant microparticles. Whole blood has been incubated with RPE-conjugated anti-GPIbα and FITC-conjugated Annexin V. Platelets and microparticles are identified by SS/FS. A larger gate ("A") is set to include all platelets and microparticles which are then analyzed for expression of GPIbα (gate "B"). GPIbα positive particles are then analyzed for binding of Annexin V, a marker of negatively charged, anionic phospholipids. Two-parameter analysis of size (FS) against Annexin V binding (FL1) is illustrated in the final figures. **(A)** shows untreated blood. Platelets in gate "A" are of normal size, express GPIbα, and show little reactivity with Annexin V. Two-parameter analysis illustrates a fairly uniform population of Annexin V-negative cells. **(B)** shows blood treated with 4 μ*M* A23187. The particles in gate "A" are much smaller than platelets but express GPIbα, albeit at lower density, as shown by the lower FL2 value, and reflecting their smaller size. These GPIbα-positive microparticles bind Annexin V very strongly as shown by the high FL1 signal. Two-parameter analysis illustrates a population of Annexin V-positive cells with a lower FS than intact platelets.

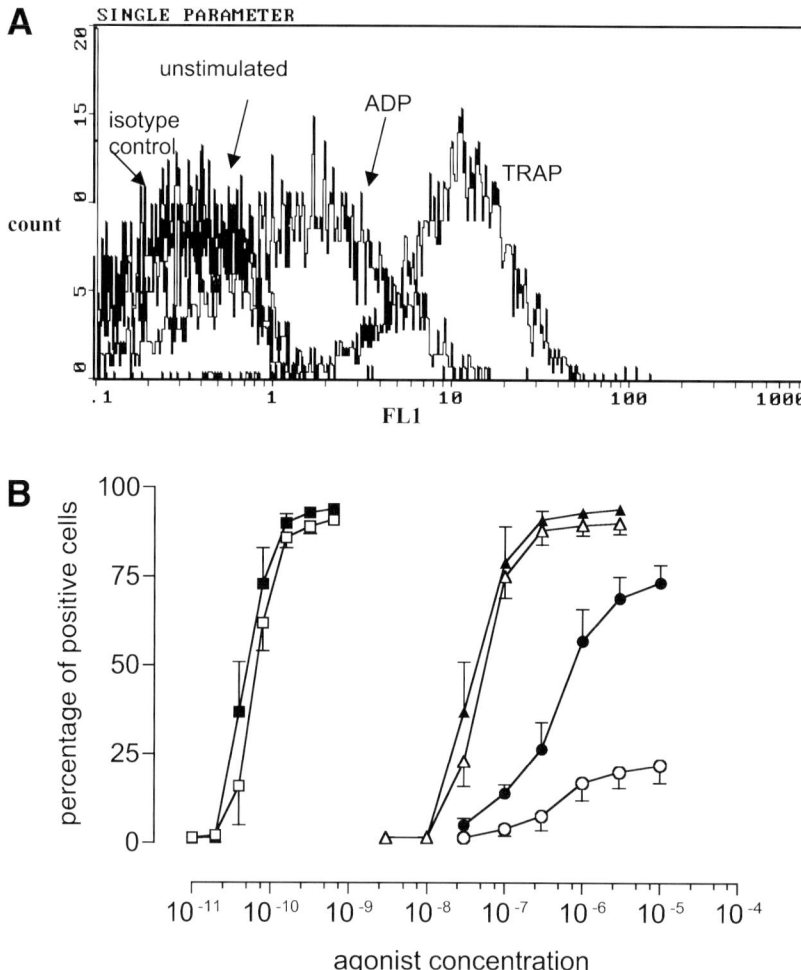

Fig. 5. Single-color analysis of P-selectin expression on platelets. Whole blood has been incubated with FITC-conjugated anti-P-selectin antibody. Platelets are identified by SS/FS characteristics and then analyzed for expression of P-selectin. **(A)** Results are shown for the isotype control and anti-P-selectin antibody on unstimulated platelets, platelets stimulated by a maximal concentration of ADP (1×10^{-5} M) and platelets stimulated by a maximal concentration of TRAP (1×10^{-4} M). **(B)** Dose-response curves for fibrinogen binding to activated GPIIb-IIIa (closed symbols) and P-selectin expression (open symbols) in platelets stimulated with thrombin (squares), TRAP (triangles), or ADP (circles). Data shown represent the mean ± s.d. from 10 normal healthy male subjects. Although thrombin is a much more potent agonist than TRAP—here generating the same effect at 3 orders of magnitude lower concentration (*see* **Note 15**)—the extent of P-selectin expression and fibrinogen binding are very similar at each dose of thrombin or TRAP, both reaching a maximum of >90% positivity with both agonists. ADP is a weaker agonist, producing fibrinogen binding on a maximum of approx 70–80% of platelets and generating P-selectin expression on a maximum of only approx 20–25% of platelets *(37)*.

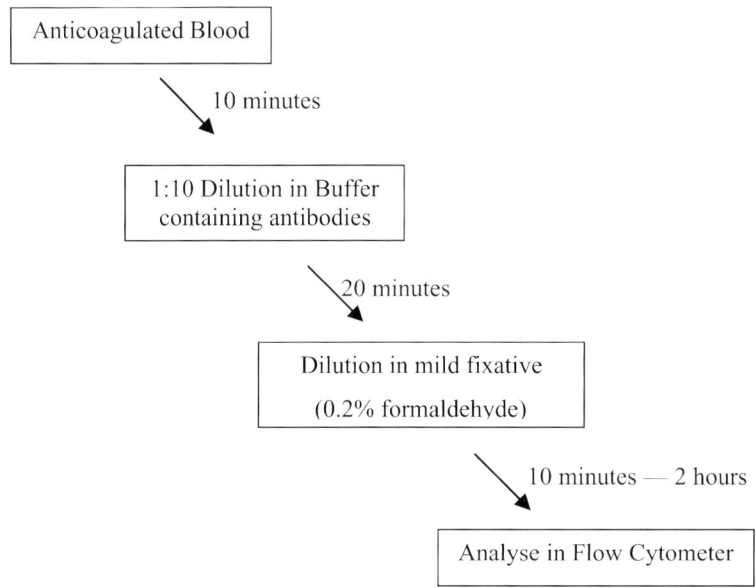

Fig. 6. Simplified flow diagram of the general method for preparing samples for whole blood flow cytometry.

- Good phlebotomy, to avoid artifactual activation of the platelets (*see* **Note 1**).
- Rapid sample processing, to avoid changes occurring in the platelets prior to analysis (*see* **Note 2**).
- Minimal sample manipulation, to avoid activation and loss of platelets (*see* **Note 3**).
- Choice of antibodies; it is important that antibody batches are checked and standardized.
- Incubation conditions designed to maximize antibody binding and minimize in vitro artifacts (*see* **Note 4**).
- Final fixation/dilution step to reduce any further platelet changes and to produce a cell suspension of an appropriate concentration for analysis in the flow cytometer (*see* **Note 5**).

1.7. Flow Cytometry

This chapter is written with the assumption that the reader has some knowledge of flow cytometry, or access to this expertise. For further information, the reader is directed to the manufacturers' guidelines or a suitable textbook (e.g., **ref. 4**). Protocols for analysis should be established before running samples. The approach given in **Subheading 3.** is based on the use of a Beckman Coulter® EPICS® (Miami, FL) XL-MCL instrument. Other manufacturers' instruments use postacquisition analysis of the samples but the principles are the same. Precise flow cytometry settings for an instrument have not been given, as they vary; the reader is advised to consult the manufacturer for specific guidance in setting up the protocols.

Some points will be common to all instruments:

- Acquisition: Because of their small size, logarithmic FS and SS acquisition is recommended for platelets. Linear FS and SS acquisition is preferred for discrimination of leukocyte subsets, which are similar in size.
- Discriminators allow data collection above a specified threshold; these should be set on the primary acquisition parameter (usually FS) to eliminate unnecessary electronic noise. Because of the small size of platelets and microparticles, a low-level discriminator should be set when identifying them by FS/SS. A higher discriminator setting is recommended for identification of leukocytes.
- Gating: Electronic gating is used (1) to identify cell populations by means of forward scatter (FS) and side scatter (SS) characteristics (i.e., by size and granularity, respectively) or by fluorescence and (2) to quantify antigen expression on the cells. Examples of a logical approach to gating have been shown in **Figs. 2–4** but other approaches can be used.
- Color compensation: This needs to be set for each type of fluorescent antibody used in multicolor analysis methods. Samples for each color should be analyzed separately and color compensation adjusted to reduce or eliminate leakage of one channel into another, without significantly reducing the positive signal. The need for color compensation can be reduced by using fluorochromes with as little overlap as possible in their emission spectra, many of which have become available in the last few years. A helpful guide to fluorochromes can be found on the Molecular Probes web site (http://www.probes.com).

Readers should also note that the methods and analyses described in this chapter are designed for the detection of antigens on human platelets and leukocytes. For details of recommended parameters and antibodies for the study of mouse cells, please refer to Chapter 20, vol. 1.

2. Materials

2.1. Blood Collection and Processing

1. Siliconized glass blood collection tubes containing 1 tenth volume trisodium citrate (3.2% w/v) (BD Vacutainer™, Franklin Lakes, NJ; 367691) (*see* **Note 6**).
2. 21-gauge butterfly needles (BD Vacutainer Systems; 367282) (*see* **Note 7**).
3. Polystyrene LP2 tubes (12 × 75 mm) (Elkay Laboratory Products; Basingstoke, UK; 2052-001).

2.2. Equipment

1. Adjustable pipets with disposable tips.
2. Flow cytometer with a laser emission at 488 nm, capable of detecting particles of ≥0.5 μm, and at least two different fluorochromes with appropriate color compensation (*see* **Note 8**).
3. 2% (v/v) sodium hypochlorite.
4. A proprietary detergent cleaning solution (e.g., Clenz™, Beckman Coulter 8546930) (*see* **Note 8**).

2.3. Analysis of Platelet Membrane Glycoprotein Expression and Activation (see Note 9)

2.3.1. Method A (In-House Method)

1. HEPES-buffered saline (HBS): 150 mM NaCl, 5 mM KCl, 1 mM MgSO$_4$, 10 mM HEPES, pH 7.4 (NaOH) (*see* **Note 10**).
2. 0.2% Formyl saline: made by dilution of 37% formaldehyde solution (Sigma F1268) in 0.85% (w/v) NaCl (Sigma 430AG-4) (*see* **Note 11**).

Table 4A
Setting Up Assay Tubes for Single-Platelet Assays

| Reagent | For analysis of constitutive antigens | | For BSS Diagnosis | | | |
	Negative control	Receptor	FITC isotype	GPIIb-IIIa	RPE isotype	GPIbα analysis
Buffer	50 µL	50 µL	50 µL	50 µL	50 µL	50 µL
Negative control	FITC isotype control	—	FITC isotype control	—	RPE isotype control	—
Antibodies (volume determined by titration)	—	Anti-receptor MAb-FITC	—	Anti-GPIIb-IIIa-FITC	Anti-GPIIb-IIIa-FITC	Anti-GPIIB-IIIa-FITC + CD42b-RPE
Agonist (10X)	Optional	Optional	Optional	Optional	Optional	Optional
Whole blood	5 µL	5 µL	5 µL	5 µL	5 µL	5 µL

Table 4B
Setting Up Assay Tubes for Analysis of Platelet Activation Markers

| Reagent | Fibrinogen binding | | Degranulation (P-selectin, CD63, etc.) | |
	Negative control	Antigen	Negative control	Antigen
Buffer	50 µL HBS	50 µL HBS	50 µL HBS	50 µL HBS
GPRP (12.5 mg/mL)	2 µL (only if thrombin used as agonist)	2 µL (only if thrombin used as agonist)	2 µL (only if thrombin used as agonist)	2 µL (only if thrombin used as agonist)
Negative control	2 µL 6-mM EDTA	—	FITC isotype control	—
Antibodies (volume determined by titration)	Rabbit anti-fibrinogen-FITC	Rabbit anti-fibrinogen-FITC	—	FITC-conjugated anti-activation
Agonist (10X)	None	None ± ADP/TRAP/Thrombin	None	None + ADP/TRAP/Thrombin
Whole blood	5 µL	5 µL	5 µL	5 µL

Table 4C
Setting Up Assay Tubes for Analysis of Platelet-Leukocyte Aggregates

Reagent	RPE-Cy5 isotype control	RPE isotype control	Platelet-leukocyte aggregates
Buffer	50 µL HBS	50 µL HBS	50 µL HBS
Blocking CD62P mAb	9E1	9E1	9E1
Blocking mouse Ig	MOPC31C	MOPC31C	MOPC31C
Negative control	RPE-Cy5 isotype control	RPE-isotype control	—
Anti-leukocyte antibody	—	CD45-RPE-Cy5	CD45-RPE-Cy5
Anti-platelet antibody	CD42b-RPE	—	CD42b-RPE
Whole blood	50 µL	50 µL	50 µL

Table 4D
Setting Up Assay Tubes for Analysis of Procoagulant Platelet Microparticles

Reagent	Negative control	RPE Isotype control	Antigen	Positive control
Buffer	35 µL HBS	35 µL HBS/c	35 µL HBS/c	35 µL HBS/c
Hirudin (100 U/mL)	5 µL	5 µL	5 µL	5 µL
Negative control	—	RPE-Isotype control	—	—
Anti-platelet antibody	CD42b-RPE	—	CD42b-RPE	CD42b-RPE
Additional reagents	None	None	None	10 µM A23187
Whole blood	5 µL	5 µL	5 µL	5 µL
Annexin V-FITC	2 µL	—	2 µL	2 µL

HBS/c is HEPES buffered saline supplemented with 2 mM CaCl$_2$.

3. Antibodies (*see* **Note 12** and **Table 4A,B**):
   a. For single-color analysis of pan-platelet markers:
      CD41/61-FITC (anti-GPIIb-IIIa) (Dako, Glostruv, Denmark; Y2/51; F0803);
      CD29/49b-FITC (anti-GPIa-IIa) (Cytomation, BD Biosciences Pharmingen, San Jose, CA; AK-7; 555498);
      CD42b-FITC (anti-GPIbα) (BD Biosciences Pharmingen; HIP-1; 555472)
   b. For diagnosing BSS:
      CD41/61-FITC (anti-GPIIb-IIIa) (Y2/51 Dako; F0803);
      CD42b-RPE (anti-GPIbα). (BD Biosciences Pharmingen; HIP-1; 555473)
   c. Antibodies to platelet-activation antigens
      Rabbit anti-fibrinogen-FITC (Dako Cytomation; F0111);
      CD62P-FITC (anti-P-selectin) (Serotec; AK-6; MCA796F).
4. Isotype controls (*see* **Note 13**):
   MOPC21-FITC (Sigma; F6397);
   MOPC21-RPE (for BSS diagnosis) (BD Biosciences Pharmingen; 555749).

5. Agonists (*see* **Note 14**):
   a. ADP (Sigma; A6646): 10 m*M* stock in distilled water, which is diluted to 0.1 m*M*, 0.03 m*M*, 0.01 m*M*, 0.003 m*M*, and 0.001 m*M* stocks in HBS and stored in aliquots at –20°C or below (preferably below –40°C).
   b. Human α-thrombin (Sigma; T9135); 10 U/mL in distilled water, which is diluted to a range of concentrations between 3.2–0.2 U/mL in HBS (equivalent to 2–0.7×10^{-9} *M*) and stored at –20°C or below (preferably below –40°C).
   c. TRAP (**T**hrombin **R**eceptor **A**gonist **P**eptide; SFLLRN; Sigma; S7152 or Calbiochem, Darmstadt, Germany; 605208); 10 m*M* in distilled water then diluted to 1 m*M*, 0.3 m*M*, 0.1 m*M*, 0.03 m*M*, and 0.01 m*M* stocks in HBS and stored in aliquots at –20°C or below (preferably below –40°C) (*see* **Note 15**).
6. GPRP peptide (Sigma; G1895); 12.5 mg/mL made in HBS and stored in aliquots at –20°C or below (preferably below –40°C) (*see* **Notes 15** and **16**).
7. EDTA: 150 m*M* Na$_2$EDTA in distilled water (*see* **Note 17**).
8. Recombinant hirudin (Pentapharm 126-05; or Sigma H0393); 100 U/mL in distilled water. Stored in aliquots at –20°C or below (preferably below –40°C) (*see* **Note 18**).
9. Flow-Set™ fluorospheres (Beckman Coulter 6607007).
10. Flow-Check™ calibration fluorospheres (Beckman Coulter 6605359).

2.3.2. Method B

Platelet Gp Screen Kit (Biocytex; 7008) (*see* **Note 19**) consisting of: Diluent buffer (10X concentrate); anti-GPIIIa mAb (CD61); anti-GPIbα mAb (CD42b); anti-GPIa mAb (CD49b); calibrated beads coated with increasing, known concentrations of mouse IgG; polyclonal anti-mouse IgG-FITC.

2.4. Analysis of Platelet-Leukocyte Aggregates

1. HEPES-buffered saline (HBS): 150 m*M* NaCl, 5 m*M* KCl, 1 m*M* MgSO$_4$, 10 m*M* HEPES, pH 7.4 (NaOH).
2. Phosphate-buffered saline (PBS): (Dulbecco's PBS without calcium, without magnesium; Invitrogen Carlsbad, CA 14190-094).
3. Blocking CD62P mAb, e.g., 9E1 (R&D Systems, Minneapolis, MN; BBA30)—to prevent platelet-leukocyte aggregates forming in vitro during the incubation period (*see* **Note 20**).
4. Blocking mouse Ig, e.g., MOPC31C (Sigma M1398)—to block Fc-binding and nonspecific binding of the MAbs to leukocytes.
5. Antibodies (*see* **Note 12** and **Table 4B,C**):
   CD45-RPE-Cy5 (Dako Cytomation T29/33; C7099) (*see* **Note 21**);
   CD42b-RPE (Pharmingen 555473).
6. Isotype controls (*see* **Note 13**):
   RPE-Cy5 IgG1 (Dako Cytomation X0955);
   MOPC21-RPE isotype control (BD Biosciences Pharmingen 555749).
7. OptiLyse®C (Immunotech, Marseille, France 1401) (*see* **Note 22**).
8. TRAP (**T**hrombin **R**eceptor **A**gonist **P**eptide; SFLLRN); 1 m*M* in HBS, stored in aliquots at –20°C or below (preferably below –40°C) (*see* **Notes 15, 23**).

2.5. Analysis of Procoagulant Platelet Microparticles

1. HEPES-buffered saline (HBS): 150 m*M* NaCl, 5 m*M* KCl, 1 m*M* MgSO$_4$, 10 m*M* HEPES, pH 7.4 (NaOH).

2. HBS with 2 m*M* CaCl$_2$, pH 7.4 (NaOH) (HBS/c).
3. Recombinant hirudin (Pentapharm 126-05, or Sigma H0393); 100 U/mL in distilled water. Stored in aliquots at –20°C or below (preferably below –40°C) (*see* **Note 18**).
4. Calcium ionophore A23187 (Sigma C7522); 2 m*M* in DMSO. Stored in aliquots at 4°C (*see* **Note 24**).
5. Antibodies/reagents (*see* **Notes 9** and **12** and **Table 4D**):
    Annexin V-FITC (BD Biosciences Pharmingen 556419);
    CD42b-RPE (BD Biosciences Pharmingen 555473).
6. Isotype control: MOPC21-RPE isotype control (BD Biosciences Pharmingen 555749).

3. Methods
3.1. Blood Collection and Storage

1. Collect blood via a 21-G butterfly needle into Becton Dickinson Vacutainers™ containing citrate anticoagulant (*see* **Notes 1**, **6**, and **7**). See also **Subheading 1.6.** for further discussion of important issues related to sample collection.
2. Mix sample immediately with anticoagulant by gentle inversion of the tube.
3. Maintain blood samples at room temperature before analysis. The maximum time for each type of analysis is critical (*see* **Note 2**).
4. Carefully remove ~500 µL blood from the tube of citrated blood and transfer to a clean screw-cap tube before use (*see* **Note 25**).

3.2. Flow Cytometers

Run cleaning and alignment programs in flow cytometers daily (*see* **Note 8**).

3.3. Sample Preparation
3.3.1. Whole Blood Analysis of Platelet-Membrane Glycoproteins (Method A)

1. For each sample set up duplicate tubes for each antigen being tested, or each treatment, plus one for the isotype (negative) control and, where appropriate, one for a positive control (*see* **Table 4A**).
2. Add 50 µL HBS to each assay tube, ensuring that the buffer is at room temperature (*see* **Note 26**).
3. Add specific antibodies to the appropriate tubes in small volumes (usually ≤5 µL), previously determined by titration (*see* **Table 4A**).
4. When measuring platelet response to agonist stimulation, add 5 µL of appropriate stock solutions of agonists (*see* **Table 4A**).
5. At this point any additional reagents (e.g., inhibitors, antiplatelet agents, etc.) are added to the tubes in small volumes (typically ≤5 µL) (*see* **Note 27**).
6. Add 5-µL aliquots of blood to the assay tubes, ensuring that the blood is delivered below the surface of the buffer. Mixing is best done by gently "flicking" the base of the tube a few times. This allows adequate mixing but avoids activation of drops of the samples or distribution of the sample up the sides of the tube.
7. Incubate undisturbed for 20 min at room temperature.
8. To a separate tube add 50 µL HBS and 5 µL Flow-Set™ calibration beads.
9. Add 0.5 mL of 0.2% (v/v) formyl saline to each assay tube and incubate for 10 min at room temperature (*see* **Note 28**).

10. Further dilute by adding 50 µL diluted sample to 450 µL 0.2% formaldehyde saline (*see* **Note 29**).
11. Analyze in the flow cytometer within 2 h.

3.3.2. Whole Blood Analysis of Platelet-Membrane Glycoprotein Expression (Method B, Biocytex Method)

1. Place 50 µL blood in a clean tube and add 150 µL of 1:10 diluted diluent buffer and vortex mix for 1–2 s.
2. Set up three tubes, one for each antigen being tested.
3. To each tube add 20 µL of one of the antibodies.
4. Add 20 µL diluted blood sample to each of these tubes.
5. Vortex mix for 1–2 s, then incubate for 10 min at room temperature.
6. To a fourth tube add 40 µL calibrated bead suspension (this needs to be vortex-mixed first to ensure an even suspension).
7. To all four tubes (blood samples and calibration beads) add 20 µL polyclonal anti-mouse IgG-FITC.
8. Vortex mix for 1–2 s and incubate for 10 min at room temperature.
9. Add 2 mL diluted assay diluent and analyze within 2 h.

3.4. Whole Blood Analysis of Platelet-Leukocyte Aggregates

1. Add 50 µL HBS to each tube (*see* **Note 26**).
2. Add the appropriate antibodies to the tubes (*see* **Table 4B**).
3. Add 50 µL citrated blood to each tube.
4. Mix gently by hand, then incubate undisturbed for 30 min at room temperature.
5. Add 250 µL OptiLyse®C solution and mix gently.
6. Allow tubes to stand at room temperature for 10 min.
7. Add 250 µL PBS and mix gently.
8. Stand tubes at room temperature for 10 min.
9. Analyze within 2 h in a flow cytometer.

3.5. Whole Blood Analysis of Procoagulant, Platelet-Derived Microparticles

1. Add 35 µL HBS + 2 mM CaCl$_2$ (HBS/c) to assay tubes (*see* **Note 30**).
2. Add the appropriate antibodies (*see* **Table 4C**).
3. In one tube replace HBS/c with HBS without calcium to act as the negative control for annexin V binding (*see* **Note 31**).
4. Add 5 µL Hirudin (10 U/mL final concentration) (*see* **Note 18**).
5. Add 5-µL aliquots of blood to each tube.
6. Mix gently by hand, by flicking the base of the tube.
7. Incubate undisturbed for 10 min at room temperature.
8. Add 2 µL annexin V-FITC and mix gently.
9. Incubate undisturbed for a further 10 min at room temperature.
10. Add 5 µL of sample to 500 µL HBS/c (HBS for negative control) buffer and run in the flow cytometer within 30 min (*see* **Note 31**).

3.6. Flow-Cytometric Analysis

3.6.1. Single-Color Analysis

1. First run the tube containing the Flow-Set beads and, if necessary, adjust the voltages for each output parameter (forward scatter, side scatter, FL1, FL2, etc.) to standardize the output signal.
2. Next, run the FITC isotype control tube.
3. Ensure that the platelet population lies within the FS/SS gate (Gate A in **Fig. 2**).
4. Set the FL1 gate/cursor/marker to the 2% level on the isotype control (Gate B in **Fig. 2**).
5. Next, run a sample labeled for a pan-platelet marker.
6. Ensure that >95% of the events in the FS/SS gate are positive for the pan-platelet marker.
7. Using these settings run each sample in turn, in ascending order of agonist concentration if analyzing platelet-agonist response (*see* **Note 32**).

3.6.2. Dual-Color Analysis for the Diagnosis of BSS

1. First run the tube containing the Flow-Set beads and, if necessary, adjust the voltages for each output parameter to standardize the output signal.
2. Next, run the FITC isotype control for the pan-platelet (GPIIb-IIIa) marker.
3. Set the FS/SS gate to encompass all the cellular events, including the red-cell and white-cell populations (*see* **Note 33**).
4. Set the fluorescence gate/cursor/marker to the 2% level on the FL1 (FITC) isotype control.
5. Next, run a sample labeled for GPIIb-IIIa.
6. Use the FLI gate to select all GPIIb-IIIa-positive cells.
7. Next, run the sample containing anti-GPIIb-IIIa-FITC and the RPE-isotype control.
8. Set the FL2 (RPE) gate/cursor/marker to the 2% level on the gated population.
9. Next, run the samples labeled for both GPIIb-IIIa (FITC) and GPIbα (RPE) and analyze the percentage of the GPIIb-IIIa positive population that is positive for GPIbα.

3.6.3. Dual-Color Analysis for Detecting Platelet-Leukocyte Aggregates

1. First run the isotype control for the pan-leukocyte marker (CD45-RPE-Cy5) (*see* **Note 21**).
2. Set three FS/SS gates to select the monocyte, lymphocyte and granulocyte populations (Gates A, B and C respectively in **Fig. 3**).
3. Set the fluorescence gate/cursor/marker to the 2% level on the isotype control for each gated leukocyte population (Gate D in **Fig. 3**).
4. Next, run a sample dual-labeled with CD45-RPE-Cy5 and with the isotype control for the platelet marker (RPE).
5. Set the FL2 (RPE) gate/cursor/marker to the 2% level on the three gated populations (junction on *y* axis between Gates J and K in **Fig. 3**).
6. Next, run the samples labeled for both CD45 (RPE-Cy5) and GPIbα (RPE) and analyze the percentage of each of the leukocyte populations that is positive for GPIbα. (**Figure 3** illustrates this just for the monocyte population).

3.6.4. Dual-Color Analysis for Detecting Procoagulant Platelet Microparticles

1. First run the isotype control tube for the pan-platelet marker (RPE).
2. Set the FS/SS gate to encompass all the cellular events, excluding the red-cell and white-cell populations (Gate A in **Fig. 4**). This is to ensure that all platelets and microparticles are included in the analysis.

3. Set the FL2 gate/cursor/marker to the 2% level on the isotype control (Gate B in **Fig. 4**).
4. Next run a sample labeled with the pan-platelet marker and annexin V-FITC in the absence of extracellular calcium (negative control for annexin V).
5. Set the FL1 gate/cursor/marker to the 2% level on the population gated through the pan-platelet marker (Gate C in **Fig. 4**).
6. Using these settings, run each sample in turn.

4. Notes

1. A standardized phlebotomy protocol should be used that involves minimal use of a tourniquet, ensures a steady flow of blood, and collects directly into anticoagulant. Repeated venipuncture should be avoided. Since platelet function can be influenced by adrenergic hormones and by physical exercise *(52)*, it is advised that the subjects should rest, preferably supine, for at least 10 min prior to venipuncture when monitoring platelet activation. Draw blood from the antecubital fossa, ideally from a vessel that has not been phlebotomized within the past 7 d. The first few milliliters of blood should be taken into a blank (nonanticoagulated) tube and discarded. The next 5-mL sample should be taken into citrate and used for flow cytometry. It is good practice when collecting multiple samples to take them in the same order within a single study.

2. Blood should be kept at room temperature and processed rapidly after collection to avoid any changes due to activation in vitro. This is particularly important when measuring markers of platelet activation or testing the platelet response to agonist stimulation, but it is also relevant for constitutively expressed antigens, such as the GPIIb-IIIa and GPIb-V-IX complexes, the levels of which can increase or decrease respectively on the platelet surface if the sample is activated. Opinions differ about the precise time scale, but our own studies indicate that significant changes can be seen 10 min after collection *(20)*. It is therefore advisable to prepare analysis tubes before the blood is collected. The maximum recommended time between blood collection and sample preparation for constitutive glycoprotein analysis is 10 h and for procoagulant microparticle analysis, 3 h.

3. Centrifugation and washing steps always result in a significant loss of platelets. For example, in excess of 30% of the platelet population may be lost in the preparation of platelet-rich plasma (PRP) and losses of at least 50% of platelets can occur during washing procedures, which may result in the loss of specific platelet subsets *(53)*. Whole blood analysis allows the full spectrum of platelets to be analyzed. If required, however, the methods described in this chapter are suitable for the analysis of PRP, which can be prepared with minimal platelet activation by centrifugation of whole blood at 170g for 20 min at room temperature.

4. The rate-limiting step for the incubation time is the rate of binding of the antibodies to the platelets. This has to be balanced against a need to minimize time-dependent platelet activation occurring in the sample. Generally, incubation periods of 20 or 30 min are used and antibody concentrations are set to allow maximum binding to occur in this time. Maximum effects of agonists and inhibitors are generally seen within 5–10 min. Most methods recommend incubation at room temperature (between 20 and 25°C). This is based on early investigations of the conditions needed to maintain platelets in a stable state, for the detection of activated platelets in clinical samples. This has been tested extensively in our laboratory *(20)*. Some methods stress the need to incubate samples in the dark. In our experience there is negligible deterioration in the fluorescence of labeled antibodies over these short incubation times, but there is no reason why incubations cannot be carried out in the absence of light.

5. Following incubation with antibodies, the final dilution step involves a mild fixative (typically, 0.2% formaldehyde), to prevent, or at least slow, any further activation occurring prior to analysis in the flow cytometer. Unfixed samples continue to become activated *(6,20)*. Some methods recommend a more aggressive fixation (e.g., with 1% formaldehyde). This has been the subject of debate, some workers maintaining that it is only suitable for the more robust antigens (e.g., P-selectin) *(2,45)* while others argue that there is little effect on either P-selectin or fibrinogen-binding measurements *(54)*.

6. The anticoagulant of choice is trisodium citrate. Heparin should be avoided, as it causes sensitization and even slight activation of platelets *(55)*; similarly, EDTA is inappropriate as the higher level of calcium chelation uncouples integrins *(56)* and modifies platelet response. If it is necessary to maintain physiological levels of calcium in the plasma, the blood can be drawn into PPACK or hirudin. Collection into Vacutainers™ is as good as, or even better than, collection into a syringe. The immediate contact of the blood with the anticoagulant minimizes any activation. The choice of manufacturer of the blood collection system is not critical; we have found both the Becton Dickinson Vacutainer and Sarstedt S-Monovette® systems to give comparable results, but it is advisable to use the same manufacturer's tubes throughout a study.

7. Collection can be made either through straight needles or "butterfly" needles, but again it is advisable to use the same system throughout a study. Concern over the potential for activation of the blood during passage through the "dead" volume of a butterfly collection tube is unfounded, as extensive comparative studies in our laboratory has found no difference either in the level of platelet activation or responsiveness.

8. All flow cytometers currently on the market are capable of analyzing platelets. When analyzing whole blood samples, care should be taken to follow the manufacturer's cleaning recommendations. In our laboratory we run tubes containing 2% sodium hypochlorite, a proprietary detergent cleaning fliud (Coulter Clenz™), and distilled water at the beginning and end of the day and between sample runs. Daily alignment of the flow cytometer with commercially available fluorescent beads (e.g., Flow-Check™ Fluorospheres; Beckman Coulter 6605359) is essential, while the use of an internal standard (e.g., Flow-Set™ beads; Beckman-Coulter 6607007) ensures day-to day standardization of the measured fluorescence. If large adjustments are required consult the manufacturer, as this indicates a fault in the instrument.

9. Standardization of the assay protocol and reagents are essential to obtaining valid data. Wherever possible, agonists should be made up in batches, checked for activity, then frozen in aliquots of suitable size for a single experiment. This not only removes a source of experimental error but also speeds up sample preparation, as reagents do not need to be prepared or diluted on that day. In addition, each batch of antibody should be titrated and used at saturation.

10. HEPES-buffered saline should be filtered through a 0.22-μm filter (to remove dust and small particles that may appear in the platelet gate) and stored at 4°C in aliquots for up to 6 wk. Solutions kept longer than this tend to give lower platelet response, especially with ADP. Use each aliquot only once. When a new batch of HBS is prepared, platelet responses to ADP should be compared directly with those in an old batch to ensure comparable results. Other buffers have been used in protocols from other laboratories (e.g., modified Tyrode's solution, PBS, etc.). We are not aware that any direct comparative studies have been carried out between buffers.

11. 0.2% Formyl saline should also be filtered through a 0.22-μm filter and stored in aliquots for up to 6 mo at room temperature. Check each batch for red-cell lysis, which can inter-

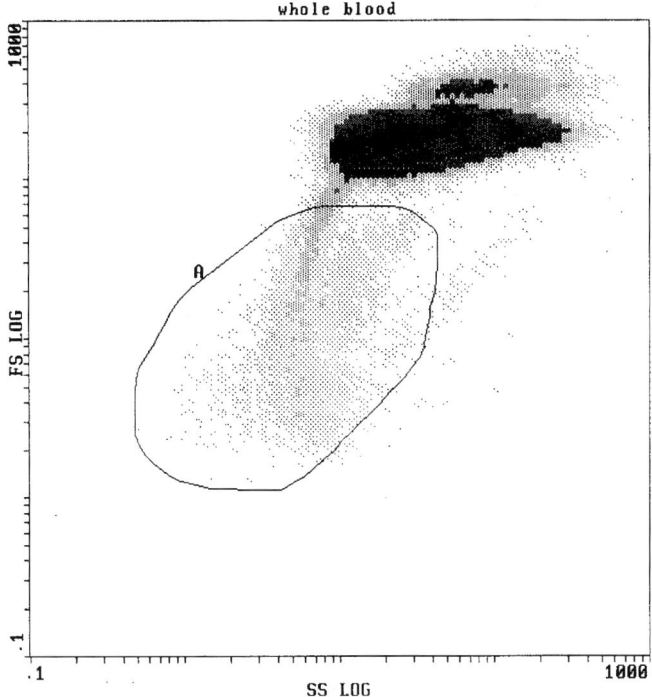

Fig. 7. Example of red-cell lysis seen in flow cytometers. This shows the SS/FS profile of a sample of blood where lysis of the red cells has occurred. There is a "tail" of red-cell ghosts entering the region occupied by the platelets. If this occurs, the percentage of platelets in gate "A" will be significantly reduced.

fere with the platelet analysis (*see* **Fig. 7**). To do this dilute 5 μL whole blood in 50 μL HBS, incubate at room temperature for 10 min, dilute 1:10 in 0.2% formyl saline, and leave at room temperature for at least 1 h before running in the flow cytometer.

12. While this chapter lists antibodies currently in use in this laboratory, many suitable antibodies to platelet antigens are available from commercial sources. Each batch of antibody should be titrated against an appropriate blood sample. For example, when testing an antibody to an activation marker it should be tested against both unstimulated and maximally stimulated samples and the dilution chosen that gives saturation binding to the stimulated platelets with low levels of nonspecific binding to the unstimulated platelets. Antibodies to constitutively expressed antigens should be used at a concentration that just reaches saturation. When running two-color analysis, appropriate color compensation needs to be set to avoid leakage of signal. Refer to manufacturers' guidelines for each instrument.

13. An isotype control is needed to set the negative controls for each specific antibody. This takes account of the nonspecific interaction of the antibody with the cells and, in particular, the interaction with Fc receptors on the cells. For mouse monoclonal antibodies the isotype control should be a mouse myeloma protein of the same isotype as the antibody to be used,

with the same fluorochrome as the antibody, and with the same fluorochrome:protein ratio as the antibody of choice. As a general rule, it is often best to purchase isotype controls from the same supplier as the specific antibody. For polyclonal antibodies an isotype control is normally non-immune serum from the same species (ideally from the same strain of animal), purified to the same degree as the antiserum that is being used and with the same fluorochrome and the same fluorochrome:protein ratio as the antiserum. Use the iso-type control at the same final protein concentration as the optimal antibody concentration. For every sample, run the negative control in the first tube to set the gate (cursor/marker) at the level of 2% positive.

14. All agonists are best prepared in batches at 10X the final concentration, tested, and stored at –80°C in aliquots sufficient for one assay. Use aliquots only once.

15. TRAP and GPRP peptides can be purchased from commercial sources or custom-made. The concentration required can vary by an order of magnitude between batches of peptide, so testing of new batches is essential.

16. GPRP is added to prevent clotting in tubes where thrombin is added or likely to be gener-ated (e.g., when calcium is present) *(38)*.

17. We have not found an isotype control for the rabbit anti-fibrinogen antibody that can reli-ably give a value that represents the level of nonspecific binding seen with the specific antibody. The negative control for this antibody therefore consists of blood plus the anti-fibrinogen antibody, without agonist, and with 6 mM EDTA (2 µL of 150 mM Na$_2$EDTA) to prevent any fibrinogen binding to GPIIb-IIIa. The EDTA disrupts the integrity of the GPIIb-IIIa complex and prevents fibrinogen from binding, thus giving a background that represents only the nonspecific binding of the antibody.

18. Recombinant hirudin is included in the procoagulant microparticle assay to inhibit thrombin generated on the PS-exposed platelet surface in HBS with 2 mM CaCl$_2$.

19. An alternative method for calibrating antigen expression, not dealt with in this chapter, is the Platelet Calibrator kit from Biocytex (7011).

20. Any MAb that blocks the interaction between P-selectin and its ligand is appropriate. Each MAb should be added at a concentration sufficient to block platelet-leukocyte aggregate formation in response to maximum TRAP stimulation of the platelets, determined by titration.

21. The pan-leukocyte marker CD45 allows identification of lymphocytes, monocytes and granulocytes. However, if just analyzing monocytes, the monocyte marker CD14 (CD14-RPE-Cy5, Serotec MCA1568C; use with an IgG2a-RPE-Cy5 isotype control, Serotec MCA929C) can be used instead. In this case, the FS/SS gates for the three leuko-cyte populations are still needed in order to identify monocytes by their light-scattering characteristics as well as CD14 positivity, as about 5% granulocytes also express CD14.

22. Lysis of red cells enriches the proportion of leukocytes in a whole blood sample, but poten-tially activates other cells for example, through the release of, ADP. A red-cell lysis reagent that contains a fixative is therefore advised. Alternative reagents exist for lysis of red cells in whole blood methods, but we find OptiLyse® to have the least effect on platelet activation.

23. TRAP provides a good positive control for the platelet-leukocyte assay.

24. A23187 provides a positive control for the procoagulant platelet-microparticle assay.

25. This is to avoid any air bubbles that may have formed in the blood tube during collection, which may activate the platelets.

26. When pipetting small volumes (≤50 µL) ensure that they are placed in the bottom of the tube. We have not found it necessary to adjust the final volume to accommodate different volumes of additional reagents, provided this does not exceed 30 µL.

27. After this point the tubes can be left for up to 30 min before the blood is added. If there is a delay in blood collection, place the tubes in a refrigerator for up to 1 h but then ensure that the tubes reach room temperature before adding blood.

28. This time is to allow re-equilibration of the antibodies in the larger volume of buffer, since 0.2% formaldehyde does not give complete fixation of the antibody-antigen interaction.

29. These dilution steps are important to ensure that single cells are analyzed in the flow cytometer. Undiluted blood contains too high a concentration of cells, resulting in coincident signals as two or more cells pass through the laser beam at the same time. The dilutions given in the following methods are based on analysis in a Beckman Coulter EPICS® XL-MCL instrument. The precise dilution required for each flow cytometer may vary and should be checked with the manufacturers, and by running controls in which parallel samples, labeled with different-color antiplatelet antibodies, are mixed and analyzed for expression of both fluorochromes. If the percentage of double-labeled particles exceeds 1%, the samples should be diluted further and/or the flow rate should be reduced.

30. Binding of annexin V to PS is highly calcium-dependent and therefore HBS with 2 mM CaCl$_2$ (HBS/c) is used in the incubation buffer when detecting PS exposure; this concentration of calcium must be maintained in the dilution stages. The calcium dependence of Annexin V binding to PS is the rationale for using calcium-free buffer as the negative control.

31. Samples are diluted in HBS/c since 0.2% formaldehyde saline permeabilizes the platelets allowing Annexin V binding to internal as well as external PS. Although the samples are stable for at least 30 min, they are not fixed and therefore should be analyzed as soon as possible.

32. If switching from strongly positive samples (e.g., a pan-platelet marker) to weakly positive (e.g., fibrinogen binding in resting samples), it may be advisable to run a tube containing sheath fluid or water between groups of sample tubes to avoid carryover of strongly fluorescent particles.

33. Although the BSS gating will include other cells, only platelets will be analysed for GPIbα, as the analysis will be performed only on cells that are positive for the pan-platelet marker GPIIb-IIIa.

References

1. Abrams, C. S., Ellison, N., Budzynski, A. Z., and Shattil, S. J. (1990) Direct detection of activated platelets and platelet-derived microparticles in humans. *Blood* **75,** 128–138.

2. Michelson, A. D. (1996) Flow cytometry: a clinical test of platelet function. *Blood* **87,** 4925–4936.

3. Michelson, A. D., Barnard, M. R., Krueger, L. A., Frelinger III, A. L., and Furman, M. I. (2002) Flow cytometry, in *Platelets* (Michelson, A. D., ed.), Academic Press, San Diego, CA pp. 297–315.

4. Ormerod, M. G. (ed.) (2000) *Flow Cytometry.* Oxford University Press, Oxford, UK.

5. Johnston, G. I., Pickett, E. B., McEver, R. P., and George, J. N. (1987) Heterogeneity of platelet secretion in response to thrombin demonstrated by fluorescence flow cytometry. *Blood* **69,** 1401–1403.

6. Shattil, S. P., Cunningham, M., and Hoxie, J. A. (1987) Detection of activated platelets in whole blood using activation-dependent monoclonal antibodies and flow cytometry. *Blood* **70,** 307–315.

7. Kunicki, T. J., Kritzik, M., Annis, D. S., and Nugent, D. J. (1997) Hereditary variation in platelet integrin α$_2$β$_1$ density is associated with two silent polymorphisms in the alpha 2 gene coding sequence. *Blood* **89,** 1939–1943.

 8. Joutsi-Korhonen, L., Smethurst, P. A., Rankin, A., Gray, E., Ijsseldijk, M., Onley, C. M., et al. (2003) The low frequency allele of the platelet collagen signalling receptor glycoprotein VI is associated with reduced functional responses and expression. *Blood* **101,** 4372–4379.

 9. Schultheiss, H. P., Tschoepe, D., Esser, J., Schwippert, B., Roesen, P., Nieuwenhuis, H. K., et al. (1994) Large platelets continue to circulate in an activated state after myocardial infarction. *Eur. J. Clin. Invest.* **24,** 243–247.

10. Gawaz, M., Neumann, F. J., Ott, I., Schiessler, A., and Schomig, A. (1996) Platelet function in acute myocardial infarction treated with direct angioplasty. *Circulation* **93,** 229–237.

11. Furman, M. I., Benoit, S. E., Barnard, M. R., Valeri, C. R., Borbone, M. L., Becker, R. C., et al. (1998) Increased platelet reactivity and circulating monocyte-platelet aggregates in patients with stable coronary artery disease. *J. Am. Coll. Cardiol.* **31,** 352–358.

12. Fijnheer, R., Modderman, P. W., Veldman, H., Ouwehand, W. H., Nieuwenhuis, H. K., Roos, D., et al. (1990) Detection of platelet activation with monoclonal antibodies and flow cytometry. Changes during platelet storage. *Transfusion* **30,** 20–25.

13. Metcalfe, P., Williamson, L. M., Reutelingsperger, C. P. M., Swann, I., Ouwehand, W. H., and Goodall, A. H. (1997) Activation during preparation of therapeutic platelets affects deterioration during storage: a comparative flow cytometric study of different production methods. *Br. J. Haematol.* **98,** 86–95.

14. Sakariassen, K. S., Holme, P. A., Orvim, U., Barstad, R. M., Solum, N. O., and Brosstad, F. R. (1998) Shear-induced platelet activation and platelet microparticle formation in native human blood. *Thromb. Res.* **92,** S33–S41.

15. Abulencia, J. P., Tien, N., McCarty, O. J. T., Plymire, D., Mousa, S. A., and Konstantopoulos, K. (2001) Comparative antiplatelet efficacy of a novel, nonpeptide GPIIb/IIIa antagonist (XV454) and abciximab (c7E3) in flow models of thrombosis. *Arterioscler. Thromb. Vasc. Biol.* **21,** 149–156.

16. Savion, N., Shenkman, B., Tamarin, I., Dardik, R., Frojmovic, M., and Varon, D. (2001) Transient adhesion refractoriness of circulating platelets under shear stress: the role of partial activation and microaggregate formation by suboptimal ADP concentration. *Br. J. Haematol.* **112,** 1055–1061.

17. Knight, C. J., Panesar, M., Wilson, D. J., Chronos, N. A., Patel, D., Fox, K., et al. (1997) Different effects of calcium antagonists, nitrates, and beta-blockers on platelet function. Possible importance for the treatment of unstable angina. *Circulation* **95,** 125–132.

18. Furman, M. I., Kereiakes, D. J., Krueger, L. A., Mueller, M. N., Pieper, K., Broderick, T. M., et al. (2001) Leukocyte-platelet aggregation, platelet surface P-selectin, and platelet surface glycoprotein IIIa after percutaneous coronary intervention: Effects of dalteparin or unfractionated heparin in combination with abciximab. *Am. Heart J.* **142,** 790–798.

19. Warkentin, T. E., Powling, M. J., and Hardisty, R. M. (1990) Measurement of fibrinogen binding to platelets in whole blood by flow cytometry: a micromethod for the detection of platelet activation. *Br. J. Haematol.* **76,** 387–394.

20. Janes, S. L., Wilson, D. J., Chronos, N. A., and Goodall, A. H. (1993) Evaluation of whole blood flow cytometric detection of platelet bound fibrinogen on normal subjects and patients with activated platelets. *Thromb. Haemost.* **70,** 659–666.

21. Zamarron, C., Ginsberg, M. H., and Plow, E. F. (1990) Monoclonal antibodies specific for a conformationally altered state of fibrinogen. *Thromb. Haemost.* **64,** 41–46.

22. Shattil, S. J., Hoxie, J. A., Cunningham, M., and Brass, L. F. (1985) Changes in the platelet membrane glycoprotein IIb.IIIa complex during platelet activation. *J. Biol. Chem.* **260,** 11,107–11,114.

23. Frelinger, A. L. 3rd., Lam, S. C., Plow, E. F., Smith, M. A., Loftus, J. C., and Ginsberg, M. H. (1988) Occupancy of an adhesive glycoprotein receptor modulates expression of an antigenic site involved in cell adhesion. *J. Biol. Chem.* **263,** 12,397–12,402.

24. Furie, B., Furie, B. C., and Flaumenhaft, R. (2001) A journey with platelet P-selectin: the molecular basis of granule secretion, signalling and cell adhesion. *Thromb. Haemost.* **86,** 214–221.

25. Nieuwenhuis, H. K., van Oosterhout, J. J., Rozemuller, E., van Iwaarden, F., and Sixma, J. J. (1987) Studies with a monoclonal antibody against activated platelets: evidence that a secreted 53,000-molecular weight lysosome-like granule protein is exposed on the surface of activated platelets in the circulation. *Blood* **70,** 838–845.

26. Michelson, A. D. and Barnard, M. R. (1987) Thrombin-induced changes in platelet membrane glycoproteins Ib, IX, and IIb-IIIa complex. *Blood* **70,** 1673–1678.

27. McEver, R. P. (2001) Adhesive interactions of leukocytes, platelets, and the vessel wall during hemostasis and inflammation. *Thromb. Haemost.* **86,** 746–756.

28. Michelson, A. D., Barnard, M. R., Hechtman, H. B., MacGregor, H., Connolly, R. J., Loscalzo, J., et al. (1996) In vivo tracking of platelets: circulating degranulated platelets rapidly lose surface P-selectin but continue to circulate and function. *Proc. Natl. Acad. Sci. USA* **93,** 11,877–11,882.

29. Michelson, A. D., Barnard, M. R., Krueger, L. A., Valeri, C. R., and Furman, M. I. (2001) Circulating monocyte-platelet aggregates are a more sensitive marker of in vivo platelet activation than platelet surface P-selectin: studies in baboons, human coronary intervention, and human acute myocardial infarction. *Circulation* **104,** 1533–1537.

30. Ott, I., Neumann, F. J., Gawaz, M., Schmitt, M., and Schomig, A. (1996) Increased neutrophil-platelet adhesion in patients with unstable angina. *Circulation* **94,** 1239–1246.

31. Li, N., Goodall, A. H., and Hjemdahl, P. (1999) Efficient flow cytometric assay for platelet-leukocyte aggregates in whole blood using fluorescence signal triggering. *Cytometry* **35,** 154–161.

32. Bevers, E. M., Comfurius, P., and Zwaal, R. F. A. (1983) Changes in membrane phospholipid distribution during platelet activation. *Biochim. Biophys. Acta* **736,** 57–66.

33. Zwaal, R. F. A., Comfurius, P., and Bevers, E. M. (1992) Platelet procoagulant activity and microvesicle formation. Its putative role in hemostasis and thrombosis. *Biochim. Biophys. Acta* **1180,** 1–8.

34. Sims, P. J., Wiedmer, T., Esmon, C. T., Weiss, H. J., and Shattil, S. J. (1989) Assembly of the prothrombinase complex is linked to the vesiculation of the platelet membrane. Studies in Scott syndrome: an isolated defect in platelet procoagulant activity. *J. Biol. Chem.* **264,** 17,049–17,057.

35. Sims, P. J., Faioni, E. M., Wiedmer, T., and Shattil, S. J. (1988) Complement proteins C5b-9 cause release of membrane vesicles from the platelet surface that are enriched in the membrane receptor for coagulation factor Va and express prothrombinase activity. *J. Biol. Chem.* **263,** 18,205–18,212.

36. Thiagarajan, P. and Tait, J. F. (1990) Binding of annexin V/placental anticoagulant protein I to platelets. Evidence for phosphatidylserine exposure in the procoagulant response of activated platelets. *J. Biol. Chem.* **265,** 17,420–17,423.

37. Janes, S. L., Wilson, D. J., Cox, A. D., Chronos, N. A., and Goodall, A. H. (1994) ADP causes partial degranulation of platelets in the absence of aggregation. *Br. J. Haematol.* **86,** 568–573.

38. Michelson, A. D. (1994) Platelet activation by thrombin can be directly measured in whole blood through the use of the peptide GPRP and flow cytometry: methods and clinical applications. *Blood Coag. Fibrinolysis* **5,** 121–131.

39. Vu, T. K., Wheaton, V. I., Hung, D. T., Charo, I., and Coughlin, S. R. (1991) Domains specifying thrombin-receptor interaction. *Nature* **353,** 674–677.

40. Faruqi, T. R., Weiss, E. J., Shapiro, M. J., Huang, W., and Coughlin, S. R. (2000) Structure-function analysis of protease-activated receptor 4 tethered ligand peptides. Determinants of specificity and utility in assays of receptor function. *J. Biol. Chem.* **275,** 19,728–19,734.

41. Knight, C. G., Morton, L. F., Onley, D. J., Peachey, A. R., Ichinohe, T., Okuma, M., et al. (1999) Collagen-platelet interaction: Gly-Pro-Hyp is uniquely specific for platelet Gp VI and mediates platelet activation by collagen. *Cardiovasc. Res.* **41,** 450–457.

42. Lanza, F., Beretz, A., Stierle, A., Hanau, D., Kubina, M., and Cazenave, J. P. (1988) Epinephrine potentiates human platelet activation but is not an aggregating agent. *Am. J. Physiol.* **255,** H1276–H1288.

43. Hjemdahl, P., Chronos, N. A., Wilson, D. J., Bouloux, P., and Goodall, A. H. (1994) Epinephrine sensitizes human platelets in vivo and in vitro as studied by fibrinogen binding and P-selectin expression. *Arterioscler. Thromb.* **14,** 77–84.

44. Rinder, C. S., Student, L. A., Bonan, J. L., Rinder, H. M., and Smith, B. R. (1993) Aspirin does not inhibit adenosine diphosphate-induced platelet alpha-granule release. *Blood* **82,** 505–512.

45. Chronos, N. A., Wilson, D. J., Janes, S. L., Hutton, R. A., Buller, N. P., and Goodall, A. H. (1994) Aspirin does not affect the flow cytometric detection of fibrinogen binding to, or release of alpha-granules or lysosomes from, human platelets. *Clin. Sci.* **87,** 575–580.

46. Ault, K. A. and Mitchell, J. (1994) Analysis of platelets by flow cytometry. *Meth. Cell Biol.* **42,** PtB:275–294.

47. Schmitz, G., Rothe, G., Ruf, A., Barlage, S., Tschope, D., Clemetson, K. J., et al. (1998) European Working Group on Clinical Cell Analysis: Consensus protocol for the flow cytometric characterisation of platelet function. *Thromb. Haemost.* **79,** 885–896.

48. Dumont, L. J., VandenBroeke, T., and Ault, K. A. (1999) Platelet surface P-selectin measurements in platelet preparations: an international collaborative study. Biomedical Excellence for Safer Transfusion (BEST) Working Party of the International Society of Blood Transfusion (ISBT). *Transfus. Med. Rev.* **13,** 31–42.

49. Johnston, G. I., Heptinstall, S., Robins, R. A., and Price, M. R. (1984) The expression of glycoproteins on single blood platelets from healthy individuals and from patients with congenital bleeding disorders. *Biochem. Biophys. Res. Comm.* **123,** 1091–1098.

50. Jennings, L. K., Ashmun, R. A., Wang, W. C., and Dockter, M. E. (1986) Analysis of human platelet glycoproteins IIb-IIIa and Glanzmann's thrombasthenia in whole blood by flow cytometry. *Blood* **68,** 173–179.

51. Jackson, C. W. and Jennings, L. K. (1989) Heterogeneity of fibrinogen receptor expression on platelets activated in normal plasma with ADP: analysis by flow cytometry. *Br. J. Haematol.* **72,** 407–414.

52. Hjemdahl, P., Larsson, P. T., and Wallen, N. H. (1991) Effects of stress and beta-blockade on platelet function. *Circulation* **84,** VI44–VI61.

53. Crook, M. and Crawford, N. (1988) Platelet surface charge heterogeneity: characterization of human platelet subpopulations separated by high voltage continuous flow electrophoresis. *Br. J. Haematol.* **69,** 265–273.

54. Hu, H., Daleskog, M., and Li, N. (2000) Influences of fixatives on flow cytometric measurements of platelet P-selectin expression and fibrinogen binding. *Thromb. Res.* **100,** 161–166.

55. Engstad, C. S., Gutteberg, T. J., and Østerud, B. (1997) Modulation of blood cell activation by four commonly used anticoagulants. *Thromb. Haemost.* **77,** 690–696.

56. Phillips, D. R., Charo, I. F., Parise, L. V., and Fitzgerald, L. A. (1988) The platelet membrane glycoprotein IIb-IIIa complex. *Blood* **71,** 831–843.

57. Gatter, K. C., Cordell, J. L., Turley, H., Heryet, A., Kieffer, N., Anstee, D. J., et al. (1988) The immunohistological detection of platelets, megakaryocytes and thrombi in routinely processed specimens. *Histopathology* **13,** 257–267.

58. Knapp, W., Dorken, B., Gilks, W. R., Rieber, E. P., Schmidt, R. E., Stein, H., et al. (eds.) (1989) *Leukocyte Typing IV: White Cell Differentiation Antigens.* Oxford University Press, Oxford, UK.

59. Berndt, M. C., Gregory, C., Kabral, A., Zola, H., Fournier, D., and Castaldi, P. A. (1985) Purification and preliminary characterization of the glycoprotein Ib complex in the human platelet membrane. *Eur. J. Biochem.* **151,** 637–649.

60. Azorsa, D. O., Moog, S., Ravanat, C., Schuhler, S., Follea, G., Cazenave, J. P., et al. (1999) Measurement of GPV released by activated platelets using a sensitive immunocapture ELISA—its use to follow platelet storage in transfusion. *Thromb. Haemost.* **81,** 131–138.

61. Giltay, J. C., Brinkman, H. J., Modderman, P. W., von dem Borne, A. E., and van Mourik, J. A. (1989) Human vascular endothelial cells express a membrane protein complex immuno-chemically indistinguishable from the platelet VLA-2 (glycoprotein Ia-IIa) complex. *Blood* **73,** 1235–1241.

62. Gralnick, H. R., Williams, S. B., McKeown, L., Shafer, B., Connaghan, G. D., Hansmann, K., et al. (1992) Endogenous platelet fibrinogen: its modulation after surface expression is related to size-selective access to and conformational changes in the bound fibrinogen. *Br. J. Haematol.* **80,** 347–357.

63. Ginsberg, M. H., Frelinger, A. L., Lam, S. C., Forsyth, J., McMillan, R., Plow, E. F., et al. (1990) Analysis of platelet aggregation disorders based on flow cytometric analysis of membrane glycoprotein IIb-IIIa with conformation-specific monoclonal antibodies. *Blood* **76,** 2017–2023.

64. Frelinger, A. L. 3rd, Cohen, I., Plow, E. F., Smith, M. A., Roberts, J., Lam, S. C., et al. (1990) Selective inhibition of integrin function by antibodies specific for ligand-occupied receptor conformers. *J. Biol. Chem.* **265,** 6346–6352.

65. Dunlop, L. C., Skinner, M. P., Bendall, L. J., Favaloro, E. J., Castaldi, P. A., Gorman, J. J., et al. (1992) Characterization of GMP-140 (P-selectin) as a circulating plasma protein. *J. Exp. Med.* **175,** 1147–1150.

66. de Bruijne-Admiraal, L. G., Modderman, P. W., Von dem Borne, A. E., and Sonnenberg, A. (1992) P-selectin mediates Ca(2+)-dependent adhesion of activated platelets to many different types of leukocytes: detection by flow cytometry. *Blood* **80,** 134–142.

67. Febbraio, M. and Silverstein, R. L. (1990) Identification and characterization of LAMP-1 as an activation-dependent platelet surface glycoprotein. *J. Biol. Chem.* **265,** 18,531–18,537.

68. Silverstein, R. L. and Febbraio, M. (1992) Identification of lysosome-associated membrane protein-2 as an activation-dependent platelet surface glycoprotein. *Blood* **80,** 1470–1475.

69. Henn, V., Slupsky, J. R., Grafe, M., Anagnostopoulos, I., Forster, R., Muller-Berghaus, G., et al. (1998) CD40 ligand on activated platelets triggers an inflammatory reaction of endothelial cells. *Nature* **391,** 591–594.

20

Flow-Cytometric Analysis of Mouse Platelet Function

Bernhard Nieswandt, Valerie Schulte, and Wolfgang Bergmeier

1. Introduction

Characterization of platelet-membrane glycoproteins and their intracellular signaling pathways has become essential to understanding platelet function not only in the context of thrombosis and hemostasis, but also other processes like inflammation, tumor metastasis, and atherosclerosis. Besides their central role in these processes in vivo, platelets are increasingly used as a convenient and physiologically relevant model for basic studies on cell adhesion and signaling processes.

Studies on human platelet function have two major limitations. First, in vivo experimentation is obviously very problematic in humans. Second, the use of genetics for studies on platelet function has been extremely difficult because platelet-membrane signaling reactions either do not occur in nucleated cells normally used for transfection studies or are insufficiently characterized. Both limitations have been overcome by the use of animal models, most importantly mice. Because of its small size, high fertility, and exceptional reproductive capacity, the common laboratory mouse (Mus musculus, Mus domesticus) has become the most frequently used inbred animal species for biological research purposes. A large number of in vivo models for platelet-related physiological and pathophysiological processes, such as arterial thrombosis, atherosclerosis, wound healing, tumor metastasis, immune thrombocytopenia, and the like have been established allowing studies on platelet function *in situ* in a large number of animals with a defined genetic background. The advent of technologies that facilitate genetic manipulations in the mouse genome has produced new ways to define protein function and is proving of value in unraveling signal transduction pathways in platelets both in vitro and in vivo.

The generation of mice with distinct mutations is well developed and can be achieved quickly and reliably. Mutations introduced into the germ line can range from null mutations to subtle changes in coding or noncoding sequences of genes, chromosomal translocations, and spatially and temporally restricted gene deletions using the Cre/loxP

From: *Methods in Molecular Biology, vol. 272:*
Platelets and Megakaryocytes, Vol. 1: Functional Assays
Edited by: J. M. Gibbins and M. P. Mahaut-Smith © Humana Press Inc., Totowa, NJ

system. The availability of knockout and transgenic mouse models has enormously improved our understanding of the hemostatic system. For example, studies with mice deficient in $G\alpha_q$ highlighted the importance of the $G\alpha_q$ subunit as an essential signal-transducing protein utilized by many platelet agonist receptors and therefore validated and extended results obtained from a single patient *(1)*. The generation of mice deficient in PAR-1 or PAR-3 has allowed the identification of a dual PAR receptor system *(2)*. Studies in the $P2Y_1$-deficient mouse *(3)* demonstrated the existence of a second ADP receptor, which is the target for antithrombotic drugs clopidogrel and ticlopidine (the recently cloned $P2Y_{12}$ receptor *[4]*). Mice deficient in GPIIIa or GPIbα have confirmed the causal relationship between a lack of certain platelet glycoproteins and a particular disease phenotype such as Glanzmann thrombasthenia or Bernard-Soulier syndrome, respectively *(5,6)*. For the extrapolation of data from mouse to human platelets, an accurate determination of the mouse hemostatic system with regard to coagulation and fibrinolytic systems, platelet structure, and platelet receptor/enzyme systems is required.

Platelet counts in mice on average are four times those of humans and mouse platelets are only approximately one-half the volume of human platelets. The coagulation and fibrinolytic systems in the mouse show striking similarities to those of the human system, with virtually every protein represented and with every cascade appearing to serve similar functions in both species. Nonetheless, differences at the molecular structural level (varying degrees of homology of proteins) and functional level (different activities of human coagulation and fibrinolytic factors) exist between both species. The hemostatic impact of these differences remains to be defined. Human and mouse platelets appear to share many of the same receptor systems and functional capacities, with the GPIIbIIIa receptor clearly playing the central role in both species *(7)*. In summary, due to the increasing number of knockout and transgenic strains, the mouse currently can be regarded as the preferable species for studies on platelet function.

1.1. Flow-Cytometric Analysis of Mouse Platelets

Compared to studies on human platelets, functional analyses of mouse platelets are restricted by the low amount of blood that can be drawn from each individual animal (0.5–1.5 mL). Flow cytometry requires only minimal amounts of cells and blood, therefore making it a powerful tool to study platelet function and morphology in mice. The power of flow-cytometric analysis lies in its ability to make quantitative multiparameter measurements—such as determination of cell size and shape, cytoplasmatic granularity, protein fluorescence, or DNA/RNA content—on a large number of individual cells. In principle, flow cytometric analysis of mouse platelets is not different from the analysis of human platelets. Therefore, for information on basic principles of flow-cytometric analysis of platelets and details cytometer calibration and color compensation the reader is referred to Chapter 9, vol. 1. However, there are differences in the procedure of blood collection and processing, and there is a need for mouse-specific reagents. This chapter will list available tools and provide protocols for the accurate analysis of platelets in whole blood, as well as more detailed functional studies on washed mouse platelets.

2. Materials
2.1. Buffers

1. Tris-buffered saline (TBS): 20 mM Tris-HCl, 137 mM NaCl, pH 7.3, containing 20 U/mL heparin (Liquemin N10,000; Roche Diagnostics, 3441242).
2. Phosphate-buffered saline (PBS): 137 mM NaCl, 2.7 mM KCl, 1.5 mM KH$_2$PO$_4$, 8 mM Na$_2$HPO$_4$, pH 7.14.
3. Tyrode's buffer (modified): 134 mM NaCl, 0.34 mM Na$_2$HPO$_4$, 2.9 mM KCl, 12 mM NaHCO$_3$, 20 mM HEPES, pH 7.0, 5 mM glucose, 0.35% (w/v) bovine serum albumin.

2.2. Equipment

1. Adjustable pipets with disposable tips.
2. Flow cytometer with a laser emission at 488 nm, capable of detecting at least two different fluorochromes with appropriate color compensation.

2.3. Blood Collection

1. Collection of 50 µL blood: 50-µL ringcaps (Hirschmann, 9600150 or Roth, Karlsruhe, Germany A761).
2. Collection of 0.5–1.0 mL blood: heparin-coated microhematocrit capillaries (Fisher Scientific, Pittsburgh, PA). Alternatively, 1.5-cm glass capillaries, prepared with a diamond cutter from Pasteur pipets, can be used.
3. 1.5-mL tubes containing 100–200 µL of TBS/heparin (20 U/mL).

2.3.1. Preparation of Washed Platelets

1. Tyrode's buffer.
2. Apyrase (Sigma, A7646); stock solution: 10 U/mL in dd H$_2$O, –20°C.
3. Prostacyclin (PGI$_2$; Calbiochem, 538925); stock solution: 1 mM in dd H$_2$O, –20°C.

2.4. Antibodies

A number of fluorophore-labeled antibodies against prominent mouse platelet-membrane glycoproteins and ligands are commercially available (*see* **Note 1**). The monoclonal antibodies are rat or hamster IgGs, the polyclonal antibodies are rabbit IgG.

2.4.1. Pan-Platelet Markers

Antigen	CD	Clone	Fluorophore	Company, cat. no.
GPIbα	42b	Xia.G5	FITC/PE	Emfret Analytics, M040-1/-2
		Xia.B2	FITC	Emfret Analytics, M043-1
GPIbβ	42c	Xia.C3	FITC	Emfret Analytics, M050-1
GPIIb/IIIa	41/61	Leo.A1	FITC	Emfret Analytics, M022-1
(α$_{IIb}$β$_3$ integrin)		Leo.D2	FITC/PE	Emfret Analytics, M020-1/-2
		MWReg30	FITC	BD Biosciences, 553848

2.4.2. Other Platelet-Membrane Glyoproteins

Antigen	CD	Clone	Fluorophore	Company, cat. no.
GPVI	n.d.	Six.E10	FITC	Emfret Analytics, M010-1
CD9	9	Nyn.H3	FITC	Emfret Analytics, M110-1
β1 integrin	29	Ha2/5	FITC	BD Biosciences, 555005
PECAM-1	31	MEC13.3	FITC	BD Biosciences, 553372
		Pec.H3	—	Emfret Analytics, M120-0
GPIX	42a	Xia.B4	FITC	Emfret Analytics, M051-1
GPV	42d	Gon.C2	FITC	Emfret Analytics, M060-1
		Gon.G6	FITC	Emfret Analytics, M061-1
α2 integrin	49b	Sam.G4	FITC	Emfret Analytics, M070-1
		Ha1/29	FITC	BD Biosciences, 554999
α5 integrin	49e	Tap.A12	FITC	Emfret Analytics, M080-1
		5H10-27	PE	BD Biosciences, 557447
α6 integrin	49f	GoH3	FITC	BD Biosciences, 555735
β3 integrin	61	Luc.A5	FITC	Emfret Analytics, M030-1
		Luc.H11	FITC	Emfret Analytics, M031-1
		2C9.G2	FITC	BD Biosciences, 553346

2.4.3. Platelet-Activation Markers

Antigen	CD	Clone	Fluorophore	Company, cat. no.
GPIIb/IIIa (activated)	41/61	JON/A	PE	Emfret Analytics, M023-2
P-selectin	62P	Wug.E9	FITC, PE	Emfret Analytics, M130-1/-2
		RB40.34	FITC	BD Biosciences, 553744
fibrinogen	—	polyclonal	FITC	Emfret Analytics, P140-1
		polyclonal	FITC	DAKO, F0111
vWf	—	polyclonal	FITC	Emfret Analytics, P150-1

2.4.4. Control Antibodies

FITC- and PE-labeled control antibodies are available (rat and rabbit IgG: Emfret Analytics; rat or hamster IgG: BD Biosciences) (*see* **Note 2**).

Isotype	Clone	Fluorophore	Company, cat. no.
Rat IgG1	R3-34	—	BD Pharmingen, 555839
Rat IgG2a	R35-95	FITC	BD Pharmingen, 555843
		PE	BD Pharmingen, 555844
Rat IgG2b	R35-38	—	BD Pharmingen, 555846
		PE	BD Pharmingen, 555848

Isotype	Clone	Fluorophore	Company, cat. no.
Rat IgG	—	FITC	Emfret Analytics, P190-1
		PE	Emfret Analytics, P190-2
Hamster IgM	G235-1	FITC	BD Pharmingen, 553960
Hamster IgG1	A19-3	FITC	BD Pharmingen, 553971
Hamster IgG2	Ha4/8	FITC	BD Pharmingen, 553964
Rabbit IgG	polyclonal	FITC	Emfret Analytics, P180-1

2.5. Agonists and Nonphysiological Activators

Different agonists/activators can be used to test the function of distinct receptors and signaling pathways in mouse platelets.

Agonist	Company, cat. no.	Stock solution	Receptor	Signaling via
ADP	Sigma, A6646	1 mM in dH$_2$O$_{dest}$, $-20°C$	P2Y$_1$ P2Y$_{12}$	Gα_q Gα_i
Convulxin	Pentapharm, 119-02	0.1 mg/mL in PBS; $-20°C$	GPVI	FcRγ/ITAM
Epinephrine	Sigma, E4375	1 mM in ddH$_2$O; $-20°C$	α_{2A}	Gα_i
Thrombin	Roche Diagnostics, 602418	20 U/mL in PBS, $4°C$	PAR3 / PAR4	Gα_i, Gα_q, G$\alpha_{12/13}$
U46619 (Thromboxane A$_2$ analog)	Alexis Biochemicals, 340-015-M001	10 mM in EtOH, $-20°C$	TPα	Gα_q, G$\alpha_{12/13}$
Botrocetin	Pentapharm, 122-01	100 U/mL in PBS, $-20°C$	GPIbα (vWf)	n.d.
PMA	Sigma, P1585	5 mg/mL in DMSO, $-20°C$	—	PKC
A23187	Sigma, C7522	10 mM in DMSO, $-20°C$	—	

2.6. Determination of Platelet Counts in Whole Blood

1. SPHERO™ rainbow-fluorescent polystyrene beads (5.5 µm diameter, RFP-50-5; Spherotech Inc., Libertyville, IL).
2. Pan-platelet marker (GPIIbIIIa-PE; Leo.D2-PE).
   Alternatively, a mouse platelet-count kit is available from Emfret Analytics.

3. Methods

3.1. Blood Collection and Processing

Blood can be drawn from the retro-orbital plexus or the vena cava or by cardiac puncture of anesthetized mice. The first method is preferable, as mice survive this procedure and can therefore be bled repeatedly. The risk of platelet activation during blood sampling is minimal with all methods. For studies on platelet activation, blood should be anticoagulated with heparin (1–10 U/mL final concentration) because calcium chelators (citrate, EDTA) will inhibit integrin activation. For retro-orbital bleeding, ether anesthesia is a convenient method but other anesthetics can also be used. Blood samples should be maintained at room temperature before analysis. Whole blood analyses should be performed within 30 min (*see* **Note 3**).

3.1.1. Preparation of Diluted Whole Blood

1. Collect 50 µL blood with a heparinized glass capillary from the retro-orbital plexus into 1.5-mL tubes containing 200 µL of TBS/heparin (20 U/mL).
2. Add 1 mL Tyrode's buffer containing 1.25 mM CaCl$_2$ directly before the start of the experiments (*see* **Note 4**).

3.1.2. Preparation of Washed Blood

1. Collect 50 µL blood with a heparinized glass capillary from the retro-orbital plexus into 1.5-mL tubes containing 200 µL of TBS/heparin (20 U/mL).
2. Add 1 mL Tyrode's buffer and centrifuge at 1300g for 5 min. Remove the supernatant and resuspend the pellet in 1.25 mL Tyrode's buffer.
3. Add 1 mM CaCl$_2$ directly before the start of the experiment.

3.1.3. Preparation of Washed Platelets

The preparation of washed platelets is a more time-consuming method that requires a larger amount of blood, but yields a platelet preparation that can be used for several hours.

1. Collect 0.5 mL blood with 1.5-cm glass capillaries from the retro-orbital plexus into a 1.5-mL tube containing 100 µL of TBS/heparin (20 U/mL).
2. Centrifuge the sample for 4 min at 500g and transfer the platelet-rich plasma (PRP) (with some red blood cells) into a new tube.
3. Centrifuge the platelet suspension for 8 min at 300g, and transfer the PRP without any red blood cells into a new tube.
4. Add 0.5 µL 1 mM prostacyclin and centrifuge at 1300g for 5 min.
5. Resuspend the platelet pellet in 1 mL Tyrode's buffer, add 2 µL 10 U/mL apyrase and 0.5 µL 1 mM prostacyclin, incubate for 5 min at 37°C, and centrifuge for 1 min at 1300g.
6. Repeat **step 5** and resuspend the platelet pellet in 0.5 mL Tyrode's buffer, add 1 µL apyrase (10 U/mL) (*see* **Note 5**) and incubate for 30 min at 37°C.
7. For flow-cytometric analysis, this platelet preparation should be used at a dilution of 1 : 25 in Tyrode's buffer containing 1 mM CaCl$_2$.

3.2. Determination of Platelet Counts in Whole Blood

A very easy and elegant way to determine platelet counts in whole blood by flow cytometry has been recently described by Alugupalli et al. *(8)*. SPHERO™ rainbow-fluorescent polystyrene beads (5.5 µm diameter, RFP-50-5; Spherotech Inc., Libertyville, IL), which emit broad-spectrum fluorescence detectable by all channels of the flow cytometer, are added to whole blood to serve as an internal standard for the cell count. Beads and platelets can easily be discriminated from other blood cells by their scatter characteristics and fluorescence. To minimize confounding "coincident events" during the analysis, the sample should be run at a relatively low flow rate (~2000 events/s) with a final dilution of the blood sample of approx 1 : 1000. To standardize the volume of the prepared sample to be analyzed, count 1000 beads per sample, which, given that the sample contained 100 beads/µL, represents 10 µL of the suspension. To calculate the number of platelets in 1 mL of blood, use the following equation:

$$\text{platelets/mL whole blood} = \text{number of platelets} \times \text{dilution factor} \times 100$$

1. Place 50 µL of diluted whole blood/platelet sample in a clean tube.
2. Add 10 µL of Leo.D2-PE (anti-$\alpha_{IIb}\beta_3$), vortex-mix, and incubate for 10 min at RT.
3. Add 100 µL of SPHERO rainbow-fluorescent polystyrene beads.
4. Add 1 mL assay diluent and analyze within 2 h.

Alternatively, a mouse platelet-count kit from Emfret Analytics can be used.

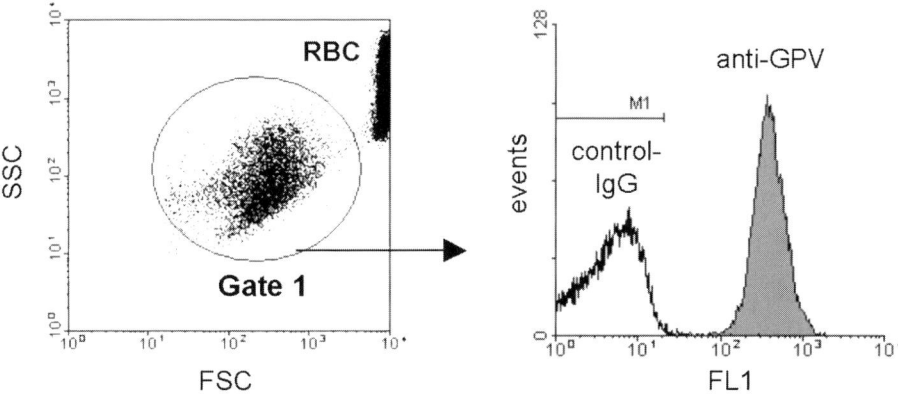

Fig. 1. Single-color staining. Whole blood was diluted 1:25 with Tyrode's buffer, incubated for 15 min with FITC-labeled control-IgG or anti-GPV, and directly analyzed on a FACScalibur (BD Biosciences). Platelets were gated by FSC/SSC characteristics (gate 1) at a high FSC amplification (E01).

3.3. Whole Blood Analysis of Platelet Membrane Glycoproteins

In principle, glycoprotein levels on platelets can be determined by single-color analysis in whole blood (**Fig. 1**). However, it is generally recommended to use the specific (directly labeled) antibody in combination with a pan-platelet marker to exclude non-platelet events (**Fig. 2**). Although agonist-induced platelet activation can also be determined in whole blood, it may be preferable to use washed platelets for such studies, if possible.

1. Add specific or negative control antibodies to the assay tube in a small volume (usually 5 µL) together with 5 µL of the pan-platelet marker.
2. When measuring platelet response to agonist stimulation, add 4 µL of 10-fold concentrates of agonists.
3. At this point, any additional reagents (e.g., inhibitors) are added in small volumes (<5 µL).
4. Add 26 µL diluted whole blood and vortex mix for 1–2 s.
5. Incubate for 15 min at room temperature.
6. Fill up with 400 µL PBS and analyze within 30 min.

Due to the presence of heparin in the blood sample, thrombin-induced platelet activation cannot be determined under these conditions. For such studies, washed blood or washed platelets should be used (*see* **Note 6**).

3.4. Two-Color Analysis of Platelet Activation

In many cases, investigators may wish to analyze platelet function in genetically modified mouse strains with defined defects in receptors or signaling pathways. Normally, such studies involve dose-response experiments with different agonists and several mice per group (wild-type and mutant) yielding a large number of samples.

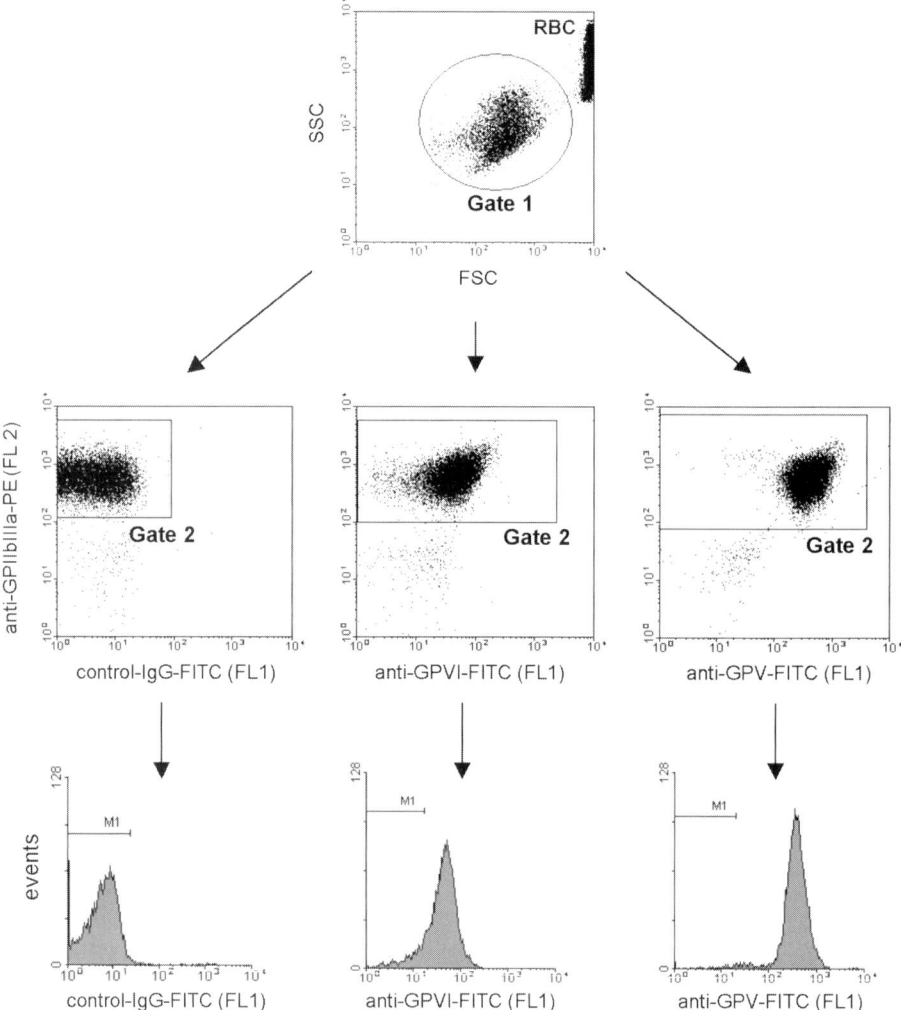

Fig. 2. Whole blood analysis of platelet membrane glycoproteins. Whole blood was diluted 1:25 with Tyrode's buffer, incubated with PE-labeled anti-GPIIbIIIa and with FITC-labeled control-IgG, anti-GPVI, or anti-GPV for 15 min and analyzed directly on a FACScalibur (BD Biosciences). Platelets were gated by FSC/SSC characteristics (gate 1) and Fl2-positivity (gate 2; pan-platelet marker, GPIIbIIIa-PE).

Such analyses are best performed with washed platelets because these can be used for several hours and undesired effects of plasma proteins on agonists, inhibitors, and antibodies are excluded. The three major steps of platelet activation can be assessed accurately by flow cytometry:

- Platelet *shape change* is easily detectable by altered FSC/SSC characteristics of the platelet population **(Fig. 3A)** (*see* **Note 7**).
- *GPIIb/IIIa activation* can be measured directly with JON/A-PE, which selectively binds to the high affinity conformation of the receptor *(9)* (Emfret Analytics) **(Fig. 3B)**. Alternatively, binding of exogenously added human fibrinogen (20 µg/mL; Sigma, F4129) can be determined using FITC-conjugated anti-fibrinogen antibodies (*see* **Subheading 2.4.3.**).
- *Release* of α-granule content is determined by measuring P-selectin expression **(Fig. 3C)**.

Principally, these antibodies can be used in single-color analysis. However, it is recommended to combine them with pan-platelet markers, which allow the exclusion of nonplatelet events **(Fig. 3B,C)**.

1. For each sample set up three assay tubes.
2. Add specific or negative control antibodies to the assay tube (5 µL of each antibody).
   a. control IgG-PE/GPIX-FITC or GPIIbIIIa-FITC
   b. JON/A-PE/GPIX-FITC
   c. P-selectin-PE/GPIIbIIIa-FITC
3. Add 4 µL of 10-fold concentrates of agonists.
4. At this point, any additional reagents (e.g., inhibitors) are added in small volumes (<5 µL)
5. Dilute washed platelets 1:25 with Tyrode's buffer containing 1 mM CaCl$_2$.
6. Add 26 µL of this dilution to the assay tube, vortex mix for 1–2 s, and incubate for 15 min at room temperature.
7. Fill up with 400 µL PBS and analyze within 30 min.

3.4.1. Two-Color Analysis for Detecting Changes in the Surface Expression of the GPIb-V-IX Complex

Von Willebrand factor (vWF) and its platelet receptor GPIb-V-IX are essential for initial platelet adhesion (tethering) to the subendothelium, especially under conditions of high shear stress as found in arteries and the microcirculation *(10–12)*. Like its human homolog, the mouse GPIb-V-IX complex consists of four different subunits: GPIbα covalently linked to GPIbβ, GPV, and GPIX. The receptor complex is expressed on the cell surface in high copy numbers and can be strongly downregulated upon cellular activation, dependent on the agonist used *(13)*. There are principally two mechanisms to downregulate the surface expression of the major functional subunit, GPIbα. First, the entire complex is translocated into the cell; second, a 130-kD fragment of GPIbα (glycocalicin) is proteolytically released into the supernatant. Using monoclonal antibodies directed against epitopes on (1) the glycocalicin portion of GPIbα, and (2) GPIX, the following flow-cytometry assay provides a rapid and easy-to-use method to discriminate between both mechanisms (modified from **ref. *13***) **(Fig. 4)**.

1. For each sample set up two assay tubes.
2. Add specific or negative control antibodies to the assay tube (5 µL of each antibody).
   a. control IgG-PE/anti-GPIX-FITC
   b. anti-GPIbα-PE/anti-GPIX-FITC
3. Add 4 µL of 10-fold concentrates of agonists.
4. At this point, any additional reagents (e.g., inhibitors) are added in small volumes (<5 µL)
5. Dilute washed platelets 1:25 with Tyrode's buffer containing 1 mM CaCl$_2$.

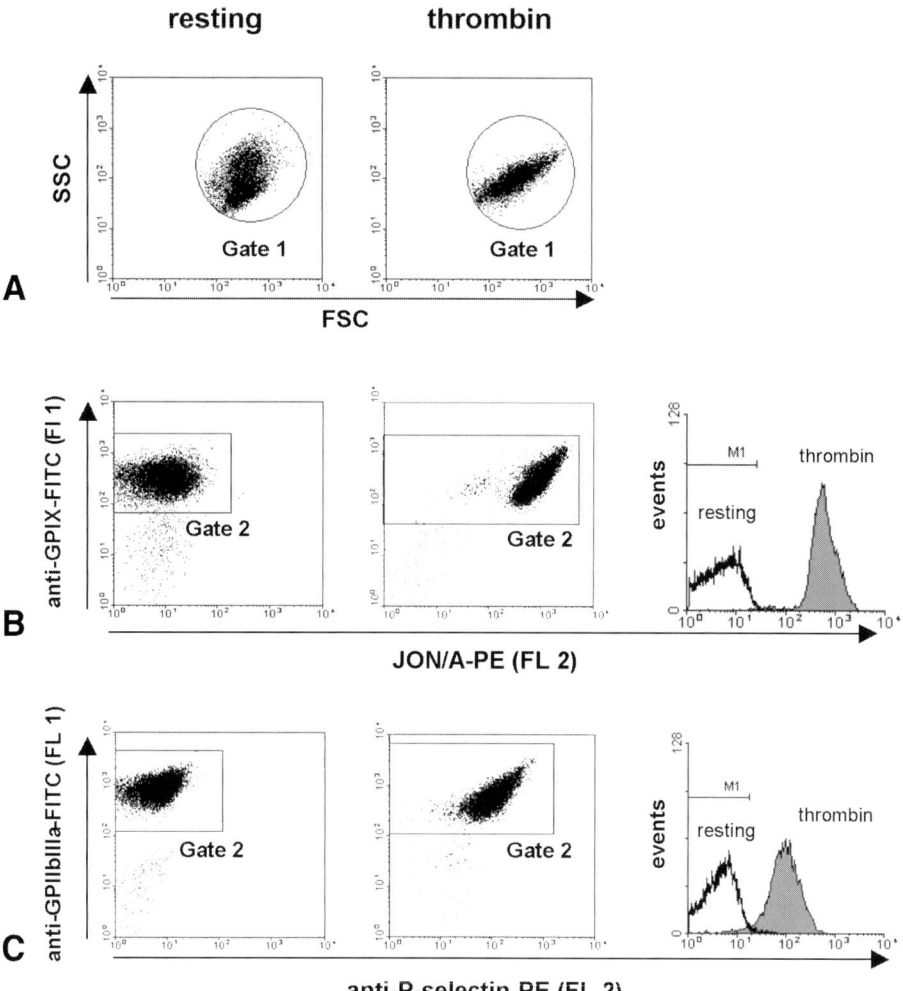

Fig. 3. Two-color analysis of platelet activation. Washed platelets were diluted 1:25 with Tyrode's buffer containing 1 mM CaCl$_2$, left unstimulated or activated with thrombin (0.1 U/mL) in the presence of the indicated antibodies. After 15 min incubation, the samples were analyzed on a FACScalibur (BD Biosciences). Platelets were gated by FSC/SSC characteristics (gate 1) and a pan-platelet marker (gate 2; **B:** GPIX-FITC; **C:** GPIIbIIIa-FITC). **(A)** The thrombin-induced shape change, is detectable by altered FSC/SSC characteristics (*see* **Note 7**). **(B)** GPIIbIIIa activation, was determined with JON/A-PE, which selectively binds to the high-affinity conformation of the integrin *(9)*. **(C)** P-selectin expression, was determined using a PE-conjugated anti-P-selectin antibody.

6. Add 26 µL of this dilution to the assay tube, vortex-mix for 1–2 s and incubate for 15 min at room temperature.
7. Fill up with 400 µL PBS and analyze within 30 min.

3.4.2. Single-Color Analysis for Studies on vWF Binding to GPIbα

Two modulating substances are used to study the binding of vWF to GPIbα on human platelets: (1) the antibiotic, ristocetin, and (2) the snake venom protein, botrocetin. However, studies on mouse platelets have demonstrated functional species-specificity for ristocetin, as it is unable to induce vWF binding to murine GPIbα. No such species specificity has been found for botrocetin. The following assay enables studies on vWF binding in murine whole blood.

1. For each sample set up two assay tubes.
2. Add specific or negative control antibodies to the assay tube (5 µL of each antibody).
   a. control IgG-FITC
   b. anti-vWf-FITC
3. Add 4 µL of botrocetin (10 U/mL).
4. At this point, any additional reagents (e.g., inhibitors) are added in small volumes (<5 µL)
5. Dilute whole blood 1:10 with Tyrode's buffer.
6. Add 10 µL of this dilution and 16 µL of Tyrode's buffer containing 5 mM EDTA (*see* **Note 8**) to the assay tube, vortex mix for 1–2 s, and incubate for 15 min at room temperature.
7. Fill up with 400 µL PBS and analyze within 30 min.

3.5. Flow-Cytometric Analysis

3.5.1. Single-Color Analysis

1. After adjusting the flow-cytometer setup (*see* Chapter 19, vol. 1), run the negative control tube.
2. Ensure that the platelet population lies within the FS/SS gate (M1 in **Fig. 1**).
3. Set the FL1 gates/cursors/markers to the 2% level on the negative control (gate 1 in **Fig. 1**).
4. Next, run a sample stained for a pan-platelet marker (GPIIbIIIa, GPIb, or GPIX).
5. Ensure that >95% of the events in the FS/SS gate are positive for the pan-platelet marker.
6. Using these settings run each sample in turn, in ascending order of agonist concentration if analyzing platelet agonist response.

3.5.2. Two-Color Analysis of Platelet-Membrane Glycoproteins in Whole Blood

1. After adjusting the flow-cytometer setup (*see* Chapter 19, vol. 1) run the tube containing the FITC-negative control antibody in combination with a pan-platelet marker (GPIIbIIIa-PE or GPIb-PE).
2. Ensure that the platelet population lies within the FSC/SSC gate (gate 1 in **Fig. 2**).
3. Use the pan-platelet marker signal to exclude nonplatelet events (gate 2 in **Fig. 2**).
4. Set the FL1 gate/cursor/marker to the 2% level on the negative control (M1 in **Fig. 2**).
5. Next, run the sample stained with specific antibody in combination with the pan-platelet marker.
6. Using these settings run each sample in turn, in ascending order of agonist concentration if analyzing platelet agonist response.

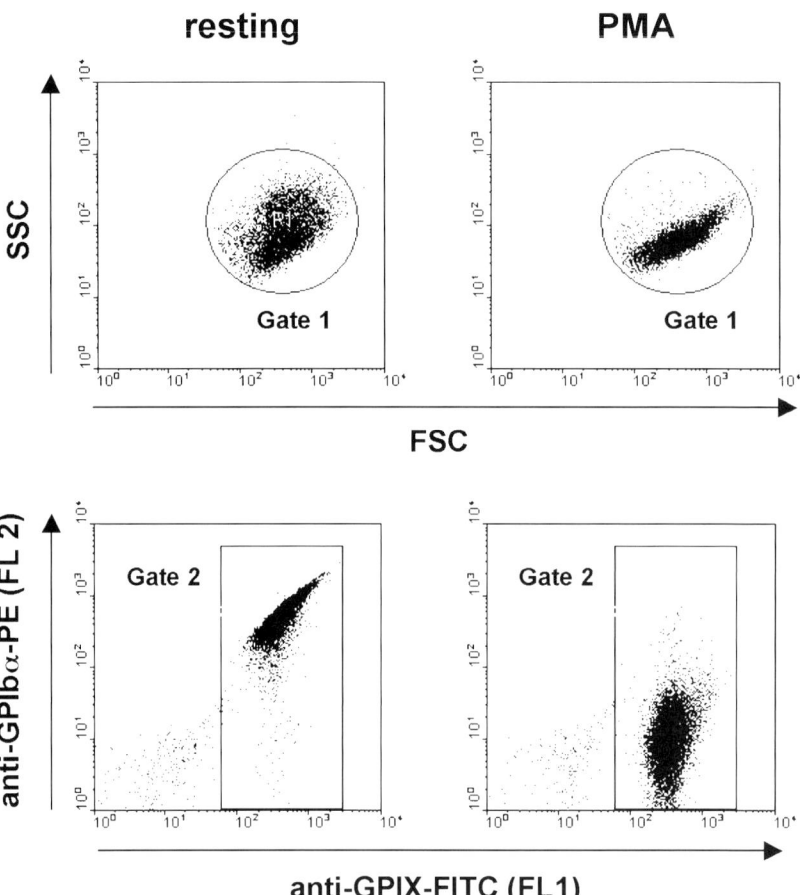

Fig. 4. Two-color analysis for detecting changes in the surface expression of the GPIb-V-IX complex. Washed platelets were diluted 1:25 with Tyrode's buffer containing 1 mM CaCl$_2$, left unstimulated or activated with PMA (50 ng/mL) in the presence of anti-GPIX-FITC and anti-GPIbα-PE. After 15 min incubation, the samples were analyzed on a FACScalibur (BD Biosciences). Platelets were gated by FSC/SSC characteristics (gate 1) and Fl1-positivity (anti-GPIX-FITC). Note that GPIbα levels decrease by >95% on PMA stimulation, whereas GPIX levels are virtually unchanged, demonstrating that PMA stimulates GPIb shedding rather than internalization of the GPIb-V-IX complex.

3.5.3. Two-Color Analysis of Platelet Activation

1. After adjusting the flow-cytometer setup (*see* Chapter 19, vol. 1) run the tube containing the negative control antibodies.
2. Ensure that the platelet population lies within the FS/SS gate (gate 1 in **Fig. 3**).
3. Use the pan-platelet marker signal to exclude nonplatelet events (gate 2 in **Fig. 3**).

4. Set the FL2 gate/cursor/marker to the 2% level on the negative control (M1 in **Fig. 3**).
5. Next run the samples stained with specific antibodies. In a resting platelet population, less than 2% of the cells should be positive for activated GPIIbIIIa (JON/A-PE) or P-selectin-PE.
6. Using these settings run each sample in turn, in ascending order of agonist concentration if analyzing platelet agonist response.

3.5.4. Two-Color Analysis for Detecting Changes in the Surface Expression of the GPIb-V-IX Complex

1. After adjusting the flow-cytometer setup (*see* Chapter 19, vol. 1) run the tube containing the negative control antibodies.
2. Ensure that the platelet population lies within the FSC/SSC gate (gate 1 in **Fig. 4**).
3. Use the GPIX-FITC signal to exclude nonplatelet events (gate 2 in **Fig. 4**).
4. Set the FL2 gate/cursor/marker to the 2% level on the negative control (M1 in **Fig. 4**).
5. Next, run the sample with resting platelets stained with specific antibodies.
6. Ensure that >98% of GPIX-positive events are postive for GPIbα (gate 2 in **Fig. 4**).
7. Using these settings run each sample in turn, in ascending order of agonist concentration if analyzing platelet agonist response.

4. Notes

1. In our experience, no significant differences in unspecific binding between different rat or hamster IgG isotype subclasses are detectable on mouse platelets. This may be explained by the fact that mouse platelets, in contrast to human platelets, do not express Fcγ receptor (FcγR) IIA, which reduces unspecific binding of IgG and the risk of antibody-induced platelet activation.
2. Antibodies from BD Biosciences or DAKO need to be titrated by the investigator before use, whereas antibodies from Emfret Analytics are supplied as ready-to-use reagents, optimized for flow cytometric applications. For further information see www.bdbiosciences.com/pharmingen; www.DakoCytomation.com; or www.Emfret.com.
3. Blood should be kept at room temperature and processed rapidly after collection to avoid any changes due to activation in vitro. This is particularly important when measuring markers of platelet activation or testing the platelet response to agonist stimulation, but it is also relevant for constitutively expressed antigens such as the GPIIbIIIa and GPIb-V-IX complexes, levels of which can increase or decrease, respectively, on the platelet surface if the sample is activated or simply ages in vitro. In whole blood, such changes become detectable after 30 min. Therefore, whole blood analyses should be performed within 30 min after blood collection. In contrast, washed platelets (*see* **Subheading 3.1.3.**) remain in a resting state for at least 2–3 h.
4. Extracellular free calcium is required for affinity regulation of integrins and other processes during platelet activation. Consequently, low levels of calcium prevent or slow down activation processes during storage of whole blood or washed platelets. Therefore, CaCl$_2$ (1 mM final concentration) should be added to the samples directly only before the start of the experiment.
5. The addition of 0.02 U/mL (final conc) apyrase prevents desensitization of the P2Y$_1$ ADP receptor by spontaneously released ADP.
6. For several reasons analysis of thrombin-induced activation of mouse platelets should not be performed in whole blood. First, thrombin activity is inhibited in heparinized blood. Second, thrombin converts plasma fibrinogen to fibrin and thereby induces clot formation.

Due to differences in the thrombin receptor system between humans and mice *(14)*, TRAP (thrombin receptor agonist peptide; SFLLRN), which is routinely used to stimulate human platelets (*see* Chapter 19, vol. 1), has no effect on mouse platelets.

7. Due to their discoid shape, resting platelets produce different side-scatter (SSC) signals in the flow cytometer, depending on their relative orientation to the laser beam. Therefore, a resting platelet population has a wide distribution in the SSC signal. Upon stimulation, platelets form pseudopods and become spherical (shape change) thereby producing a characteristic SSC signal irrespective of their relative orientation to the laser beam. Therefore, an activated platelet population appears more condensed on a FCS/SSC plot.

8. EDTA is added to the assay tubes to exclude vWF binding to GPIIbIIIa.

References

1. Offermanns, S., Toombs, C. F., Hu, Y. H., and Simon, M. I. (1997) Defective platelet activation in Gαq-deficient mice. *Nature* **389,** 183–186.

2. Kahn, M. L., Zheng, Y. W., Huang, W., Bigornia, V., Zeng, D., Moff, S., et al. (1998) A dual thrombin receptor system for platelet activation. *Nature* **394,** 690–694.

3. Leon, C., Hechler, B., Freund, M., Eckly, A., Vial, C., Ohlmann, P., et al. (1999) Defective platelet aggregation and increased resistance to thrombosis in purinergic P2Y$_1$ receptor-null mice. *J. Clin. Invest.* **104,** 1731–1737.

4. Hollopeter, G., Jantzen, H. M., Vincent, D., Li, G., England, L., Ramakrishnan, V., et al. (2001) Identification of the platelet ADP receptor targeted by antithrombotic drugs. *Nature* **409,** 202–207.

5. Hodivala-Dilke, K. M., McHugh, K. P., Tsakiris, D. A., Rayburn, H., Crowley, D., Ullman-Cullere, M., et al. (1999) Beta3-integrin-deficient mice are a model for Glanzmann thrombasthenia showing placental defects and reduced survival. *J. Clin. Invest.* **103,** 229–238.

6. Ware, J., Russell, S., and Ruggeri, Z. M. (2000) Generation and rescue of a murine model of platelet dysfunction: the Bernard-Soulier syndrome. *Proc. Natl. Acad. Sci. USA* **97,** 2803–2808.

7. Tsakiris, D. A., Scudder, L., Hodivala-Dilke, K., Hynes, R. O., and Coller, B. S. (1999) Hemostasis in the mouse *(Mus musculus)*: a review. *Thromb. Haemost.* **81,** 177–188.

8. Alugupalli, K. R., Michelson, A. D., Barnard, M. R., and Leong, J. M. (2001) Serial determinations of platelet counts in mice by flow cytometry. *Thromb. Haemost.* **86,** 668–671.

9. Bergmeier, W., Schulte, V., Brockhoff, G., Bier, U., Zirngibl, H., and Nieswandt, B. (2002) Flow cytometric detection of activated mouse integrin α$_{IIb}$β$_3$ with a novel monoclonal antibody. *Cytometry* **48,** 80–86.

10. Tschopp, T. B., Weiss, H. J., and Baumgartner, H. R. (1974) Decreased adhesion of platelets to subendothelium in von Willebrand's disease. *J. Lab. Clin. Med.* **83,** 296–300.

11. Sakariassen, K. S., Bolhuis, P. A., and Sixma, J. J. (1979) Human blood platelet adhesion to artery subendothelium is mediated by factor VIII-Von Willebrand factor bound to the subendothelium. *Nature* **279,** 636–638.

12. Savage, B., Saldivar, E., and Ruggeri, Z. M. (1996) Initiation of platelet adhesion by arrest onto fibrinogen or translocation on von Willebrand factor. *Cell* **84,** 289–297.

13. Bergmeier, W., Rackebrandt, K., Schroder, W., Zirngibl, H., and Nieswandt, B. (2000) Structural and functional characterization of the mouse von Willebrand factor receptor GPIb-IX with novel monoclonal antibodies. *Blood* **95,** 886–893.

14. Coughlin, S.R. (2001) Protease-activated receptors in vascular biology. *Thromb. Haemost.* **86,** 298–307.

21

Platelet Microparticles

Shosaku Nomura and Shirou Fukuhara

1. Introduction

One of the responses of activated platelets to certain stimuli is the shedding of microparticles. Microparticles released from platelets (PMPs) may play a role in the normal hemostatic response to vascular injury, as these particles exhibit prothrombinase activity *(1)*. It is also possible that local generation of PMPs in small atherosclerotic arteries or arterioles may promote acute arterial occlusion by providing and expanding a catalytic surface for the coagulation cascade.

PMPs carry several antigens characteristic of intact platelets, chiefly glycoproteins (GP) IIb/IIIa (integrin $\alpha_{IIb}\beta_3$) and GPIb/IX. PMPs cannot be detected by standard platelet counting methods but they can be detected by other means. PMPs were first described by Wolf *(2)*; Warren and Vales *(3)* demonstrated the release of vesicles from platelets following the adhesion of platelets to vessel walls. Platelet-derived procoagulant activity was previously called platelet factor 3 *(4)*.

Pathologic levels of fluid-shear stress may occur in small arteries or arterioles partially obstructed by atherosclerosis or vasospasm and may induce activation and aggregation of circulating platelets *(5–8)*. This type of platelet aggregation may play a crucial role in thrombogenesis in various pathological states *(6,7,9)*. High shear stress can initiate both platelet aggregation and shedding of procoagulant-containing microparticles *(10,11)*, suggesting the possibility that microparticles are generated by high shear stress in small diseased arteries and arterioles *(12)*.

PMPs can range in size from 0.02 μm to 0.1 μm, and they have no clear definition. It is unclear whether PMPs arise from complete conversion of a few platelets or from partial conversion of many or most platelets, but it is likely that both scenarios occur. There is a growing body of evidence that platelets comprise a heterogeneous population that is not attributable solely to senescence *(13–15)*. George et al. *(16)* quantified many different GPs on PMPs, many of which are present routinely, notably GPIIb/IIIa and GPIb/IX. Sims et al. *(17)* characterized PMPs and reported the presence

From: *Methods in Molecular Biology, vol. 272:*
Platelets and Megakaryocytes, Vol. 1: Functional Assays
Edited by: J. M. Gibbins and M. P. Mahaut-Smith © Humana Press Inc., Totowa, NJ

of GPIIb/IIIa, GPIb/IX, and α-granule membrane protein-140 (P-selectin or CD62P). In addition, an activation-dependent epitope of GPIIb/IIIa was found on complement-activated platelets but not on PMPs *(18)*. Other researchers have also reported differences in the composition of membrane proteins between activated platelets and PMPs *(18–20)*.

Current methods for studying PMPs include quantifying assays, functional assays, and morphologic assays. Flow cytometry is now the most widely used method for studying PMPs because of its simplicity and the wealth of information that can be gleaned from the population under study *(21–23)*. However, this method is not sufficiently sensitive to produce highly accurate, consistent PMP counts *(24)*. Thus, an easier and more reproducible PMP assay is needed. We recently described a new method to accurately measure PMPs with an enzyme-linked immunosorbent assay (ELISA) method *(25)*. In this chapter we describe the use of this ELISA as well as flow cytometry to measure the PMP content of samples.

2. Materials

1. 20-*g* needle.
2. 3.8% (w/v) sodium citrate.
3. Centrifuges.
4. Washing buffer: 9 mM Na$_2$EDTA, 140 mM NaCl, and 26 mM Na$_2$HPO$_4$, pH 7.2.
5. HEPES-Tyrode's buffer: 129 mM NaCl, 8.9 mM NaHCO$_3$, 0.8 mM KH$_2$PO$_4$, 0.8 mM MgCl$_2$, 5.6 mM glucose, and 10 mM HEPES, pH 7.4.
6. 2% (v/v) paraformaldehyde.
7. Stock solution: 9 mM Na$_2$EDTA, 26.4 mM Na$_2$HPO$_4$, 140 mM NaCl, 0.1% (w/v) NaN$_3$, and 2% (v/v) fetal bovine serum, pH 7.2.
8. ACD/EDTA: 1.0 g Na$_2$EDTA, 2.2 g trisodium citrate, 0.807 g citric acid, 2.2 g dextrose in 100 mL of distilled water.
9. EDTA/saline: 9 mM Na$_2$EDTA and 140 mM NaCl.
10. Antibodies against platelet GPIb (e.g., NNKY5-5) *(26)*, GPIIb/IIIa (e.g., NNKY2-11) *(27)*, GPIX (e.g., KMP-9) *(28)*, and anti-CD9 (e.g., NNKY1-19) *(29)*.
11. Biotinylated anti-CD41 (Cosmo Bio, Tokyo, Japan).
12. Protein biotinylation kit (Pierce Chemical Co., Rockford, IL).
13. Internal standard, 30 µL (1000 beads/µL) of microbeads (Flow-Count; Coulter, Miami, FL).
14. Flow cytometer (e.g., FACS Calibur, Becton Dickinson, Mountain View, CA).
15. FITC-conjugated mouse IgG.
16. 96-well microtiter plates (Nunc MaxiSorp, Nalge Nuno International, Tokyo, Japan).
17. Tris-saline: 50 mM Tris-HCl containing 140 mM NaCl, pH 7.6.
18. 1% (v/v) Triton X-100.
19. Plate shaker (200 rpm).
20. Phosphate-buffered saline (PBS) containing 0.05% (v/v) Tween-20.
21. 50 µL of peroxidase-conjugated avidin (Vector Laboratories, Burlingame, CA) diluted 1:20,000 in 1% (w/v) nonfat dry milk, PBS.
22. 100 µL of peroxidase substrate solution (ScyTek, Logan, UT).
23. Assay stop solution (ScyTek).
24. EIA reader (e.g., Model 550, Microplate Reader, Bio-Rad Laboratories, Tokyo, Japan) at 450 nm.

3. Methods

3.1. Blood Samples

To minimize platelet activation during sample collection and fixation, the following procedures should be used for flow-cytometric analysis.

1. Blood is carefully drawn from an antecubital vein through a 20-*g* needle and collected in tubes containing 3.8% (w/v) sodium citrate (9:1 vol blood:vol citrate).
2. Platelet-rich plasma (PRP) is prepared by centrifugation at 200*g* for 10 min at room temperature.
3. Washed platelets are prepared by centrifuging PRP at 1400*g* for 10 min at room temperature.
4. The resultant pellet is washed twice with washing buffer and resuspended in HEPES-Tyrode's buffer.
5. Following treatment of platelets as required in specific experiments, an equal volume of 2% (v/v) paraformaldehyde is added to washed platelets and incubated for 15 min at room temperature.
6. Platelets are washed twice as described above, resuspended in stock solution, and stored at 4°C until analysis.

3.2. Preparation of PMP

1. Draw blood samples into a syringe, and mix with 1/10 volume of ACD/EDTA.
2. Centrifuge at 150*g* for 10 min and remove PRP.
3. To PRP, add EDTA/saline (to a final concentration of 60% (v/v) PRP) and centrifuge at 1500*g* for 20 min (*see* **Note 1**).
4. Remove the buffer, which contains platelet microparticles (PMP). PMP solutions may be subjected to flow cytometry (*see* **Subheading 3.4.**); for ELISA assays (*see* **Subheading 3.5.**), samples are further diluted with 1% (w/v) EDTA/saline (to a final concentration of 50% (v/v) PMP).

3.3. Antibodies

Where required, antibodies may be labeled with biotin using a protein biotinylation kit (e.g., from Pierce, Biotechnology Inc., Rockford, IL) following the manufacturer's instructions.

3.4. Flow Cytometry Assay

1. To distinguish PMP from background noise, microparticles are immunocytochemically stained with an antibody to GPIb. The concentrations of antibody give are for NNKY5-5, and alternative antibodies may require optimization. Add 3 µL FITC-conjugated NNKY5-5 (1 µg/mL of final concentration) to 50 µL of sample and incubate for 30 min at 4°C.
2. As an internal standard, add 30 µL (1000 beads/µL) of microbeads to each sample and mix well.
3. Dilute samples with 250 µL of phosphate-buffered saline (pH 7.5), and measure the fluorescence level of 300 beads using the flow cytometer. To exclude background scatter, samples treated with nonspecific FITC-conjugated mouse IgG should first be run to determine the threshold FITC fluorescence.

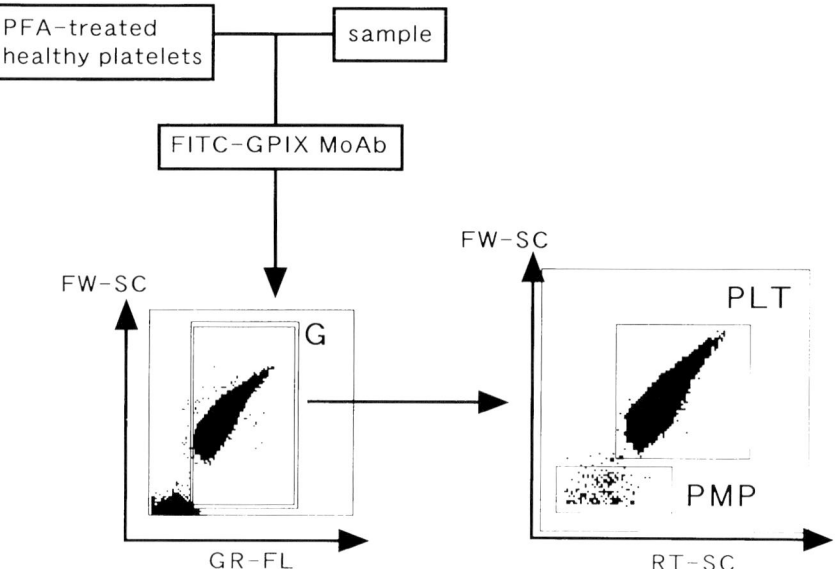

Fig. 1. Flow-cytometric measurement of PMPs. Washed intact platelets from healthy subjects were added to samples and incubated with FITC-labeled anti-GPIX monoclonal antibody (KMP-9), followed by dilution with HEPES-Tyrode's buffer containing 5 nmol/L EGTA. Only cells and particles positive for GPIX were gated, to distinguish platelets and PMPs from noise. To differentiate between platelets and PMPs, the lower limit of the platelet gate was set at the left-hand border of the forward scatter profile of resting platelets. PFA, paraformaldehyde; FW-SC, forward scatter; GR-FL, green fluorescence; RT-SC, right scatter.

4. The population of particles solely positive for FITC but smaller than platelets are gated as microparticles. As illustrated in **Fig. 1**, 10,000 FITC-positive particles in the microparticle gate may then counted to determine the number of microparticles released per 10,000 platelets.

3.5. ELISA

1. To antibody-coat microtiter plates, add 50 µL of purified antibodies (anti-GPIX; 1 µg/mL) to each well of 96-well microtiter plates and incubate for 18 h at 4°C.
2. Wash the plates three times with Tris-saline (pH 7.6).
3. To block wells add 350 µL of PBS containing 1% (w/v) BSA to each well and incubate for at least 8 h at 4°C. Pool PRP samples from several healthy volunteers and adjust to 200,000 platelets/µL to be used as standards for the ELISA.
4. Centrifuge 1 mL of platelet suspension at 1500g for 20 min and solubilize pellet with 1 mL of 1% (v/v) Triton X-100. One unit/mL of PMP is defined as 24,000 platelets/mL of solubilized platelets in this ELISA. Pipet 50 µL of diluted PMP samples or standards into each well and incubate for 18 h at 25°C on a plate shaker (200 rpm).

Table 1
Conditions of Centrifugation for PMP Preparation

	PRP dilution (%)			
	0	20	30	40
PMP	3876.5 ± 847.6	2981.0 ± 538.1	2401.0 ± 319.6	2596.5 ± 318.5
Platelets	2473.3 ± 639.5	1542.5 ± 1263.2	774.0 ± 632.7	346.8 ± 260.6

PRP was centrifuged at 150g for 10 min, and the pellet was diluted with 0.2, 0.3, or 0.4 volumes 0.1% EDTA/saline as described in the Methods section. The platelet suspension was centrifuged at 1500g for 20 min, and the PMP fraction was subjected to flow cytometry. Data are PMP counts/μL.

5. Wash each well of the plates three times with 350 μL/well of wash buffer (0.05% (v/v) Tween-20 in PBS).
6. Add 50 μL of biotinylated antibody (anti-GPIb; 0.2 μg/mL in 1% (w/v) nonfat milk/PBS) to each well and incubate for 2 h at 25°C on a plate shaker.
7. Wash each well three times with 350 μL of wash buffer.
8. Add 50 μL of peroxidase-conjugated avidin (diluted 1:20,000 in 1% [w/v] nonfat dry milk) to each well and incubate for 2 h at 25°C with shaking.
9. Wash each well three times with 350 μL of wash buffer.
10. Add to each well 100 μL of peroxidase substrate solution and incubate for 20 min at room temperature.
11. Add 100 μL of stop solution (ScyTek) to each well, and measure the absorbance with an EIA reader at 450 nm.
12. Using a range of standards, draw a standard curve that may be used to determine the concentrations of the samples. The results are expressed arbitrary units per mL (U/mL) (*see* **Notes 2–4**).

4. Notes

1. We have found that the recovery of PMPs from PRP diluted with 0.2 volumes of 0.1% EDTA/saline is equivalent to, but more contaminated than that from PRP diluted with 0.4 volumes of 0.1% EDTA/saline (**Table 1**). It is therefore advisable to dilute PRP with 0.4 volumes of 0.1% EDTA/saline. To establish optimum centrifugation conditions for preparing PMPs for ELISA, PMPs were solubilized with Triton X-100, centrifuged at either 1000g for 10 min, 1500g for 10 min, 1500g for 20 min, or 2000g for 10 min, and then assayed with the ELISA described in **Subheading 3.5.** Centrifugation conditions had no effect on ELISA optical density (OD) among PMPs receiving no Triton X-100 treatment. However, ELISA OD of PMPs solubilized with Triton X-100 was lowest when centrifuged at 1500g for 20 min, and therefore these conditions are recommended for use.
2. PMPs (1500g 20 min supernatant) were mixed (1:1) with platelets and subjected to PMP ELISA. Shaking had no effect on ELISA OD of samples containing PMPs and no platelets. However, among samples containing PMPs and platelets, ELISA ODs were higher without shaking than with shaking (**Fig. 2**).
3. PMPs were prepared by activation of platelets with 3 μg/mL of collagen and recovered by centrifugation. PMPs were serially diluted with 0.1% (w/v) EDTA/saline and sub-

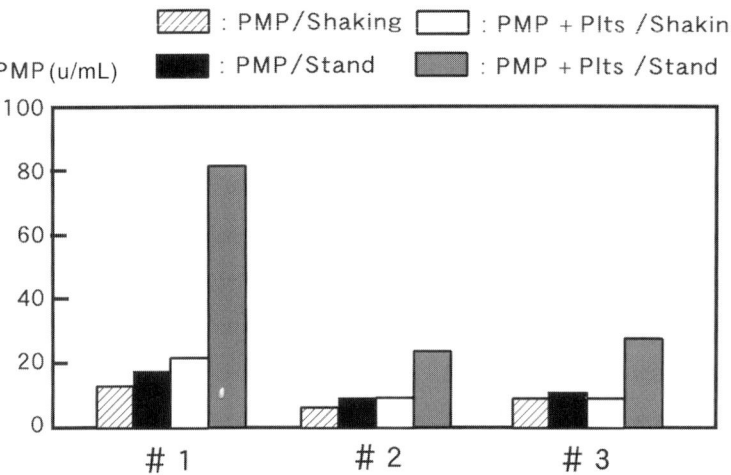

Fig. 2. PMPs (1500 g supernatant) were mixed with platelets (2000 platelets/μL) and subjected to PMP ELISA with or without shaking (200 rpm).

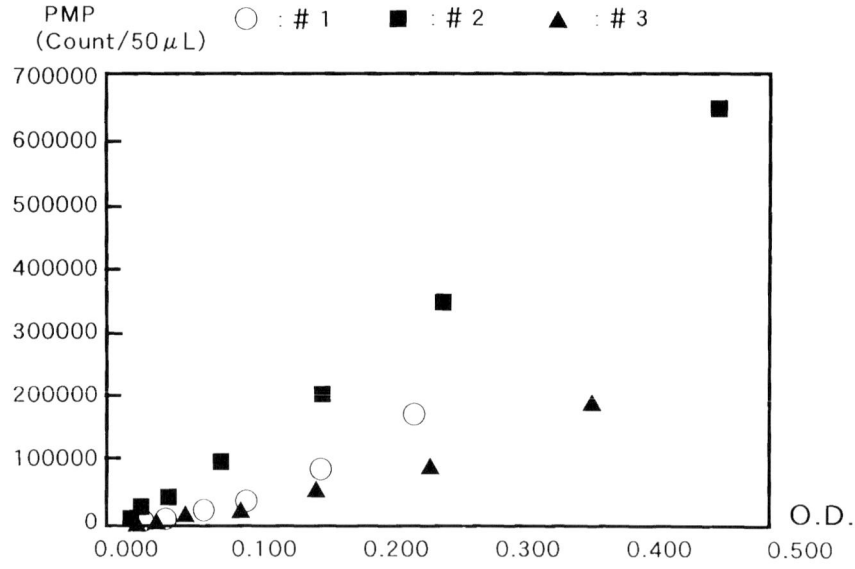

Fig. 3. Platelets were activated with 3 μg/mL of collagen, and PMPs were recovered by centrifugation. PMPs were serially diluted with EDTA/saline and subjected to FCM or ELISA.

jected to FCM and ELISA. Good correlation between FCM and ELISA methods was observed **(Fig. 3)**.
4. Activated PMPs were prepared by stimulation with collagen. Activated or circulating PMPs were filtered with 0.8-μL filters and PMP numbers were counted by flow cytometry.

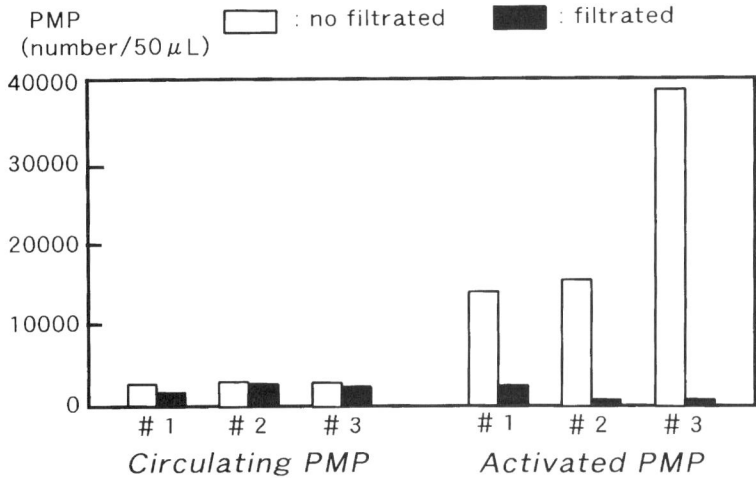

Fig. 4. Platelets were treated with or without 3 µg/mL of collagen, and PMPs were recovered by centrifugation. PMPs were filtered thought a 0.8-µm disposable filter and the PMP numbers were counted by FCM.

Circulating PMPs were not absorbed by the filter, but activated PMPs were absorbed by the filter **(Fig. 4)**.

References

1. Sims, P. J., Wiedmer, T., Esmon, C. T., Weiss, H. J., and Shattil, S. J. (1989) Assembly of the platelet prothrombinase complex is linked to vesiculation of the platelet plasma membrane. *J. Biol. Chem.* **264,** 17,049–17,057.
2. Wolf, P. (1967) The nature and significance of platelet products in human plasma. *Br. J. Haematol.* **13,** 269–288.
3. Warren, B. A. and Vales, O. (1972) The relase of vesicles from platelets following adhesion to vessel walls in vitro. *Br. J. Exp. Pathol.* **53,** 206–215.
4. Hardisty, R. M. and Hutton, R. A. (1966) Platelet aggregation and the availability of platelet factor 3. *Br. J. Haematol.* **12,** 764–776.
5. Moake, J. L., Turner, N. A., Stathopoulos, N. A., Nolasco, L. H., and Hellums, J. D. (1986) Involvement of large plasma von Willebrand factor (vWF) multimers and unusually large vWF forms derived from endothelial cells in shear stress-induced platelet aggregation. *J. Clin. Invest.* **78,** 1456–1461.
6. O'Brien, J. R. (1990) Shear-induced platelet aggregation. *Lancet* **335,** 711–713.
7. Ikeda, Y., Handa, M., Kawano, K., Kamata, T., Murata, M., Araki, Y., et al. (1991) The role of von Willebrand factor and fibrinogen in platelet aggregation under varying shear stress. *J. Clin. Invest.* **87,** 1234–1240.
8. Ruggeri, Z. M. (1993) Mechanisms of shear-induced platelet aggregation. *Thromb. Haemost.* **70,** 119–123.
9. Butler, J. (1995) Shear stress platelet activation. *Lancet* **346,** 841.

10. Miyazaki, Y., Nomura, S., Miyake, T., Kagawa, H., Kitada, C., Taniguchi, H., et al. (1996) High shear stress can initiate both platelet aggregation and shedding of procoagulant containing microparticles. *Blood* **88,** 3456–3464.

11. Holme, P. A., Orvim, U., Hamers, M. J. A. G., Solum, N. O., Brosstad, F. R., Barstad, R. M., et al. (1997) Shear-induced platelet activation and platelet microparticle formation at blood flow conditions as in arteries with a severe stenosis. *Arterioscler. Thromb. Vasc. Biol.* **17,** 646–653.

12. Nomura, S. (2001) Function and clinical significance of platelet-derived micropartricles. *Int. J. Hematol.* **74,** 397–404.

13. Johnston, G. I., Pickett, E. B., McEver, R. P., and George, J. N. Heterogeneity of platelet secretion in response to thrombin demonstrated by fluorescence flow cytometry. *Blood* **69,** 1401–1403.

14. Behnke, O. and Forer, A. (1993) Blood platelet heterogeneity: Evidence for two classes of platelets in man and rat. *Br. J. Haematol.* **84,** 686–693.

15. Jaremo, P. and Sandberg-Gertzen, H. (1996) Platelet density and size in inflammatory bowel disease. *Thromb. Haemost.* **75,** 560–561.

16. George, J. N., Pickett, E. B., Saucerman, S., et al. (1986) Platelet surface glycoproteins: Studies on resting and activated platelets and platelet membrane microparticles in normal subjects, and observations in patients during adult respiratory distress syndrome and cardiac surgery. *J. Clin. Invest.* **78,** 340–348.

17. Sims, P. J., Faioni, E. M., Wiedmer, T., and Shattil, S. J. (1988) Complement proteins C5b-9 cause release of membrane vesicles from the platelet surface that are enriched in the membrane receptor for coagulation factor Va and express prothrombinase activity. *J. Biol. Chem.* **263,** 18,205–18,212.

18. Tschoepe, D., Spangenberg, P., Esser, J., Yamaguch, K., Fukuroi, T., Yanabu, M., et al. (1990) Flow-cytometric detection of surface membrane alterations and concommitant changes in the cytoskeletal actin status of activated platelets. *Cytometry* **11,** 652–656.

19. Nomura, S., Suzuki, M., Kido, H., et al. (1992) Differences between platelet and microparticle glycoprotein IIb/IIIa. *Cytometry* **13,** 621–629.

20. Nomura, S., Nakamura, T., Cone, J., Tandon, N. N., and Kambayashi, J. (2000) Cytometric analysis of high shear-induced platelet micro-particles and effect of cytokines on microparticle generation. *Cytometry* **40,** 173–181.

21. Bode, A. P., Orton, S. M., Frye, M. J., and Udis, B. J. (1991) Vesiculation of platelets during in vitro aging. *Blood* **77,** 887–895.

22. Jy, W., Horstmann, L. L., Arce, M., and Ahn, Y. S. (1992) Clinical significance of platelet microparticles in autoimmune thrombocytopenias. *J. Lab. Clin. Med.* **119,** 334–345.

23. Abrams, C. S., Ellison, N., Budzynski, A. Z., and Shattil, S. J. (1990) Direct detection of activation platelet and platelet-derived micro-particles in humans. *Blood* **75,** 128–138.

24. Miyamoto, S., Marcinkiewicz, C., Edmunds, L. H., Jr., and Niewiarowski, S. (1998) Measurement of platelet microparticles during cardiopulmonary bypass by means of capture ELISA for GPIIb/IIIa. *Thromb. Haemost.* **80,** 225–230.

25. Osumi, K., Ozeki, Y., Saito, S., Nagamura, Y., Ito, H., and Kimura, Y. (2001) Development and assessment of enzyme immunoassay for platelet-derived microparticles. *Thromb. Haemost.* **85,** 326–330.

26. Yanabu, M., Ozaki, Y., Nomura, S., Miyake, T., Miyazaki, Y., Kagawa, H., et al. (1997) Tyrosine phosphorylation and p72[syk] activation by an anti-glycoprotein Ib monoclonal antibody. *Blood* **89,** 1590–1598.

27. Hamamoto, K., Nomura, S., Suzuki, M., Ohga, S., and Fukuhara, S. (1995) Internalization of an anti-glycoprotein IIb/IIIa antibody by HEL cells. *Thromb. Haemost.* **75,** 291–296.

28. Miyake, T., Nomura, S., Komiyama, Y., Miyazaki, Y., Kagawa, H., Masuda, M., et al. (1997) Effect of a new monoclonal anti-glycoprotein IX antibody, KMP-9, on high shear-induced platelet aggregation. *Thromb. Haemost.* **78,** 902–909.

29. Ozaki, Y., Satoh, K., Kuroda, K., Qi, R., Yatomi, Y., Yanagi, S., et al. (1995) Anti-CD9 monoclonal antibody activates p72^{syk} in human platelets. *J. Biol. Chem.* **270,** 15,119–15,124.

II

MEGAKARYOCYTE FUNCTIONAL ASSAYS

22

Isolation of Primary Megakaryocytes and Studies of Proplatelet Formation

Robert M. Leven

1. Introduction

Bone marrow megakaryocytes were first described well over one hundred years ago *(1,2)* and it is almost one hundred years since their role in platelet formation was first appreciated *(3,4)*. Prior to the development of megakaryocyte isolation techniques, a great deal had been learned about megakaryocyte structure and megakaryocytopoiesis using electron microscopy and in vivo experimentation. However, the development of isolation techniques opened up entirely new areas of research on megakaryocytes. Megakaryocyte isolation has been a challenge due to the fragile nature of megakaryocytes and their relative rarity, constituting less than 1% of the nucleated cells in mammalian bone marrow. Nevertheless, techniques including density gradient centrifugation, centrifugal elutriation, selective aggregation, and immunomagnetic bead isolation have been described for megakaryocyte isolation from murine, rat, guinea pig, bovine, and human tissue *(5–23)*.

The first successful isolation of megakaryocytes was based on separation with density gradients. We can understand how these methods work by examining the forces that determine the sedimentation rate of particles.

The rate of sedimentation *(V)* of an ideal particle in a centrifugal field is:

$$V = \frac{\alpha^2(D_p - D_m)\omega^2 r}{18\eta}$$

Where α = particle diameter, D_p = particle density, D_m = density of the medium, η = viscosity of the medium, ω = angular velocity, r = radial distance from the axis of rotation.

For the isolation of megakaryocytes there are two important points to make from this equation. When separating a mix of different cell types in a single suspension, α and D_p are the only characteristics that vary between cell types (assuming all cells to be

From: *Methods in Molecular Biology, vol. 272:*
Platelets and Megakaryocytes, Vol. 1: Functional Assays
Edited by: J. M. Gibbins and M. P. Mahaut-Smith © Humana Press Inc., Totowa, NJ

spherical). The fact that V is a function of the square of the cell diameter means that the large size of megakaryocytes is an important and effective characteristic for their separation from smaller cells. In addition, we see that when $D_p = D_m$, the velocity of particle sedimentation is zero (density equilibrium). Therefore megakaryocytes (or any cell) can be separated from cells of different density, since each cell will come to rest in the gradient at a point where the cell and medium density are the same. Application of these two characteristics is the basis for nonimmunologic megakaryocyte separation techniques. Although not the first publication on megakaryocyte isolation, the technique of Levine and Fedorko (5) was the first to provide consistent preparations of large numbers of megakaryocytes with a relatively high degree of purity (~70%) and a high degree of viability. In this technique megakaryocytes are first separated from cells of greater density in a density equilibrium gradient. A subsequent unit velocity ($1g$) gradient of low density is then used. In this second gradient, cell separation will be primarily due to size differences, since all of the cells are of greater density than the medium. Consequently, megakaryocytes are separated by settling more quickly than the other cells.

The drawback to this scheme is that it does not allow for recovery of smaller, more immature megakaryocytes. The introduction of antibody-based separation techniques has provided a solution to this problem. Targeting of megakaryocyte-specific antigens (e.g., CD41 or CD42) with antibodies conjugated directly or indirectly to microscopic magnetic beads allows cells to be isolated independently of their size and density. Although in theory one should be able to isolate a pure population of megakaryocytes in a one-step process using immunologic selection, in practice it is generally necessary to first separate out the large number of high-density cells to get a high megakaryocyte purity. This is due to the tendency of cells to stick to one another and to the relatively low percentage of megakaryocytes.

2. Materials

1. Bone marrow: As indicated in the introduction, bone marrow megakaryocytes have been isolated from a variety of species. Regardless of the species used, the age of the animal from which the tissue is obtained is most important. This is due to the decrease in hematopoietic tissue in the marrow of older animals. Therefore young adult animals should be used. Rats of 100–200 g or guinea pigs 250–300 g are most suitable for megakaryocyte isolation.
2. Dissection tools: Scissors, forceps, #10 scalpel, scissors-style dog nail clipper, small weighing spatula (see **Note 1**).
3. Sterile tissue culture plastics and accessories: 35- and 100-mm diameter tissue culture dishes, 10–15- and 50-mL polypropylene tubes, sterile Nitex (nylon mesh) filter (200-μm mesh; Tetko, Elmsford, NY), 1.5-mL plastic tubes (see **Note 1**). For the albumin density gradient, 50-mL round-bottom tubes must be used.
4. 10X Calcium-magnesium-free Hank's salt solution (CMFH): Dissolve the following in 100 mL of water and adjust the pH to 7.4 with NaOH: 0.4 g KCl, 0.06 g KH_2PO_4, 8.0 g NaCl, 0.35 g $NaHCO_3$, 0.048 g Na_2HPO_4, 1.0 g glucose.
5. CATCH buffer: Combine 100 mL 10X CMFH, 850 mL H_2O, 376 mg adenosine, 494 mg theophylline, 3.8 g sodium citrate. Adjust pH to 7.4 with 1.0 N NaOH or 1.0 N HCl as necessary and adjust volume to 1000 mL. This solution is sterilized by filtration and stored for up to 2 wk at 4°C.

Table 1
Bovine Serum Albumin Gradient Solutions

Density (g/mL)	Refractive index	Stock BSA solution (mL)	CATCH buffer (mL)
1.050	1.3697	25	2
1.045	1.3662	30	6
1.040	1.3630	30	12
1.035	1.3598	24	12.5
VG stock solution	1.3430	25	80
2/3 VG solution	20 mL VG stock solution + 10 mL CATCH buffer		
1/3 VG solution	10 mL VG stock solution + 20 mL CATCH buffer		

6. Siliconized pipets: Glass Pasteur pipets and Sigmacote (Sigma Chemical Co., St. Louis, MO) (*see* **Note 2**).

7. Albumin: Bovine serum albumin is commonly used as a density gradient medium for megakaryocyte separation. We use electrophoresis-grade bovine serum albumin, minimum 98% from Sigma Chemical Co.

8. Digital refractometer: We have used an Abbe Mark II digital refractometer from Cambridge Instruments, Buffalo, NY.

9. Bovine serum albumin (BSA) stock solution: To 200 mL water in a 600-mL beaker, add 15.5 mL 10X CMFH, 97.2 mg adenosine and 128.4 mg theophylline. Add 58 g bovine serum albumin, but do not stir or mix. Cover the beaker and leave overnight at 4°C to allow albumin to dissolve. Once all the albumin has dissolved, adjust the pH to 7.4 with 1.0 *N* NaOH, using slow, continuous stirring to avoid protein denaturation. Then centrifuge the solution at a minimum of 25,000g for 30 min at 4°C to remove insoluble material. If this is not done, filter sterilization of the albumin solutions will be extremely difficult.

10. Bovine serum albumin gradient solutions: The gradient solutions are made by mixing the bovine serum albumin stock solution with the CATCH buffer and adjusting the solution to the appropriate refractive index. The refractive index must be monitored with a digital refractometer (item 8 above). The volumes indicated in **Table 1** will give solutions close to the required refractive index. The refractive index must be adjusted by addition of more stock BSA solution or more CATCH buffer until the correct refractive index is achieved. In our laboratory we adjust the refractive index to within ± 0.0003 units. It is not necessary to adjust the refractive index of the 2/3 VG solution or the 1/3 VG solution. All the bovine serum albumin gradient solutions are filter-sterilized and stored at 4°C for up to two weeks.

11. Ficoll 400: is used as a velocity gradient medium. It is commercially available from several suppliers, such as Promega Corp. (Madison, WI), Amersham Biosciences (Piscataway, NJ), and United States Biological (Swampscott, MA).

12. Ficoll solution: 2% and 4% solutions are prepared by dissolving 2 g and 4 g Ficoll in 100 mL CATCH buffer. The solutions are filter-sterilized and stored at 4°C for up to two weeks.

13. Ficoll gradient construction: Dual-chamber gradient mixer (Model SG30 from Hoefer Scientific Instruments, San Francisco, CA), magnetic stirrer, 15-mL conical-bottom tube, peristaltic pump.

14. Antibodies: When performing immunomagnetic bead separation, the most critical factor in successful megakaryocyte isolation is the primary antibody to be used. Clearly the antibody must be specific for a megakaryocyte-specific protein such as glycoprotein IIb (integrin αIIb) or glycoprotein Ib. We have had consistently excellent results for guinea pig

megakaryocyte isolation using a monoclonal antibody to glycoprotein Ib from Dako (Dako Corporation, Carpenteria, CA, catalog no. MO719). This antibody can be used for rat megakaryocyte isolation, but the purity is much lower than when using guinea pig marrow. Since the commercial antibodies are almost always to human proteins, individual monoclonal antibodies and different antibody batches must be tested for specificity and cross-reactivity for the species being used for megakaryocyte isolation. Even if the antibody recognizes antigen of the species being used for megakaryocyte isolation, each antibody must be tested for its effectiveness in cell selection.

15. Paramagnetic beads: Paramagnetic beads are available from different manufacturers. We have had greatest success using beads manufactured by Dynal Biotech, Inc. (Lake Success, NY). The larger 4.5-μm diameter beads should be used and can be purchased with secondary antibody already conjugated. M-450 goat anti-mouse magnetic Dynabeads are suitable for use with the monoclonal antibody to glycoprotein Ib from Dako.

16. Magnetic bead separator: Dynal MPC-1 magnetic bead separator (Dynal Biotech).

17. Proplatelet culture medium: Dulbecco's modified Eagle medium (DMEM) with 10% fetal-calf or newborn-calf serum and appropriate antibiotics.

18. Matrigel: Matrigel is commercially available from BD Biosciences, San Jose, CA.

19. Collagen gel: For the study of platelet formation we have used type I, rat-tail-tendon collagen. We have had our best results using a solution of Type I rat-tail-collagen from Upstate Biotechnology (Lake Placid, NY). DMEM (10X and 1X) and 0.1 N NaOH are also required to prepare the collagen gel for proplatelet formation.

20. Other reagents: Other reagents such as adenosine, theophylline, PGE_1, sodium citrate, and cell-culture reagents can be obtained from standard laboratory supply companies.

3. Methods

The techniques detailed below are best applied to either rat or guinea pig megakaryocytes. We have had success using a four-step BSA density gradient followed by either a continuous Ficoll velocity gradient or a three-step BSA unity velocity gradient. A successful isolation should yield approx 250,000 megakaryocytes from a guinea pig and 150,000 megakaryocytes from a rat (but *see* **Notes 3–7**). Purity for both species should be at least 70–80% using the two-gradient technique and at least 90% from using the immunomagnetic-bead technique.

3.1. Two-Stage Gradient Method (Based on Levine and Fedorko [5])

1. After sacrifice of the animals, dissect out the humeri, femurs, and tibiae and remove attached muscle and connective tissue. This is most easily done by holding the bones with a pair of forceps and scraping with a No. 10 scalpel in a 100-mm culture dish (*see* **Notes 1** and **4**).

2. Collect the scraped bones in a 50-mL tube containing enough CATCH buffer to cover the bones. Remove the marrow from the bones by cracking the bones open one at a time in a 100-mm culture dish containing 5–10 mL of CATCH buffer. A scissors-style dog nail clipper is suggested for cracking the bones open. Use a small weighing spatula to scrape the marrow off the bone fragments and discard the scraped bone fragments (*see* **Note 4**).

3. Use a siliconized glass Pasteur pipet to repeatedly pipet the bone marrow and break up the marrow pieces (*see* **Note 5**). Cover a 100-mm culture dish with a sterile piece of Nitex (nylon mesh) filter (200-μm mesh) and pour the bone marrow suspension over the mesh into the dish. Remove the filtered cell suspension from the culture dish and put into a 10–15-mL polypropylene tube for centrifugation. Pellet the cells by centrifugation at 200*g* for 5 min (*see* **Note 6**).

4. During centrifugation of the cells, prepare the bovine serum albumin density gradient in a 50-mL polypropylene tube. The gradient consists of four 7.5-mL layers, going from the most dense at the bottom to the least dense at the top of the tube (*see* **Table 1** and **Note 6**). A clear boundary between each of the layers should be visible. Each tube can be used for the marrow from one to two guinea pigs or one to three rats. Prepare additional gradients if more animals are used.

5. Resuspend the bone-marrow cell pellet from **step 3** in 1.8 mL of CATCH buffer for each gradient tube and gently layer on top of the BSA density gradient. Centrifuge the gradient at 10,000g for 30 min at 10°C in a swing-out bucket rotor (*see* **Note 7**). We have used the SW27 rotor in Beckman centrifuges or the HB-4 rotor in Sorvall centrifuges. Automatic acceleration controls should be set at the lowest setting. If there is no acceleration control, the acceleration must be controlled manually, with a gradual increase of velocity up to 10,000g. Any brake on the centrifuge should be turned off.

6. After centrifugation, remove the entire supernatant (thus combining cells from all four albumin solution densities) and mix with an equal volume of CATCH buffer to give a total volume of about 50–60 mL. Invert several times to mix the BSA solution with the CATCH buffer then centrifuge the tubes for 10 min at 300g to pellet the cells. Resuspend the cell pellet in 2.5 mL of CATCH buffer. Pellet the cells again by centrifugation at 200g for 5 min and resuspend in 1.0 mL of CATCH buffer.

7. BSA Unit Velocity Gradient: Prepare the unit velocity gradient in a 10–15-mL polypropylene tube with 3.6 mL of the VG stock solution as the bottom step. Gently layer 1.8 mL of 2/3 VG solution over the VG stock solution and then layer 1.8 mL of the 1/3 VG solution over the 2/3 VG Solution. Clear boundaries should be seen between layers. Layer the cells from the end of **step 6**, suspended in 1.0 mL of CATCH buffer, on top of the BSA unit velocity gradient (use cells from one density gradient tube for each unit velocity gradient) and allow to settle on the benchtop for 30 min. After 30 min the top layers are discarded. The bottom VG stock solution layer and cells at the interface with the 2/3 VG layer are kept. The tube is filled with CATCH buffer, mixed gently and centrifuged at 200g for 8 min. The cell pellet is the final megakaryocyte preparation.

Ficoll gradient: Prepare the Ficoll gradient with a dual-chamber gradient mixer. Place 6.5 mL of the 4% Ficoll solution into the outlet chamber of the gradient mixer and 6.5 mL of the 2% Ficoll solution into the other chamber. Add a stirrer bar to the 4% solution and arrange to stir continuously. Transfer the solutions to a 15-mL conical-bottom tube with a peristaltic pump to form a continuous gradient of increasing density from bottom to top (*see* **Note 8** for further details). Layer the cells from the BSA density gradient (end of **step 6**, suspended in 1 mL CATCH buffer) on top of the Ficoll gradient and centrifuge for 5 min at 100g. The cell pellet after centrifugation is the enriched megakaryocyte fraction.

3.2. Immunomagnetic Bead Method (Based on Leven and Rodriguez [17])

1. Perform **steps 1–6** as described in **Subheading 3.1.** Place the cells from the end of **step 6**, suspended in 1 mL CATCH buffer, in a 1.5-mL plastic tube.

2. Add megakaryocyte-specific primary antibody to the cell suspension. For guinea pig megakaryocyte isolation we have had the greatest success with mouse monoclonal antibody to human platelet glycoprotein Ib from Dako Corporation (Carpinteria, CA) at a concentration of 20 µg/mL. After antibody addition, place the cell suspension on a rotary mixer for 60 min at room temperature.

3. At the end of the 60 min add 5.0 µL of Dynabeads (e.g., M-450 goat anti-mouse magnetic beads) to the cell suspension and mix the cells for an additional 30 min.

4. Pull the beads and attached cells out of the suspension using a Dynal MPC-1 magnetic bead separator. While on the magnetic bead separator, remove the CATCH buffer in the tube, then remove the magnet and resuspend the selected cells in 1.5 mL of CATCH buffer. Repeat this extraction/wash/resuspension cycle three further times to yield an enriched megakaryocyte fraction.

3.3. Culture for Proplatelet Formation

Observation of proplatelet formation in vitro has been reported with nonpurified marrow cultures and isolated megakaryocyte cultures *(24–29)*. Proplatelet formation in nonpurified marrow cultures as described by Radley appears *(24,25)* the same as proplatelet formation by isolated megakaryocytes. Lecine et al. have also demonstrated proplatelet formation in cultures of fetal mouse liver stimulated with thrombopoietin *(30)*. In our laboratory we have been successful in stimulating proplatelet formation with both rat and guinea pig megakaryocytes. In all studies we have used DMEM with 10% fetal calf or newborn calf serum and appropriate antibiotics. We have also used HEPES-buffered culture medium with no deleterious effect on the cells. All cultures were maintained in a 37°C, 100% humid, 5% CO_2:95% air atmosphere. In earlier studies we found that by simply adding a thrombopoietin-enriched fraction of thrombocytopenic rabbit plasma to a liquid culture with isolated guinea pig megakaryocytes, proplatelet process formation was stimulated *(26,27)*.

There are two drawbacks to using this method to stimulate proplatelet formation. The first is the considerable effort and cost of obtaining thrombocytopenic rabbit plasma and the subsequent fractionation of the plasma. The second is that the activity of different preparations of thrombopoietin-enriched thrombocytopenic rabbit plasma is quite inconsistent, making experimentation more difficult. If this approach is used, each batch of thrombocytopenic plasma must be tested for its activity in a dose-response experiment (*see also* **Note 9**). In contrast we have found that megakaryocytes from guinea pigs and rats can be more consistently stimulated to form proplatelets by simply culturing the cells on the appropriate matrix material (collagen gel or Matrigel) (*see also* **Note 4**).

3.3.1. Guinea Pig Proplatelet Formation

We have had the best proplatelet response from guinea pig megakaryocytes cultured on a hydrated type I collagen gel.

1. To prepare the gel, mix 0.1 *N* NaOH, 10X DMEM, and rat-tail-collagen solution in a 1:1:10 volume ratio (1 mL is required for each culture dish).
2. Add 1.0 mL of the gel solution to each 35-mm diameter culture dish and evenly distribute over the surface.
3. Allow the gel to set in a tissue culture incubator for 30 min prior to use.
4. Rinse the gel gently with 1X DMEM three times before addition of the megakaryocyte cell suspension.

3.3.2. Rat Proplatelet Formation

Although rat megakaryocytes do form proplatelets when cultured on a hydrated rat-tail collagen gel, we have observed a more consistent response, with a greater number of cells forming proplatelets, when rat megakaryocytes are cultured on Matrigel.

1. Pipet Matrigel into a culture dish and allow to gel at 37°C for approx 10 min. The volume of Matrigel should be enough to evenly cover the culture dish (1.0 mL in a 35 mm dish).
2. Add the megakaryocytes, in culture medium, onto the solidified Matrigel.

When using either the collagen gel or Matrigel, the morphological changes that culminate in proplatelet formation do not generally begin until at least 12 h in culture. By 48 h in culture, megakaryocytes seem to have undergone the full extent of their morphological change. Examples of various stages and patterns of proplatelet formation from guinea pig megakaryocytes cultured on collagen gel are shown in **Fig. 1**. Similar patterns are observed for cultured rat megakaryocytes cultured on Matrigel.

4. Notes

1. Glassware, solutions, dissection tools, culture dishes, tubes, etc.: These must be sterile. Although it is preferable to perform all steps after removal of bones in a laminar-flow culture hood, it is possible to perform all steps on an open bench and maintain sterility if cells are cultured for short periods (up to 48 h).
2. Siliconized glass Pasteur pipets: It is much easier to handle the cells with Pasteur pipets. One can purchase sterilized plastic pipets. We have always used siliconized pipets. The pipets are immersed in a 1% solution of Sigmacote (Sigma Chemical Co., St. Louis, MO) to wet all surfaces. The Sigmacote currently available is sold to be used without dilution. The pipets are then allowed to air-dry. After drying the pipets are sterilized in an autoclave.
3. Maximum yield and viability: In order to maximize the viability and yield of mega-karyocytes, the points in **Notes 4–7** should be taken into consideration.
4. Marrow collection: We have described our method for harvesting marrow. It is tedious, but we find that by carefully scraping marrow from the bone as extensively as possible we get a higher yield. Nevertheless, a certain balance must be maintained with the time spent on the procedure. At some point extending the time excessively by trying to scrape every last bit of marrow from the bone can be detrimental. An alternative to scraping the marrow from the bone is to cut off the ends of the bones and flush the marrow out by squirting CATCH buffer into the marrow space with a syringe. This is much faster, but yield may be somewhat lower since less marrow is recovered using this technique.
5. Pipetting technique: If the procedures are followed carefully as described there should be little difficulty in obtaining relatively pure populations of megakaryocytes with good viability. In general one must remember that megakaryocytes are fragile cells. Pipetting of cell suspensions should always be performed as gently as possible. The tip of the pipet should be kept in the liquid in the tube to avoid spraying cell suspensions. The albumin solutions can foam up easily and this should be avoided. Gentle pipetting will avoid foaming of the albumin solutions.
6. Centrifugation technique: Care must be taken when making both the density and velocity gradients. The gradient solutions must be pipetted very gently over one another. If a clear boundary cannot be seen between layers, then too much mixing has occurred. We suggest some practice preparing the gradients before an actual cell separation is done. One alternative that we have used with similar results is to use a two-step density gradient instead of a four-step gradient. In the two-step gradient, the bottom layer is the same as described in the methods (1.05 g/mL), while the top layer is a volume equivalent to the top three layers combined (22.5 mL) of the 1.04 g/mL solution. It is somewhat simpler to prepare the two-step gradient, but we have found our purity to be poorer than with a four-step gradient.

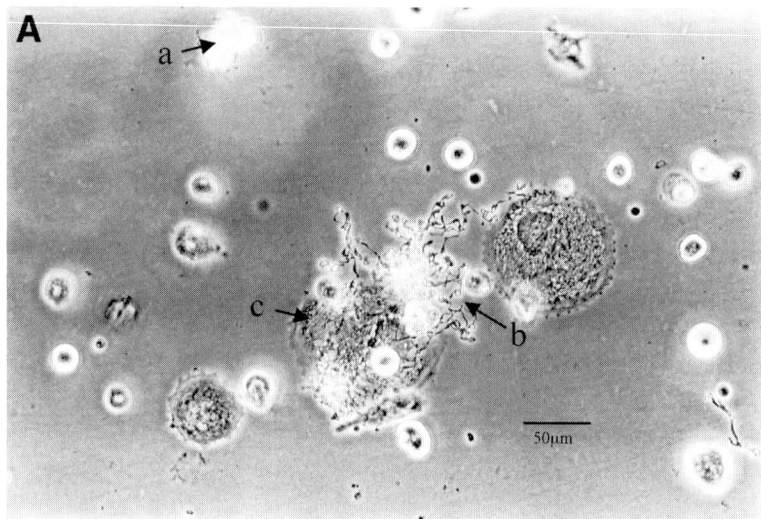

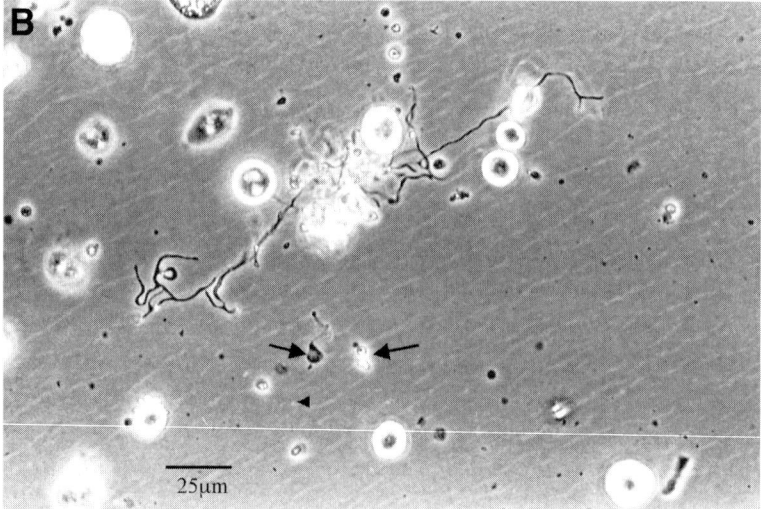

Fig. 1. Examples of proplatelet formation from isolated guinea pig megakaryocytes cultured on collagen gel. (**A**) Phase-contrast image showing (a) a cell that is beginning to alter its morphology and form proplatelets and (b) a cluster of proplatelets that probably originates from a single megakaryocyte. The latter overlies a megakaryocyte that has spread (c) rather than form proplatelets. (**B**) A single megakaryocyte that has formed elongated, branching proplatelets is seen in this micrograph. A few small released fragments can also be seen (arrows).

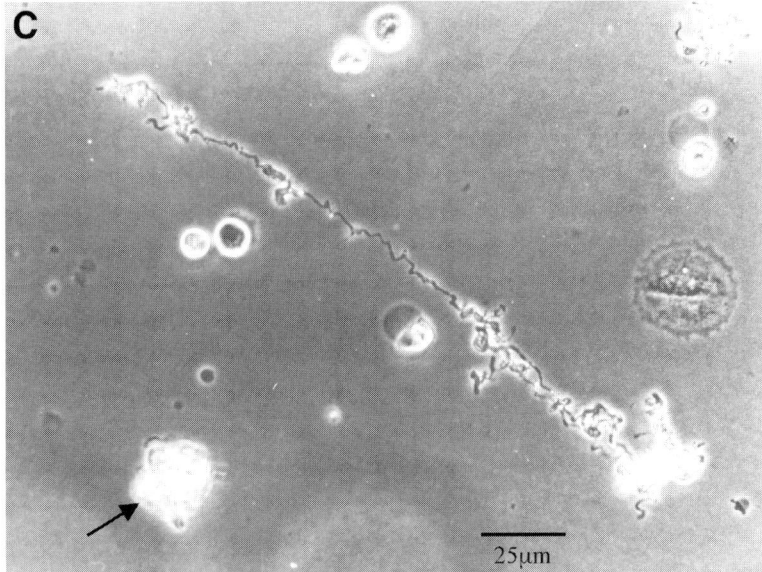

Fig. 1. **(C)** In this image one megakaryocyte has almost entirely developed into a single large, slightly branched proplatelet. Another megakaryocyte (arrow) can be seen in the early stage of proplatelet formation.

7. Density gradient centrifugation must be done at low acceleration. If manual control of acceleration must be done, one should increase the centrifuge speed very slowly, no more than by 500 rpm at a time until the speed to reach 10,000*g* is achieved.

8. Ficoll density gradient: To create the continuous-density Ficoll gradient, tape the outlet tube from the gradient mixer at the top of a 15-mL conical-bottom tube. The solutions are pumped at 2.0 mL/min. After pumping 5 mL of the 4% solution open the valve between the two solutions and continue until both Ficoll solutions have been transferred.

9. Proplatelet formation: As mentioned previously, a significant amount of work is required to produce and test thrombocytopenic plasma for stimulation of proplatelet formation. We have found that purified thrombopoietin or interleukin-6 may also stimulate proplatelet formation, although the response of any given megakaryocyte preparation is unpredictable. For reasons still unknown, different preparations of megakaryocytes isolated from the same age and species of animal with the identical reagents may respond quite differently in regard to proplatelet formation. Some cultures will form proplatelets quite vigorously, while others will not. Another important issue in the culture of megakaryocytes for proplatelet formation is that using soluble factors to stimulate proplatelet formation will leave the megakaryocytes only minimally adherent to the culture dish. This is advantageous if one wishes to remove the cells from culture. For morphological studies where adherence is often desired, use of collagen or Matrigel keeps the megakaryocytes adherent to the gel.

References

1. Howell, W. H. (1890) Observations upon the occurrence, structure, and funtion of the giant cells of the marrow. *J. Morphol.* **4,** 117–130.
2. Heidenhan, M. (1894) Neve Ontersuchungen Über die zentralkolrper udn ihre Beziehungen zum kern-und Zellerprotoplasma. *Arch. Mikrosk. Anat.* **43,** 423–758.
3. Wright, J. H. (1906) The origin and nature of the blood plates. *Boston Med. Surg. J.* **154,** 643–645.
4. Wright. J. H. (1910) The histogenesis of the blood platelets. *J. Morphol.* **21,** 265–278.
5. Levine, R. F. and Fedorko, M. (1976) Isolation of intact megakaryocytes from guinea pig femoral marrow. Successful harvest made possible with inhibitors of platelet aggregation; enrichment achieved with a two-step separation technique. *J. Cell Biol.* **69,** 159–172.
6. Levine, R. F. (1980) Isolation and characterization of normal human megakaryocytes. *Br. J. Haematol.* **45,** 487–497.
7. Seitz, R. and Wesemann, W. (1980) Studies on megakaryocytes: isolation from rat and guinea pig and incorporation of 5-hydroxytryptamine. *Eur. J. Cell Biol.* **21,** 183–187.
8. Leven R. M. and Nachmias, V. T. (1982) Cultured megakaryocytes: Changes in the cytoskeleton after ADP-induced spreading. *J. Cell Biol.* **92,** 313–323.
9. Sitar, G. (1984) Isolation of normal human megakaryocytes. *Br. J. Haematol.* **58,** 465–472.
10. Berkow, R. L., Straneva J. E., Bruno, E., Beyer, G. S., Burgess, J. S., and Hoffman, R. (1984) Isolation of human megakaryocytes by density centrifugation and counterflow centrifugal elutriation. *J. Lab. Clin. Med.* **103,** 811–818.
11. Weseman, W., Raha, S., and McDonald, T. P. (1985) Isolation of mouse megakaryocytes. II. Functional and metabolic aspects of two different maturational stages. *Eur. J. Cell. Biol.* **37,** 117–121.
12. Saigo, K., Ryo, R., Nakaya, Y., and Yamaguchi, N. (1985) Isolation of megakaryocytes by a combination of density gradient centrifugation and velocity sedimentation, and centrifugal elutriation. *Kobe J. Med. Sci.* **31,** 251–261.
13. Tanaka, H., Ishida, Y., Kaneko, T., and Matsumoto, N. (1989) Isolation of human megakaryo-cytes by immunomagnetic beads. *Br. J. Haematol.* **73,** 18–22.
14. Shoff, K. and Levine, R. F. (1989) Elutriation for isolation of megakaryocytes. *Blood Cells* **15,** 285–305.
15. Mazur, E. M., Basilico, D., Newton, J. L., Cohen, J. L., Charland, C., Sohl, P. A., et al. (1990) Isolation of large numbers of enriched human megakaryocytes from liquid cultures of normal peripheral blood progenitor cells. *Blood* **76,** 1771–1782.
16. Shikama, Y. (1990) Isolation of rat megakaryocytes by immunomagnetic beads. *Fukushima J. Med. Sci.* **36,** 59–70.
17. Leven, R. M. and Rodriguez, A. (1991) Immunomagnetic bead isolation of megakaryocytes from guinea-pig bone marrow: effect of recombinant interleukin-6 on size, ploidy and cytoplasmic fragmentation. *Br. J. Haematol.* **77,** 267–273.
18. Van Pampus, E. C. M., van Geel, B. J. M., Huijgens, P. C., Wijermans, P. W., Ossenkoppele, G. J., Rodriguez, F., et al. (1991) Combining counterflow centrifugal elutriation and glycoprotein Ib-dependent purification of human megakaryocytes: Efficacy and selectivity. *Eur. J. Haematol.* **47,** 299–304.
19. Kuter, D. J., Gminski, D., and Rosenberg, R. D. (1992) Botrocetin agglutination of rat megakaryocytes: a rapid method for megakarycoyte isolation. *Exp. Hematol.* **20,** 1085–1089.
20. Schmitz, B., Radbruch, A., Kümmel, T., Wickenhauser, C., Korb, H., Hansmann, M. L., et al. (1994) Magnetic activated cell sorting (MACS)—a new immunomagnetic method for

megakaryocytic cell isolation: Comparison of different separation techniques. *Eur. J. Haematol.* **52,** 267–275.

21. Park, S. K., Olson, T. A., Ercal, N., Summers, M., and O'Dorsio, M. S. (1996) Characterization of vasoactive intestinal peptide receptors on human megakaryocytes and platelets. *Blood* **87,** 4629–4635.

22. Miyazaki, R., Ogata, H., Iguchi, T.,Sogo, S., Kushida T., Ito, T., et al. (2000) Comparative analyses of megakaryocytes derived from cord blood and bone marrow. *Br. J. Haematol.* **108,** 602–609.

23. Nagata Y., Oda, M., Nakata, H., Shozaki, Y., Kozasa, T., and Todokoro, K. (2001) A novel regulator of G-protein signaling bearing GAP activity for Gαi and Gαq in megakaryocytes. *Blood* **97,** 3051–3060.

24. Radley, J. M. and Scurfield, G. (1980) The mechanism of platelet release. *Blood* **56,** 996–999.

25. Radley, J. M. and Haller, C. J. (1982) The demarcation membrane system of the megakaryocyte: A misnomer? *Blood* **60,** 213–219.

26. Leven R. M. and Yee, M. K. (1987) Megakaryocyte morphogenesis stimulated *in vitro* by whole and partially fractionated thrombocytopenic plasma: A model system for the study of platelet formation. *Blood* **69,** 1046–1052.

27. Leven, R. M. (1987) Megakaryocyte motility and platelet formation. *Scanning Microscopy* **1,** 1701–1709.

28. Hunt, P., Hokom, M. M., Wiemann, B., Leven, R. M., and Arakawa, T. (1993) Megakaryocyte proplatelet-like process formation in vitro is inhibited by serum prothrombin, a process which is blocked by matrix-bound glycosaminoglycans. *Exp. Hematol.* **21,** 372–381.

29. Ishida, Y., Yano, K., Ito, T., Shigematsu, H., Sadaki, K., Kondo, S., et al. (2001) Purification of proplatelet formation (PPF) stimulating factor: Thrombin/antithrombin III complex stimulates PPF of megakaryocytes in vitro and platelet production in vivo. *Thromb. Haemost.* **85,** 349–355.

30. Lecine, P., Villeval, J. L., Vyas, P., Swencki, B., Xu, Y., and Shivdasani, R. A. (1998) Mice lacking transcription factor NF-E2 provide in vivo validation of the proplatelet model of thrombocytopoiesis and show a platelet production defect that is intrinsic to megakaryocytes. *Blood* **92,** 1608–1616.

23

Isolation and Culture of Megakaryocyte Precursors

Najet Debili, Fawzia Louache, and William Vainchenker

1. Introduction

Megakaryocyte (MK) precursor cells correspond to a spectrum of cells extending from an early progenitor to the promegakaryoblast, a 2N cell that switches from a mitotic to an endomitotic process *(1)*. The MK progenitors express the CD34$^+$ antigen and are either CD38$^-$ or CD38$^+$, depending upon their maturation stage. The most primitive progenitors (BFU-MK and the mixed erythro-MK progenitors) are negative for CD38, while the others are CD38 positive *(2)*. Other differentiation markers, such as HLA-DR or AC133 *(3,4)*, have also been used to study MK differentiation. In the adult, CD41 (platelet GPIIb) appears during differentiation and can be used to select a subset of MK progenitors that essentially correspond to the more mature MK progenitors and promegakaryoblasts. In contrast, CD41 is more widely exprsssed on neonatal hematopoietic progenitors. CD42 has a slightly later expression than CD41 (5), although after the beginning of CD42 synthesis, expression levels of CD41 and CD42 are well correlated. Thus, MK differentiation may proceed by different stages: CD34$^+$CD38$^-$CD41$^-$, CD34$^+$CD38$^+$CD41$^-$, CD34$^+$CD38$^+$CD41$^+$CD42$^-$, CD34$^+$CD41$^+$CD42$^+$, CD34$^-$CD41$^+$CD42$^+$, CD34$^-$CD41^{+++}CD42^{+++} **(Fig. 1)**.

In the marrow, MK progenitors and precursors are extremely rare. Thus, it is much easier to study their differentiation after induction and amplification in vitro in the presence of thrombopoietin (TPO), allowing the selection of different cell populations *(6)*. However, purification of MK progenitors or precursors from adult blood, cord blood, and leukapheresis is not easy. Indeed, activated platelets or platelet microparticles adhere to CD34$^+$ cells and thus give an artefactual phenotype *(7)*. MK progenitors can be tested either by semisolid assays, which allow an easy quantification, or by liquid culture. Liquid cultures for the MK lineage have many advantages because they can provide an easy manner to study MK maturation by flow cytometry (antigen expression, ploidy; *see* Chapter 24, vol. 1) or by ultrastructural studies (*see* Chapter 25, vol. 1). They are usually not quantitative but use of individual cell culture may overcome this limitation.

From: *Methods in Molecular Biology, vol. 272:*
Platelets and Megakaryocytes, Vol. 1: Functional Assays
Edited by: J. M. Gibbins and M. P. Mahaut-Smith © Humana Press Inc., Totowa, NJ

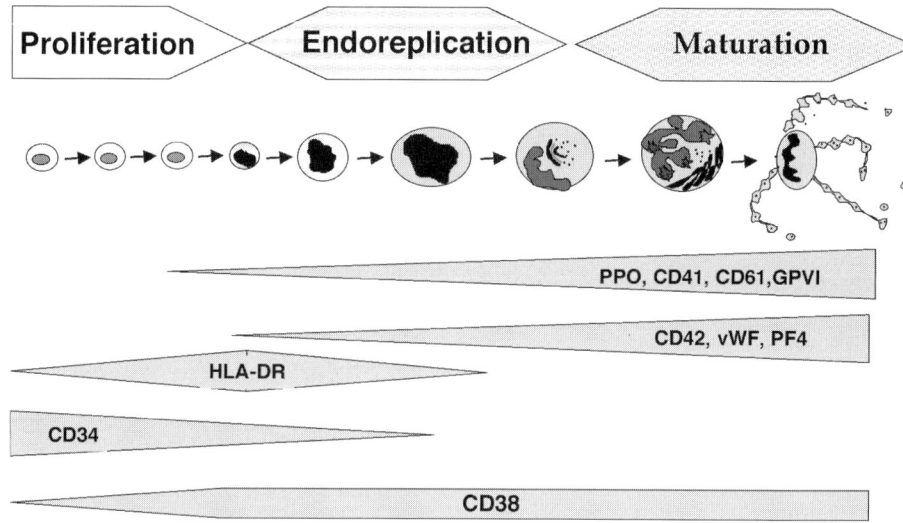

Fig. 1. Expression of different markers during MK differentiation. See introduction for further explanation.

This chapter describes the purification, culture, and assessment of MK precursor cells derived from blood or bone marrow.

2. Materials

2.1. Isolation of CD34⁺ Cells and MK Progenitors (see Note 1)

1. Cells: CD34⁺ cells can be isolated from peripheral blood or marrow. Three sources of peripheral blood cells are possible: (a) normal or patient blood, (b) leukapheresis samples obtained from patients undergoing autologous peripheral blood stem-cell transplantation, or (c) umbilical human blood cells obtained from full-term deliveries. Bone marrow cells are usually obtained from normal adult donors undergoing hip surgery or from donors by aspiration. The disadvantages of samples obtained from aspiration is that they are likely to be slightly contaminated by blood and thus by platelets. All blood and marrow samples must be obtained under guidelines established by a local ethical committee. Separation of mononuclear cells, purification of progenitors, and all culture steps must be performed in a sterile atmosphere using a laminar-flow hood.
2. Minimum essential medium (MEM) alpha medium (Gibco, UK).
3. DNAse: 10 mg/mL (Sigma; St Louis, MO), stock solution prepared in PBS and stored at –20°C.
4. Phosphate-buffered saline (PBS) (Sigma).
5. PBS containing 0.1% (1 mg/mL) EDTA, pH 7.2 adjusted with NaOH (PBS:EDTA). The EDTA dissolves completely once the pH has been adjusted.
6. Ficoll, isotonic aqueous solution of density 1.077 g/cm³ (Lymphoprep; Nycomed Pharma, Norway). This is a sterile solution that maintains the viability of the hematopoietic progenitors and is sold ready to use for density centrifugation.

7. Mini or Midi MACS magnetic cell sorting system (Miltenyi Biotec GmbH; Bergisch Gladbach, Germany) consisting of custom metal stand, magnet, and appropriate column. For up to 2×10^8 cells cells use "MS" columns in the Mini MACS system and for up to 2×10^9 cells use "LS" columns in the Midi MACS system.

8. 30-μm sterile pore nylon mesh (Miltenyi Biotec GmbH).

9. Antibodies for immunomagnetic sorting: Anti-CD34 antibody directly conjugated to magnetic beads (Clone QBEND10) and FcR-blocking reagent IgG to inhibit nonspecific or Fc-receptor-mediated binding, provided by Milyenyi Biotec.

10. Antibodies for flow cytometry: Directly conjugated monoclonal antibodies (MoAb) R-phycoerythrin-(PE)-HPCA2 or APC HPCA2 anti-CD34 (clone 8G12, Class II epitope, Becton Dickinson, Mountain View, CA), fluorescein isothiocyanate (FITC) or R-PE/Cyanine 5 (R-PE/Cy5) anti CD34 (clone 581, Class III epitope, Pharmingen, San Diego, CA, or Immunotech-Beckman Coulter), FITC anti-CD38 (Immunotech-Beckman Coulter) or PE anti CD38 (Becton Dickinson) and FITC or R-PE anti-CD41a (clone HIP8, Becton Dickinson) are used for cell sorting. Anti-CD42a MoAb FITC-(clone FMC25) and R-PE-conjugated IgG$_1$ MoAb controls can be obtained from Becton Dickinson.

11. Flow cytometer: A cell sorter such as the FACS Vantage (Becton Dickinson) equipped with (a) an argon laser (Coherent Radiation, Palo Alto, CA) tuned to 488 nm and operating at 500 mW, (b) a helium-neon laser operating at 633 nm and at 30 mW, and (c) a 100-μm nozzle is used to sort the cells.

12. Elastase (Elastin Products, Pacific, MO).

2.2. Liquid Culture

1. Human cytokines: Several recombinant cytokines can be used, especially recombinant human (rh) interleukin-3 (rhIL-3) (R&D, Oxon, UK), rh interleukin-6 (rhIL-6, from Dr. S. Burstein, Oklahoma City, OK), rh stem-cell factor (rhSCF) (Amgen, Thousand Oaks, CA) and rh TPO (either the complete cytokine or the pegylated-Megakaryocyte Growth and Differentiating Factor (Peg-rhMGDF) (Kirin, Tokyo, Japan), and erythropoietin (Epo) (from Janssen-Cilag, Issy les Moulineaux, France). G-CSF is from from Amgen-Roche.

2. Bovine serum albumin (BSA), Cohn's fraction V; powder purchased from Sigma and stored at 4°C.

3. Detoxification resin AG501-X8D, 20×50 mesh (Bio-Rad, Hercules, CA).

4. NaHCO$_3$ (Sigma).

5. Iscove's modified Dulbecco medium (IMDM) purchased as liquid medium with NaHCO$_3$ or as powder without NaHCO$_3$ (Gibco, UK). Store at 4°C. The IMDM powder is used only for the iron-saturated human transferrin, BSA, and mixed lipid preparations (*see* **Subheadings 2.3.1.**, **3.2.1.**, and **3.2.2.**). Addition of NaHCO$_3$ to the powder form is necessary only for the IMDM 2X preparation for the BSA preparation (**Subheading 3.2.1.**).

6. 0.22-μm filters (Sterivac gp10, Millipore) (*see* **Note 2**).

7. Lipids: Oleic acid, cholesterol, and 3 L-α-phosphatidylcholine dipalmytoyl are all purchased from Sigma *(8–10)*.

8. Vibra Cell sonicator (Bioblock, Illkirch, France).

9. Insulin selenium transferrin-X supplement (100X liquid) from Gibco™ Invitrogen Corporation (Cergy poutrise, France) (*see* **Note 3**).

10. Antibiotics (penicillin/streptomycin solution; Gibco Invitrogen Corp).

11. 6-, 24-, and 96-well or Terazaki tissue culture plates.

2.3. Assessment of Megakaryocyte Progenitors

2.3.1. Colony Formation: The Serum-Free Fibrin Clot Assay

1. Iron-saturated human transferrin preparation: Prepare a stock solution of 7.9×10^{-3} M iron chloride, which also contains 1 μL/mL of 1 N HCl; for example, dissolve 64 mg FeCl$_3$ 6H$_2$O (Sigma) in 30 mL pure H$_2$O and add 30 μL 1 N HCl. Dissolve 500 mg Apotransferrin (Sigma) in 5.5 mL reconstituted 1X IMDM without NaHCO$_3$, add 1.5 mL of the iron chloride solution, filter (0.2-μm pore), divide into 130-μL aliquots in sterile plastic tubes, and store at –20°C. Immediately prior to use add 2.9 mL IMDM. The final concentration of iron-saturated human transferrin preparation in culture is 300 μg/mL.
2. Insulin preparation: Dissolve 1 mg of bovine pancreatic insulin (Sigma) in 1 mL 0.01 N HCl, filter, divide into 10-μL aliquots and store at –20°C. For culture, dilute the 10 μL in 1 mL IMDM and use 10 μL/mL of culture. The final concentration in culture will be 100 ng/mL.
3. CaCl$_2$ stock (100X): Dissolve 370 mg CaCl$_2$ (Merck, Strasbourg, France) in 100 mL H$_2$O millipore. Filter and store at 4°C.
4. *Asparagine stock (100X):* Dissolve 2 mg asparagine (Sigma) in 1 mL IMDM. Filter, aliquot into small quantities (50–200 μL), and store at –20°C.
5. Fibrinogen fraction I from bovine serum (Sigma): Dissolve 10 mg fibrinogen in 1 mL PBS at 37°C and use immediately. Do not store after use.
6. H-ε amino-n-caproic acid (Sigma): Dissolve 140 mg ε amino-n-caproic acid in 1 mL PBS.
7. α-thioglycerol (Sigma).
8. L-glutamine, 200 mM (Sigma).
9. Horse thrombin (6 mU/mL final concentration in culture; Stago, Asnières, France).
10. 35-mm sterile Petri dishes (Corning #430165).

2.3.2. Immuno-Alkaline Phosphatase Labeling Technique

1. 32-mm diameter filter papers (Whatman, UK).
2. Methanol.
3. Tris-buffered saline (TBS), 0.05 M, pH 7.6. To prepare, mix 100 mL of 0.5 M Tris (Tris[hydroxymethyl]methylamine, Merck), titrated to pH 7.6 with HCl, 100 mL of 1.5 M NaCl, pH 7.6, and 800 mL distilled water.
4. TBS 0.1 M, pH 8.2. To prepare, mix 100 mL 1 M Tris, pH 8.2 with HCl, and 900 mL distilled water.
5. Monoclonal antibodies against MK-specific markers such as an anti-GPIIIa, clone Y2/51 from Dako.
6. Levamisole stock solution. Dissolve 240 mg levamisole (Sigma) in 1 mL of distilled water. Store at –20°C in 130-μL aliquots.
7. Enzymatic reaction solution: 20 mg Naphtol AS-TR phosphate, free acid (Sigma), 2 mL of N, N-dimethyl-formamide (Sigma), 100 mL TBS 0.1 M, pH 8.2, 130 μL stock solution of levamisole, 100 mg Fast Red TR salt (4-chloro-2-methylbenzenediazonium salt, Sigma). This complete enzymatic reaction solution must be made in this order immediately before use.
8. Goat F(ab′)2 anti-mouse IgG antibody conjugated to alkaline phosphatase (Caltag, Burlingame, CA).
9. Harris hematoxylin (BioLyon-Unipath, Dardilly, France).

2.3.3. Colony Formation in Methylcellulose Culture

1. Methylcellulose from Stem Cell Technology (MethoCult H4100). It is supplied as a stock solution (40 mL/bottle) composed of 2.6% methylcellose in IMDM without serum and cytokines and should be stored at –20°C.

2. 16 g blunt-end needle.
3. Methylcellulose culture medium: After thawing the methylcellulose (overnight at 4°C or for immediate use at either room temperature or 37°C), add the following to each 40-mL bottle: 12 mL 10 % BSA preparation (*see* **Subheading 3.2.1.**), 8 mL iron-saturated transferrin (*see* **Subheading 2.3.1.**; after dilution of 130-μL aliquots with 2.9 mL IMDM, combine aliquots to give 8 mL), 800 μL insulin preparation (*see* **Subheading 2.3.1.**), 1 mL of 200 m*M* L-glutamine, 1 mL of 0.01 *M* β-mercaptoethanol, 20 mL IMDM supplemented with L-glutamine (2 m*M*) and penicillin/streptomycin (100 U/mL and 100 μg/mL, respectively). Shake the bottle vigorously to uniformly mix all the components. For triplicate experiments, aliquot into tubes (3 mL each) using a syringe and a 16-gauge blunt-end needle. Store at –20°C.
4. 35- and 100-mm Petri dishes.

2.3.4. Chemotaxis Assay

1. Transwell, 24-well cell clusters, with 5-μm pore filters (Costar, Cambridge, MA).
2. Human SDF-1α (R&D systems, Oxon, UK).
3. Pertussis toxin (Sigma).
4. Liquid serum-free medium as described in **Subheading 3.2.3.**
5. May-Grunwald Giemsa stain (VWR International, Fontenay sous Bois, France).

3. Methods
3.1. Purification of CD34+ Cells and Subsets From Bone Marrow, Cord Blood, and Peripheral Adult Blood

3.1.1. Mononuclear Cell (MNC) Preparation

1. Collect *bone marrow cells* by vigorous shaking of bone fragments containing marrow in 15 mL MEM supplemented with 100 ng/mL of DNAse and penicillin/streptomycin (100 U/mL and 100 μg/mL, respectively). Recover the medium and repeat this procedure twice. Centrifuge the medium from all three washes and resuspend the cells without counting in 10 mL MEM medium supplemented with DNase and penicillin/streptomycin. *Peripheral blood cells from leukapheresis* are diluted to a concentration of approx 5×10^6/mL in PBS:EDTA, centrifuged, and resuspended in PBS:EDTA for direct CD34 separation (*see* **Subheading 3.1.2.**). For other samples of blood (e.g., from normal or patient samples), collect in acid citrate dextrose anticoagulant and isolate platelet-rich plasma.
2. Separate mononuclear cells (MNC) from medium or plasma using a Ficoll gradient (1.077) at room temperature with centrifugation at *400g* for 20 min. After centrifugation, the mononuclear cells (i.e., low-density cells; <1.077 g/cm³) are located in a band at the interface between the Ficoll and upper layer of plasma or medium.
3. Recover the mononuclear cells with a pipet and wash with either PBS:EDTA (for blood cells) or MEM (for bone marrow cells) and centrifuge at *200g* for 10 min. Resuspend the cells in PBS:EDTA or MEM for a second wash, count the cells, centrifuge again, and then use for isolation of CD34+ cells by an immunomagnetic technique using the Miltenyi magnetic cell sorting system as described in **Subheading 3.1.2.**

3.1.2. Isolation of CD34+ Cells

See **Fig. 2**.

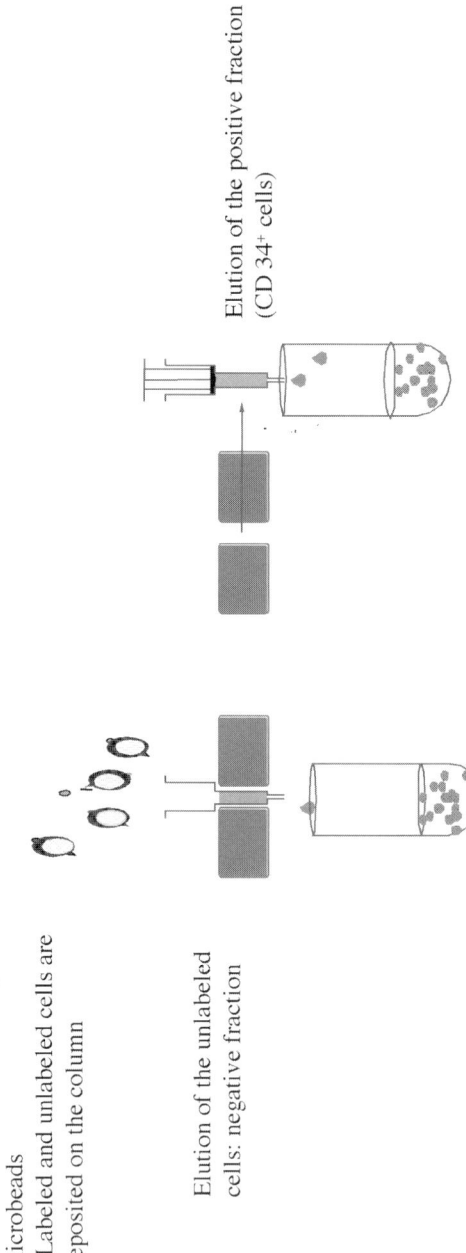

- Labeling performed with QBEND10 anti -CD34 coupled to microbeads
- Labeled and unlabeled cells are deposited on the column

Elution of the unlabeled cells: negative fraction

Elution of the positive fraction (CD 34+ cells)

Fig. 2. Schematic representation of the CD34+ cell purification using the Milyenyi Biotec technique.

1. Resuspend the cell pellet from **Subheading 3.1.1., step 3** in PBS:EDTA and adjust to give 100×10^6 mononucleated cells (MNCs) in either 300 µL (for marrow, peripheral-blood-derived MNCs, and leukapheresis) or 150 µL (for cord blood).

2. For marrow-derived cells, peripheral-blood-derived MNCs, and leukapheresis, add 100 µL of anti-CD34 (clone QBEND10) directly conjugated to microbeads and 100 µL of FcR-blocking reagent IgG to inhibit nonspecific or Fc-receptor-mediated binding of CD34 microbeads to nontarget cells, and incubate at 4°C for 30 min. For cord-blood-derived MNCs add 50 µL of anti-CD34 conjugated beads and 50 µL of FcR-blocking reagent.

3. Wash once ($200g$, 10 min) in PBS:EDTA and resuspend MNC in either 500 µL of PBS:EDTA for $<2 \times 10^8$ MNC or 3 mL of PBS:EDTA for between 2×10^8 and 2×10^9 MNCs.

4. Select either the MS column ($<2 \times 10^8$ cells) or LS column ($<2 \times 10^9$ cells). Place the column in the appropriate size magnet (Mini or Midi MACS), which is then supported by the custom metal stand.

5. Place a 30-µm pore nylon mesh over the top of the column and pass 500 µL or 3 mL of PBS:EDTA (depending on the selected column type) through this filter to wet it, followed by the MNC suspension (*see* **Note 4**).

6. Wash with 3×500 µL (MS column) or 3×3 mL (LS column) of PBS:EDTA, remove the column from the magnet, and place the column at the top of a suitable tube.

7. Pipet 1 mL (MS column) or 3 mL (LS column) of medium (PBS:EDTA or serum-free culture medium) on the top of the column and flush out retained (CD34$^+$) cells in the tube with pressure using the plunger supplied with the column.

8. To obtain a higher purity, repeat **steps 5–7** using a new column (prefiltering is unnecessary with the second column, but it is advisable to pass 500 µL or 3 mL of medium before the cells to wet the column) (*see* **Note 5**).

9. When dealing with very small samples, such as a blood sample from a patient (especially a child), it is preferable to couple immunomagnetic antibody separation and flow-cytometric cell sorting in order to get a better yield of CD34$^+$ cells. Incubate MNCs with the anti-CD34 antibody coupled to immunomagnetic beads and an anti-CD34 antibody coupled to a fluorochrome such as PE or FITC for 30 min. After one wash in PBS:EDTA, pass the MNC only once through the column (without the use of the mesh filter), which may give a poor purification after passing through the column; then directly purify the CD34$^+$ cells by cell sorting. This enhances the percentage of the CD34 cell population after the column separation and thereby reduces the time taken for cell sorting.

3.1.3. Purification of CD34$^+$CD38$^+$ and CD34$^+$CD38$^-$ Subsets From Bone Marrow

In order to purify the CD34$^+$CD38$^-$ and CD34$^+$CD38$^+$ subsets, the purified CD34$^+$ cells are labeled with anti-CD34 and -CD38 antibodies and sorted. In these experiments, in order to better distinguish between CD38$^-$, CD38^{low}, and CD38$^+$ subsets, it is preferable to use an R-PE labeled anti-CD38. The FITC anti-CD34 (clone 8G12 MoAb) gives a clear but often weak labeling. Thus, better results are obtained with the FITC-anti-CD34 clone 581 from Pharmingen or the same clone but coupled with R-PE/CY5 from Immunotech (Beckmann Coulter), which gives a brighter labeling. The labeling of cells is performed as follows:

1. Incubate 2×10^6 CD34$^+$ immunomagnetic sorted cells (from **Subheading 3.1.2., step 7**) in 100 µL PBS containing 0.5% BSA with 20 µL of anti-CD34 FITC and 20 µL of anti-

CD38 PE. If an RPe/Cy5 anti-CD34 MoAb is used, 10 µL of RPe/Cy5 anti-CD34 MoAb is added with 20 µL of R-PE anti-CD38 MoAb.
2. Sort the cells on a FACS Vantage by gating on the mononuclear cells on the FCS and SSC parameters (*see* Chapter 19, vol. 1 for further details of flow cytometry). The CD34+CD38- cells usually correspond to 2–5% of the entire CD34+ cell population, the CD34+CD38low to 15–20%, and the CD34+CD38+ to 75%.

3.1.4. Purification of the CD34+CD41+ and CD34+CD41- Subsets From Fresh Bone Marrow CD34+ Cell

CD41 is expressed on ~2% of fresh bone marrow CD34+ cells. They can be sorted in one step by flow cytometry directly from low-density bone marrow cells or in two steps after a CD34+ purification by the immunomagnetic bead technique. The two-step technique permits a marked shortening of the flow-cytometric sorting stage. Cells are processed as described for the CD34+CD38+ cell purification using a FACS Vantage cytometer equipped with an argon laser and a 100-µm nozzle.

1. Incubate 2×10^6 bone marrow-derived CD34+ cells (in 100 µL MEM medium containing 0.5% BSA) with 20 µL FITC anti-CD41a (clone HIP8, Pharmingen) and 10 µL R-PE CY5 anti-CD34 (clone 581, Immunotech, Beckman Coulter) MoAbs for 30 min at 4°C.
2. After one wash in MEM, resuspend the cells at a concentration of 4×10^6 cells mL in MEM medium and sort CD34+CD41+ cells as shown in **Fig. 3A**.

3.1.5. Purification of the CD34+CD41+ and CD34+CD41- Subsets From Leukapheresis Products or Cord Blood

The sorting of CD34+CD41+ cells from leukapheresis products or cord blood is more difficult due to platelet adherence to CD34+ cells, resulting in a high level (2–90%) of platelet antigens (e.g., CD41) on the CD34+ cell population. Therefore, when using leukapheresis products or cord blood it is necessary to treat the cell population with elastase to remove the platelet fragments stuck on the CD34+ cells.

1. Incubate CD34+ cells in 100 µL PBS with 0.2% BSA and 10 µg/mL of elastase at 37°C for 30 min.
2. Wash the cells and proceed to antibody labeling and separation with anti-CD34 and anti-CD41 antibodies as described in **Subheading 3.1.4.**

3.1.6. Purification of the CD34+CD41+ Subsets From Liquid Culture

In order to obtain different MK precursor subsets, CD34+ cells are first cultured in liquid culture medium for six to eight days in the presence of cytokines, then incubated with antibody combinations to allow purification.

Fig. 3. *(see facing page)* FACS dot blot of sorting of the different populations of CD41 cells. (**A**) Bone marrow CD34+ cells are gated for forward/side scatter properties (FSC, SSC), and a gate for FSC-W/CD34 in order to determine a gate for the singlets and eliminate the aggregates. (**B**) day 6 MKs obtained from a liquid leukapheresis culture.

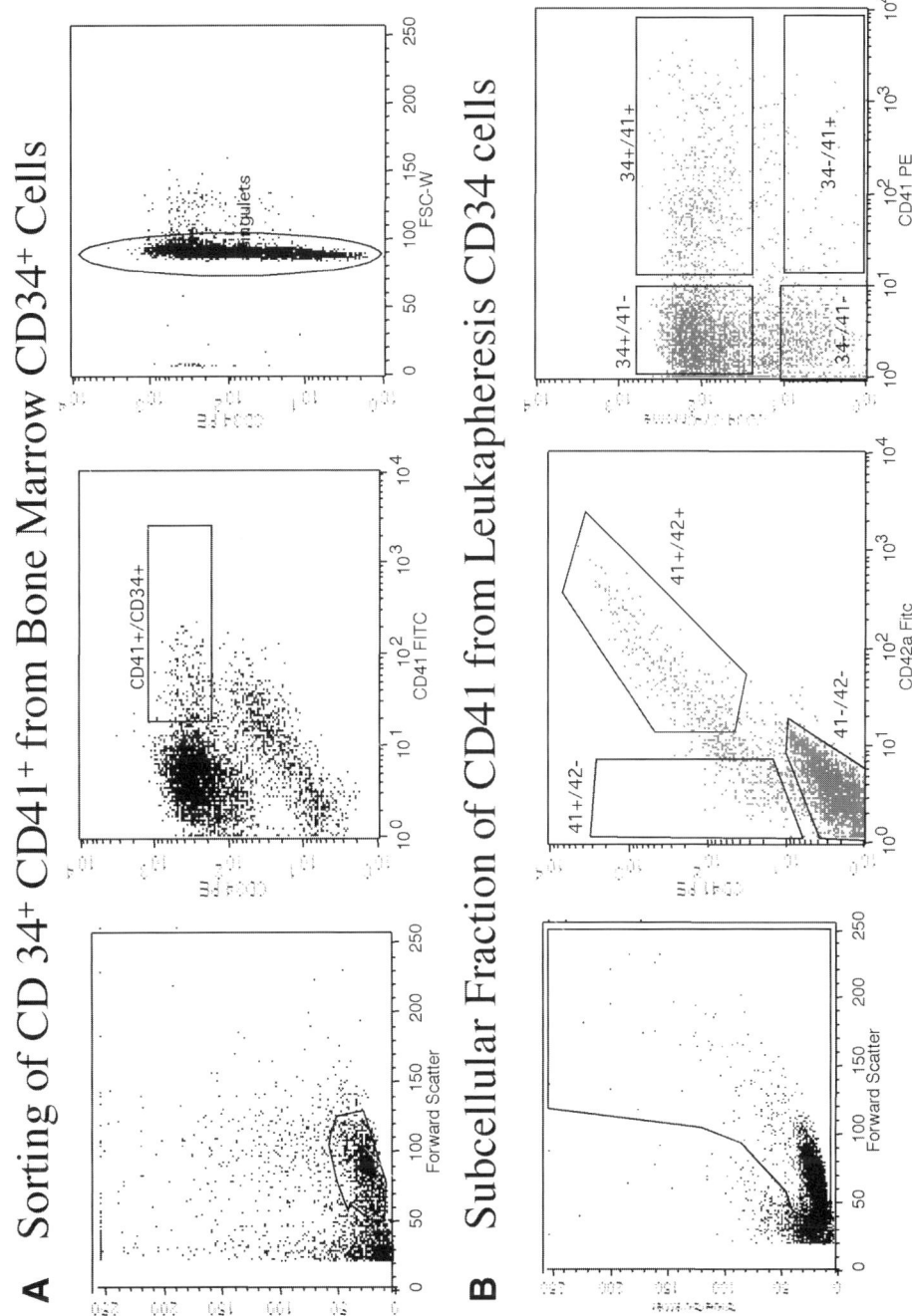

A Sorting of CD 34+ CD41+ from Bone Marrow CD34+ Cells

B Subcellular Fraction of CD41 from Leukapheresis CD34 cells

1. Incubate CD34$^+$ cells with a combination of TPO (10 ng/mL) and stem cell factor (50 ng/mL) for 6–8 d (*see* **Subheading 3.2.4.** for further details of culturing conditions).
2. Recover the cells and wash twice in ice-cold MEM medium supplemented with 0.5% BSA.
3. Add to 2×10^6 cells in 100 µL of medium, 20 µL FITC anti-CD42a (clone FMC25, Pharmingen), 20 µL R-PE anti-CD41a (Pharmingen), and 10 µL R-PE/CY5 anti-CD34 MoAbs (Beckman-Coulter) and incubate for 30 min at 4°C.
4. Wash the cells once and resuspend in MEM with 0.5% BSA at 4×10^6 cells/mL.
5. Using a FACS Vantage cytometer equipped with a 100-µm nozzle (*see* **Note 6**), sort the cells according to their immuno-phenotype into three (CD34$^+$CD41$^+$, CD34$^+$CD41$^+$, and CD34$^-$CD41$^+$) or four (CD34$^+$CD41$^-$CD42$^-$, CD34$^+$CD41$^+$CD42$^-$, CD34$^-$CD41$^+$CD42$^-$, and CD34$^-$CD41$^+$CD42$^+$) different populations (*see* **Fig. 3B**). Controls include double specific labeling and a control isotype for each color as well as unlabeled cells.

3.2. Liquid Culture of Megakaryocyte Progenitors

3.2.1. 10% BSA Preparation

1. In a 1000-mL beaker, place a large magnetic stir bar and 440 mL millipore H$_2$O.
2. Add 100 g BSA, cover beaker with parafilm and agitate or stir slowly overnight at 4°C.
3. When the BSA has been dissolved, add 15 g detoxification resin AG501-X8D, 20×50 mesh (Bio-Rad). The resin will change from a blue to a yellow color.
4. Add an additional 15 g of resin and leave again overnight at 4°C.
5. Repeat **step 4** until the resin remains blue.
6. Centrifuge the suspension at 200*g* for 10 min to eliminate the resin, transfer the solution into a 500-mL graduated cylinder, and note the volume.
7. Add an equal volume of 2X concentrated IMDM (supplemented with NaHCO$_3$) and filter.
8. Divide the BSA preparation into 10–20-mL aliquots and store at –20°C.
9. For culture, thaw and add 0.5 mL NaHCO$_3$ (from a stock solution of 7.5%) for 20 mL of 10% BSA preparation. Addition of NaHCO$_3$ is necessary since the deionized BSA has a low pH.

3.2.2. Mixed Lipid Preparation

1. In a plastic tube dissolve the following in 4 mL of 100% ethanol at 56°C: 62 mg oleic acid, 78 mg cholesterol, 74 mg 3 L-α-phosphatidylcholine dipalmytoyl.
2. After complete dissolution of the mixed lipid, transfer the mixed solution to a plastic beaker and evaporate it under a flux of nitrogen gas.
3. When the mixture is completely dried, it forms a thin white pellicle in the bottom of the plastic beaker.
4. Add 90 mL of reconstituted 1X IMDM without NaHCO$_3$ and 10 mL of the 10% BSA mixture from **Subheading 3.2.1.** Sonicate the mixture in an ice bath (cycle 50%, pulse 6–7 in a Vibra Cell sonicator).
5. Centrifuge at 400*g* for 10 min, filter, and aliquot in 10, 20, or 50 mL. Store in the dark at 4°C.

3.2.3. Complete Medium for Serum-Free Liquid Culture (see **Note 7**)

1. In a sterile plastic tube mix the following components: 150 µL 10% BSA (**Subheading 3.2.1.**), 10 µL insulin selenium transferrin-X (commercial, from Gibco Invitrogen Corp.), and 20 µL mixed lipid preparation (**Subheading 3.2.2.**).
2. Adjust the volume to 1 mL with 820 µL IMDM supplemented with penicillin/streptomycin and 11.5 µ*M* α-thioglycerol (Sigma).

3.2.4. Liquid Culture in Serum-Free Medium

1. Cell density: Seed the cells in flasks or 6-, 24-, or 96-well plates, depending on the quantity of the cells and of the type of experiments. (a) CD34$^+$ cells: culture at a concentration of approx 100,000 cells/mL in 5–8 mL in flasks, in 3–4 mL in 6-well tissue culture plates, or 1 mL in 24-well tissue culture plate. (b) CD34$^+$CD41$^+$ cells: grow in 96-well plates in a 100-μL volume or in 24-well tissue plates, usually at a concentration of less than 100,000 cells/mL. Either progenitor can be also grown at one cell per well using either 96-well or Terazaki tissue plates in 100- and 20-μL volume, respectively. In this case, the cells are directly deposited with an automatic cell deposit unit of the flow cytometer.
2. Cytokines: The combination of the cytokines depends greatly on the purpose of the experiments. When growth of pure MKs populations is required, cultures can be performed in TPO alone (10 ng/mL). However, higher expansion can be obtained by a combination of SCF (50 ng/mL) + TPO or SCF (25 ng/mL) + IL-3 (100 IU/mL) + TPO (10 ng/mL). Larger combinations of cytokines can be used with a slight improvement in the number of MKs obtained.
3. Cells are incubated at 37°C in a fully humidified atmosphere containing 5% CO_2 in air. The cultures are examined with an inverted microscope at 40 and 100X magnification. When starting with the entire CD34$^+$ cell population, optimum days range from day 9 to day 12; with the CD34$^+$CD41$^+$ cell population, optimum growth is obtained around day 5.

3.3. Assessment of Megakaryocyte Progenitors

Several techniques can be used to assay MK progenitors, including measurements of MK colony formation or studies of cellular migration that may represent movement out of the marrow. MK colony-forming assays are normally carried out in semisolid medium—for example, using methylcellulose as the gelling agent. Methylcellulose is widely used in the investigation of hematopoietic progenitors. One clear limitation to the identification of the MK colonies based on morphological criteria is that the technique requires a lot of training, since MKs are not always evident. Thus, techniques permitting direct identification of the colonies after labeling with antibodies to MK-specific antigens appear more adapted to the MK lineage. In our laboratory we use a derivative of the plasma-clot technique, the serum-free fibrin clot assay *(8,11,12)* using cultures in the presence of cytokines *(2,3)*.

3.3.1. Megakaryocyte Colony Formation:
The Serum-Free Fibrin Clot Assay

1. Prepare culture medium in 1-mL aliquots as follows: 150 μL BSA 10%, 10 μL $CaCl_2$ 100X, 10 μL asparagine 100X, 10 μL insulin preparation (from 10 μL of stock solution diluted in 1 mL IMDM), 100 μL iron-saturated transferrin preparation (from 130 μL stock solution diluted with 2.9 mL IMDM), 10 μL ε amino caproic acid of a stock solution (140 mg/mL dissolved in 1X PBS), 20 μL mixed lipids, 100 μL fibrinogen (from 10 mg stock solution fibrinogen dissolved immediately prior to use at 37°C in 1 mL 1X PBS), 490 μL IMDM (IMDM sold in liquid form containing $NaHCO_3$) (*see* **Note 8**).
2. Filter the medium and add 100 μL of a cellular suspension with the adequate cytokines (*see* **Subheading 3.2.4.**).
3. For each tube, add 6 mU/mL thrombin, mix, and immediately deposit the fibrinogen-cell mixture into a Corning 35-mm culture dish. Gently rotate the dish and place it at 37°C in a fully humidified atmosphere containing 5% CO_2 in air (*see* **Note 9**).

4. Plate the cells in triplicate at a concentration ranging from 500 to 1×10^3 cells/mL (which permits easy counting of the number of growing colonies) in the presence of PEG-rh MGDF (10 ng/mL) and SCF (50 ng/mL) for the growth of MK colonies. For other lineages, a much larger combination of cytokines is used, such as IL-6 (100 U/mL) G-CSF (2 ng/mL) and erythropoietin (Epo) (1 U/mL).

5. After 10–12 d, score the cultures. MK colonies are enumerated by an indirect immuno-alkaline phosphatase labeling technique using an anti-platelet glyoprotein MoAb (CD41, CD42) *(13)*, as described in **Subheading 3.3.2.**

3.3.2. Immuno-Alkaline Phosphatase Labeling of Megakaryocyte-Lineage Cells

1. Preparation for immunostaining: Dry the fibrin clot with 32-mm diameter filter papers by depositing in a cumulative manner on top of the clot until the top filter is nearly dry. This step is necessary to adsorb excess liquid.

2. Gently remove the filters, fix with 0.5–1 mL methanol per Petri dish, and leave for 5 min at room temperature.

3. Wash with 0.05 *M* TBS, pH 7.6.

4. Add 0.5 mL/dish of diluted mouse monoclonal antibody in 0.05 *M* TBS, pH 7.6, against megakaryocytic-specific markers (for example, an antibody against CD41 or CD42). Incubate at room temperature for 30 min to 1 h.

5. Wash four times with 0.05 *M* TBS, pH 7.6, leaving in each saline wash for 5 min.

6. To each Petri dish, add 0.5 mL of diluted goat F(ab')2 anti-mouse IgG antibody conjugated to alkaline phosphatase at a final dilution of 1:200 in 0.05 *M* TBS, pH 7.6, and incubate for 30 min at room temperature.

7. Wash once in 0.05 *M* TBS, pH 7.6, then twice in 0.1 *M* TBS, pH 8.0.

8. Prepare the enzymatic reaction solution immediately prior to use (*see* **Subheading 2.3.2.**).

9. Add 1 mL of this solution to each Petri dish; incubate for 30 min in the dark at room temperature.

10. Wash with distilled water and counterstain with Harris hematoxylin solution for 1 min, then wash extensively with tap water and keep the Petri dishes open to evaporate all the water.

11. Cover the dishes with microscope immerson oil and count colonies under an inverted microscope (*see* **Note 10**).

3.3.3. Megakaryocyte Colony Formation: The Methylcellulose Assay

Colonies are also grown in serum-free medium.

1. Thaw the methylcellulose culture medium (**item 3**, **Subheading 2.3.3.**) overnight at 4°C the day before use or on the day of the experiment at either room temperature or 37°C.

2. To each tube containing 3 mL of methylcellulose culture medium, add 60 μL mixed lipids and 300 μL of IMDM containing cells with the adequate cytokines.

3. Mix with a syringe or vortex to uniformly mix all the components, let stand for a few minutes to allow the bubbles to rise to the top, and then using the same syringe with a 16-gauge blunt end needle dispense 1-mL aliquots of the mixture to 35-mm Petri dishes.

4. Gently tilt and rotate each Petri dish to uniformly distribute the methylcellulose and cells.

5. Place triplicate 35-mm culture dishes in a 100-mm covered Petri dish with a fourth, smaller uncovered dish containing 2 mL distilled water and place them at 37°C in a fully humidified atmosphere containing 5% CO_2 in air.

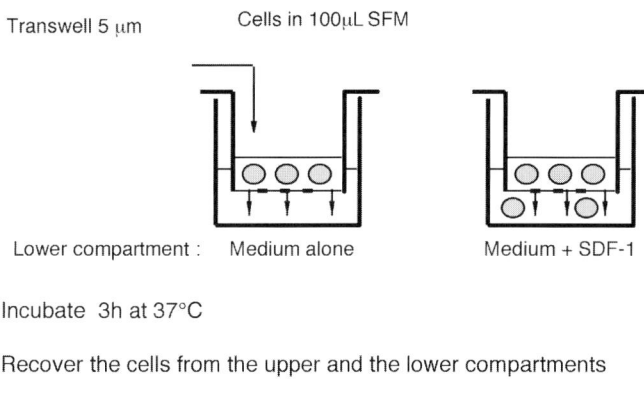

Fig. 4. Schematic representation of the migration assay.

6. After 12 d, count the MK colonies under an inverted microscope on the basis of the unique morphology of the megakaryocyte—that is, a large size, spherical shape, round contour, and high refringence (producing a clearly defined cell border) (*see* **Note 11**).

3.3.4. Chemotactic Assay

Megakaryocyte migration from the bone marrow microenvironment to the blood is an essential step for platelet production. Among the chemokines that may play a central role in cell migration, the stromal cell-derived factor-1α (SDF-1α) has recently been described to act as a potent chemoattractant for megakaryocytes *(18,19)*. This biological effect is mediated by the chemokine receptor CXCR4 (Fusin, LESTR), which is expressed on hematopoietic stem cells, megakaryocytes, and platelets. The biological significance of CXCR4 expression by platelets is actually not well understood, as platelets are devoid of chemotaxis. On the other hand, despite a high level of expression of CXCR4 on megakarocytes, only a fraction of these cells are induced to migrate by SDF-1α. This biological effect depends greatly on the stage of MK development *(20)*. The protocol of the chemotaxis/migration assay that we use is performed as follows (*see also* **Fig. 4** and **Note 12**).

1. Place 500 μL of SDF-1α diluted at different concentration (50–300 ng/mL) in serum-free medium in the lower wells of the transwell cell clusters. For controls, add serum-free medium without agonist.
2. Deposit 100 μL of cells at a concentration of 1×10^6 to 5×10^6/mL in serum-free medium to the upper wells.
3. Incubate for 1–3 h at 37°C in a fully humidified atmosphere containing 5% CO_2 in air.
4. Carefully remove the upper chambers and recover in the same volume the cells from the upper and the bottom chambers for counting. Label both cell fractions with a PE-anti-CD41a antibody and FITC anti-CD42a antibody (at the dilutions recommended by the manufacturer; lower antibody levels can be used if experience shows these to be adequate) and analyze by flow cytometry.

5. The chemotactic response of SDF-1 via its receptor CXCR4 is mediated by a pertussis-toxin-sensitive G-protein; thus, this toxin can act as a control. Preincubate cells for 2 h at 37°C with pertussis toxin (100 ng/mL) before conducting the migration assay.

6. All assays should be conducted in triplicate. Data are presented either as the chemotaxis index calculated as the ratio of number of cells migrating to SDF-1/number of cells migrating to medium, or as the percentage of migrated cells calculated as follows: 100 × number of migrated cells/number of input cells (*see* **Fig. 4**). For morphological studies, the different cell fractions obtained are spun on cytocentrifuge slides and observed at light microscopy after May-Grunwald Giemsa staining.

4. Notes

1. All glassware, plastics, solutions, etc. should be sterile and cells isolated in as sterile an environment as possible.

2. Unless stated otherwise, filtering refers to the use of these 0.22-μm diameter pore filters.

3. Tests of the insulin-selenium-transferrin preparation from Gibco:Invitrogen show that this is a good component for serum-free medium. However, the transferrin concentration is lower than that required for stimulation of erythroid and mixed progenitors in culture and we therefore use our own preparation of iron-saturated transferrin (**Subheading 2.3.1.**).

4. It is important to filter the suspension of MNCs through the 30-μm nylon mesh filter to eliminate any "clumps" of cells before passing through the separation column.

5. After two passages on the column, the purity as judged by flow cytometry using the R-PE conjugated HPCA2 is usually higher than 90%. In most cases, this level of purity is sufficient and the CD34+ cell population can be directly used for cultures.

6. The use of a large-size nozzle (100 μm) is useful because the size of MK precursors is larger than that of the CD34+ cell population.

7. A commercial preparation of serum-free liquid medium is available from Stem Cell Technologies (Vancouver, BC, Canada) and Recherches et Techniques Moderne (RTM) (Tourcoing, France), and semisolid collagen assay from Stem Cell Technologies. We have tested these commercials products which give satisfactory results.

8. Failure to obtain gel formation in fibrin-clot assay may be due to omission of one of the products, such as calcium or thrombin.

9. A problem with all semisolid cultures is a tendency to dry out after a long period of incubation. To minimize this risk, it is recommended to place three Petri dishes containing culture together with a fourth open Petri dish (35 mm or slightly smaller) containing distilled water in a larger covered dish.

10. *Quantification in the serum fibrin clot assay:* There are no difficulties with identifying megakaryocytes due to the intense staining of GPIb or IIb positive cells produced by the alkaline phosphatase technique. However, there are two problems in the assay: (a) The number of cells present to score a colony: In the literature, the usual number is three. However, one polyploid MK has undergone the same number of DNA replications as a CFU-E derived colony or a granulo-macrophage cluster. In addition, when CD34+ cells are plated individually in a well, they can give rise to individual or more MKs. Thus it seems important to also score the "one-cell" and "two-cell" colonies *(16,17)*. (b) In the fibrin-clot assay, many colonies are dispersed and the limit of each colony is not always easy to assess. It is important to seed a low number of cells (around 500 CD34+ cells per well). CFU-MK-derived colonies are usually enumerated at day 10–12 of culture, whereas BFU-MK derived colonies are scored at day 16–18. The latter are colonies of more than

50 cells and composed of several clusters, but in fact many large MK colonies may be composed of only one cluster.

11. *Quantification of MK colonies in methyl cellulose:* MK colonies are identified by the unique morphology of the megakaryocyte, that is the large size of the cells, their spherical shape, their round contour, and their refringence (clearly defined cell borders). Colonies are composed of only a few cells. Colonies can be either relatively dispersed but can also be tight. These colonies are easily identified when cultures are performed with a small combination of cytokines. It is much more difficult when large combinations of cytokines are used and errors may occur from the presence of macrophage colonies. Mixed MK colonies can be recognized by the presence of some MKs inside erythroid, granulocytic, or mixed colonies *(2,14,15)*.

12. This chemotaxis assay can also be performed after coating the transwell inserts with an extracellular matrix protein such as fibronectin or collagen, or with endothelial cells. Coating with BSA is used as the control *(18,21–23)*.

Acknowledgments

We thank Drs. Jonathan Dando and Françoise Wendling for reading and greatly improving the English of the manuscript.

References

1. Jackson, C. W., Arnold, J. T., Pestina, T. I., and Stenberg, P. E. (1997) In Kuter, D. J., Hunt, P., Sheridan, W., and Zucker-Franklin, D. (eds.), *Thrombopoiesis and Thrombopoietins. Molecular, Cellular, Preclinical, and Clinical Biology.* Humana Press Inc., Totowa, N.J., pp. 3–39.
2. Debili, N., Coulombel, L., Croisille, L., Katz, A., Guichard, J., Breton-Gorius, J., et al. (1996) Characterization of a bipotent erythro-megakaryocytic progenitor in human bone marrow. *Blood* **88,** 1284–1196.
3. Briddell, R. A., Brandt, J. E., Straneva, J. E., Srour, E. F., and Hoffman, R. (1989) Characterization of the human burst-forming unit-megakaryocyte. *Blood* **74,** 145–151.
4. Murray, L. J., Bruno, E., Uchida, N., Hoffman, R., Nayar, R., Yeo, E. L., et al. (1999) CD109 is expressed on a subpopulation of CD34+ cells enriched in hematopoietic stem and progenitor cells. *Exp. Hematol.* **27,** 1282–1294.
5. Debili, N., Issaad, C., Masse, J. M., Guichard, J., Katz, A., Breton-Gorius, J., and Vainchenker, W. (1992) Expression of CD34 and platelet glycoproteins during human megakaryocytic differentiation. *Blood* **80,** 3022–3035.
6. Debili, N., Robin, C., Schiavon, V., Letestu, R., Pflumio, F., Mitjavila-Garcia, M. T., et al. (2001) Different expression of CD41 on human lymphoid and myeloid progenitors from adults and neonates. *Blood* **97,** 2023–2030.
7. Dercksen, M. W., Weimar, I. S., Richel, D. J., Breton-Gorius, J., Vainchenker, W., Slaper-Cortenbach, C. M., et al. (1995) The value of flow cytometric analysis of platelet glycoprotein expression of CD34+ cells measured under conditions that prevent P-selectin-mediated binding of platelets. *Blood* **86,** 3771–3782.
8. Mitjavila, M. T., Vinci, G., Villeval, J. L., Kieffer, N., Henri, A., Testa, U., et al. (1988) Human platelet alpha granules contain a non specific inhibitor of megakaryocyte colony formation: its relationship to type b transforming growth factor (TGF-b). *J. Cell Physiol.* **134,** 93–100.

9. Guilbert, L. J. and Iscove, N. N. (1976) Partial replacement of serum by selenite, transferrin, albumin and lecithin in haemopoietic cell cultures. *Nature* **263,** 594–595.

10. Iscove, N. N., Guilbert, L. J., and Weyman, C. (1980) Complete replacement of serum in primary cultures of erythropoietin-dependent red cell precursors (CFU-E) by albumin, trans-ferrin, iron, unsaturated fatty acid, lecithin and cholesterol. *Exp. Cell Res.* **126,** 121–126.

11. Berthier, R., Valiron, O., Schweitzer, A., and Marguerie, G. (1993) Serum-free medium allows the optimal growth of human megakaryocyte progenitors compared with human plasma supplemented cultures: role of TGF beta. *Stem Cells* **11,** 120–129.

12. McLeod, D. L., Shreve, M. M., and Axelrad, A. A. (1976) Induction of megakaryocyte colonies with platelet formation in vitro. *Nature* **261,** 492–494.

13. Mazur, E. M., Basilico, D., Newton, J. L., Cohen, J. L., Charland, C., Sohl, P. A., et al. (1990) Isolation of large numbers of enriched human megakaryocytes from liquid cultures of normal peripheral blood progenitor cells. *Blood* **76,** 1771–1782.

14. Vainchenker, W., Guichard, J., and Breton-Gorius, J. (1979) Growth of human mega-karyocyte colonies in culture from fetal, neonatal, and adult peripheral blood cells: ultrastructural analysis. *Blood Cells* **5,** 25–42.

15. Longmore, G. D., Pharr, P., Neumann, D., and Lodish, H. F. (1993) Both megakaryo-cytopoiesis and erythropoiesis are induced in mice infected with a retrovirus expressing an oncogenic erythropoietin receptor. *Blood* **82,** 2386–2395.

16. Mintern, J., Williams, N., and Jackson, H. (1997) The relative population sizes of megakaryo-cytic cells in mouse bone marrow as determined by mpl ligand responsiveness. *Exp. Hematol.* **25,** 1233–1239.

17. Burstein, S. A., Adamson, J. W., Thorning, D., and Harker, L. A. (1979) Characteristics of murine megakaryocytic colonies in vitro. *Blood* **54,** 169–179.

18. Hamada, T., Mohle, R., Hesselgesser, J., Hoxie, J., Nachman, R. L., Moore, M. A., et al. (1998) Transendothelial migration of megakaryocytes in response to stromal cell-derived factor 1 (SDF-1) enhances platelet formation. *J. Exp. Med.* **188,** 539–548.

19. Wang, J. F., Liu, Z. Y., and Groopman, J. E. (1998) The alpha-chemokine receptor CXCR4 is expressed on the megakaryocytic lineage from progenitor to platelets and modulates migration and adhesion. *Blood* **92,** 756–764.

20. Riviere, C., Subra, F., Cohen-Solal, K., Cordette-Lagarde, V., Letestu, R., Auclair, C., et al. (1999) Phenotypic and functional evidence for the expression of CXCR4 receptor during megakaryocytopoiesis. *Blood* **93,** 1511–1523.

21. Giet, O., Van Bockstaele, D. R., Di Stefano, I., Huygen, S., Greimers, R., Beguin, Y., et al. (2002) Increased binding and defective migration across fibronectin of cycling hemato-poietic progenitor cells. *Blood* **99,** 2023–2031.

22. Aiuti, A., Webb, I. J., Bleul, C., Springer, T., and Gutierrez-Ramos, J. C. (1997) The chemokine SDF-1 is a chemoattractant for human CD34+ hematopoietic progenitor cells and provides a new mechanism to explain the mobilization of CD34+ progenitors to peripheral blood. *J. Exp. Med.* **185,** 111–120.

23. Pelletier, A. J., van der Laan, L. J., Hildbrand, P., Siani, M. A., Thompson, D. A., Dawson, P. E., et al. (2000) Presentation of chemokine SDF-1 alpha by fibronectin mediates directed migration of T cells. *Blood* **96,** 2682–2690.

24

Assays of Megakaryocyte Development
Surface Antigen Expression, Ploidy, and Size

Anthony Mathur, Ying Hong, Guosu Wang, and Jorge D. Erusalimsky

1. Introduction

Mature megakaryocytes (MKs) are large cells, having an approximate diameter in humans of 20–40 µm. They develop from $CD34^+$ multipotent hematopoietic progenitors through a complex differentiation process driven primarily by the hormone thrombopoietin (TPO) (reviewed in **refs. *1,2***). The cellular hierarchy of the megakaryocytic lineage comprises three types of cells *(3,4)*: MK progenitors, immature MKs or promegakaryoblasts, and mature MKs **(Fig. 1)**. MK progenitors (HPP-CFU, BFU and CFU in **Fig. 1**; *see* caption for definitions) are a functionally heterogeneous group of cells, endowed with varying degrees of proliferative capacity, all of which express the surface antigen CD34. Promegakaryoblasts are transitional cells, intermediate between the proliferating progenitor cells and the mature, differentiated MKs *(5)*. They are also a heterogeneous group of cells, which undergo polyploidization during development and increase their size and cytoplasmic complexity. Mature MKs are polyploid cells that no longer proliferate but have the unique ability to shed their cytoplasm *(6)*, and as a result, produce in the order of 2000–3000 platelets/cell. In addition to TPO, other pleiotropic growth factors and cytokines (*see* **Fig. 1**) can act synergistically on hematopoietic progenitors to promote the growth and maturation of MK *(7–9)*.

A characteristic of cells of the megakaryocytic lineage is the presence of the surface antigens CD41 and CD61 *(10)*. These antigens correspond to the integrins α_{IIb} (CD41) and β_3 (CD61), which form a heterodimeric receptor complex, also known as glycoprotein (GP) IIb/IIIa *(11)*. CD41 and CD61 are expressed on cells of the megakaryocytic lineage, from the progenitor cell through to the platelet *(12,13)*. Their expression level is low in MK progenitor cells and increases substantially as the cells differentiate *(13)*. GPIIb/IIIa functions as a receptor for four adhesive proteins—fibrinogen, fibronectin, vitronectin, and von Willebrand factor—and plays an important role in hemostasis *(14)*. Several monoclonal antibodies are available that recognize the presence of GPIIb/IIIa on

From: *Methods in Molecular Biology, vol. 272:*
Platelets and Megakaryocytes, Vol. 1: Functional Assays
Edited by: J. M. Gibbins and M. P. Mahaut-Smith © Humana Press Inc., Totowa, NJ

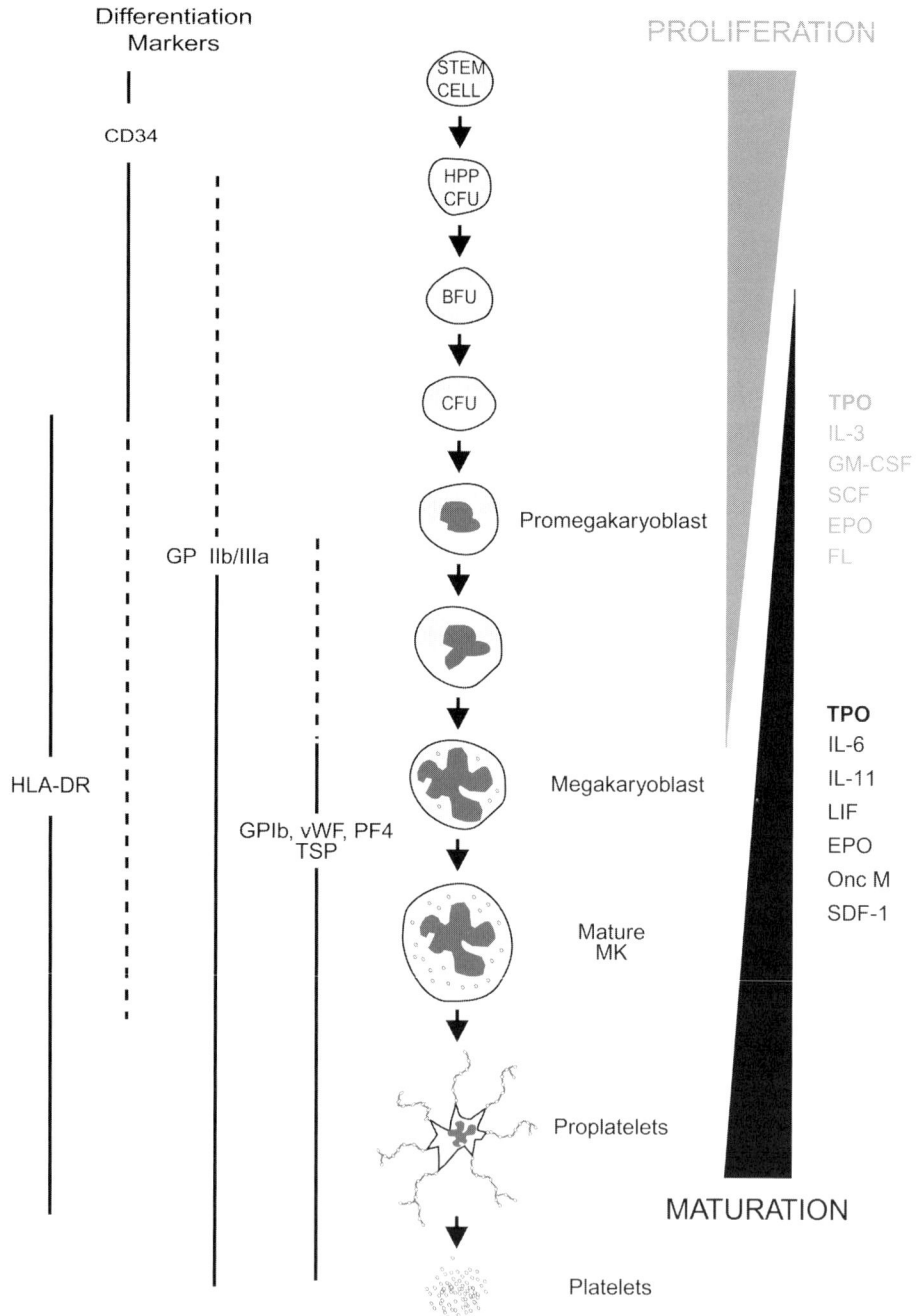

the cell surface *(15–17)*. One of these, clone Y2/51, which recognizes the GPIIIa subunit (CD61), has been widely used to follow the process of MK differentiation in culture, to distinguish MKs from other cell types, and to purify MKs from heterogeneous mixtures of nucleated cells *(18–21)*.

Mature MKs can be obtained from bone-marrow aspirates. In addition, MKs can be produced in liquid cultures of hematopoieitic progenitor cells that may be obtained from a variety of sources, including bone marrow, umbilical cord blood, and the harvest of peripheral blood leukaphoresis *(22–24)*. Such cultures can also be used to investigate the biology of MK differentiation. In this chapter we will describe (1) the immuno-magnetic purification of CD34$^+$ progenitor cells from human umbilical cord blood, (2) the culture of these cells in liquid medium supplemented with TPO for up to two weeks, and (3) the assessment of MK differentiation by flow cytometry. A similar flow-cytometric technique can also be used to evaluate the presence of MKs in bone marrow aspirates *(19)*.

2. Materials
2.1. Purification of CD34$^+$ Progenitor Cells

1. Heparin sodium (CP Pharmaceuticals Ltd., Wrexham, UK): dispense in aliquots of 200 IU into 50-mL sterile polypropylene centrifuge tubes (Falcon) and store at room temperature.
2. Butterfly-21ST needle (Abbot Ireland, Sligo, Ireland).
3. Human umbilical cord blood, obtained from scheduled Caesarean births.
4. 20-mL plastic syringes.
5. Ficoll-paque™ PLUS (Amersham Biosciences, Bucks, UK).
6. MiniMACS separation unit (Miltenyi Biotec GmbH, Bergisch Gladbach, Germany, 130-042-102).
7. MS MACS separation columns (Miltenyi Biotec, 130-042-201).
8. CD34$^+$ progenitor cell isolation kit (Miltenyi Biotec, 130-046-701) containing FcR-blocking reagent, hapten-conjugated anti-CD34 monoclonal antibody (clone QBEND/10), and colloidal super-paramagnetic MACS MicroBeads conjugated to an anti-hapten antibody. For storage details, follow the manufacturer's instructions.
9. Fluorescein isothiocyanate (FITC)-conjugated anti-human progenitor-cell antigen (HPCA-2) monoclonal antibody (clone 8G12, Becton Dickinson, Oxford, UK).
10. Dulbecco's phosphate-buffered saline (PBS), pH 7.4 (Gibco, BRL, Paisley, UK).
11. PBS/EDTA: PBS containing 2 mM EDTA (added from a stock solution of 0.5 M disodium EDTA, titrated to pH 7.5 with NaOH). Sterilize by autoclaving at 126°C for 30 min.

Fig. 1. *(see opposite page)* Overview of megakaryocyte development and expression of differentiation markers. Broken lines indicate low levels of antigen expression. Abbreviations: TPO, thrombopoietin; IL, interleukin; GM-CSF, granulocyte-macrophage colony-stimulating factor; SCF, stem cell factor; EPO, erythropoietin; FL, flt ligand; LIF, leukemia inhibitory factor; Onc M, oncostatin M; SDF-1, stromal cell derived factor 1; HPP CFU, high-proliferative potential colony-forming unit; BFU, burst-forming unit; CFU, colony-forming unit; vWF, von Willebrand factor; PF4, platelet factor 4; TSP, thrombospondin; GP, glycoprotein.

12. PBS/EDTA/BSA: PBS/EDTA supplemented with 0.5% bovine serum albumin (BSA, Sigma, Gillingham, UK A4503). Sterilize by filtering through a 0.2-μm pore filter unit (e.g., Nalgene 151-4020, Nalge Nunc International, New York, NY). Store at 4°C.

13. PBS/BSA (cell-surface marker staining buffer): PBS containing 1% BSA. Filter through 0.2-μm pore filter unit and store at 4°C.

14. MK basal culture medium (MKBM): Iscove's modified Dulbecco's medium (Sigma, 13390) supplemented with 0.2% (w/v) BSA (fraction V, Sigma A8412), 2 mM glutamine, 1 mM sodium pyruvate, MEM non-essential amino acids (Gibco BRL, diluted 1:100), MEM vitamins (Gibco BRL, diluted 1:100), 0.1 mM 2-mercaptoethanol, 100 U/mL penicillin, 0.1 mg/mL streptomycin. Store at 4°C for up to one month.

15. Polypropylene centrifuge tubes, 15- and 50-mL capacity, sterile (Falcon).

16. Polystyrene round-bottom tubes, 5-mL capacity (Becton Dickinson).

2.2. Culture of CD34+ Cells

1. CD34+ cell suspension (obtained as described in **Subheading 3.1.**).

2. Human umbilical cord plasma: prepared from heparinized cord blood obtained from Caesarean births (*see* **Notes 1** and **2**). Dispense in aliquots of 2 mL under sterile conditions and store at –20°C for up to 4 mo.

3. 0.4% Trypan blue solution (Sigma).

4. Hemocytometer, Abingdon, UK.

5. MKBM: as listed in **Subheading 2.1.**

6. Recombinant human TPO (R&D Systems), 10 μg/mL: dissolve in PBS containing 0.1% BSA and store in aliquots at –20°C for up to 6 mo. Once thawed, do not refreeze; keep at 4°C for up to 2 wk.

7. 24-well tissue culture plates.

8. Polypropylene centrifuge tubes, 50 mL capacity, sterile (Falcon).

2.3. Analysis of Megakaryocytic Differentiation by Flow Cytometry

1. Cell culture suspension (**Subheading 3.2.**).

2. FITC-conjugated anti-human CD61 monoclonal antibody (clone Y2/51, Dako UK).

3. FITC-conjugated mouse IgG$_1$ control antibody (Dako, Ely, UK).

4. PBS: Dulbecco's phosphate-buffered saline, pH 7.4. Before use, filter through a 0.2-μm pore filter to remove any insoluble material.

5. PBS/BSA: as listed in **Subheading 2.1.**

6. 1% paraformaldehyde (BDH, Poole, UK 29447): dissolve 0.5 g in 50 mL PBS at 60°C, adding at the same time a few drops of 1 M NaOH to help in the solubilization (this procedure should be carried out in a fume hood). After the solution has cooled down to room temperature, adjust the pH to 7.4. Store at 4°C and use within one week. Before use filter through a 0.2-μm pore filter to remove any insoluble material.

7. 1000 U/mL RNase A, DNase free: Dissolve protein in 10 mM Tris-HCl/1 mM EDTA, pH 7.5, heat at 95°C for 15 min to inactivate any contaminating DNase, and store in aliquots at –20°C.

8. 1 mg/mL propidium iodide (PI) (Sigma): dissolve in PBS and store at 4°C protected from light. This substance is a mutagen and must be handled according to local safety regulations.

9. DNA staining solution: PBS containing 2 mM MgCl$_2$, 0.05% saponin, 0.01 mg/mL PI, and 10 U/mL RNase A. PI and RNase A are added just prior to use from the concentrated stock solutions.

10. FACSflow (isotonic flow cytometry solution from Becton Dickinson).

11. FACScan™ flow cytometer (Becton Dickinson) (or similar flow cytometer equipped with a wide nozzle of at least 70 μm diameter).
12. CELLQUEST software (Becton Dickinson).
13. Polystyrene round-bottom tube, as listed in **Subheading 2.1.**
14. Polypropylene centrifuge tubes, 15 mL capacity (Falcon).

3. Methods

3.1. Purification of CD34⁺ Progenitor Cells

CD34 is a surface antigen strongly expressed by progenitor cells of all hematopoietic lineages *(25)*. Its expression declines as lineage differentiation progresses, being virtually absent from terminally differentiated blood cells *(26)*. Hence, the presence of CD34 on the surface of hematopoietic progenitor cells allows their separation from other bone marrow or blood cells.

Unless otherwise indicated, perform all steps at room temperature under sterile conditions. Once the blood is transported from the labor ward to the laboratory for processing, all the remaining steps are carried out under Level II containment standards, ensuring that local safety regulations relating to the handling of human biological material are observed at all times.

3.1.1. Isolation of Low-Density Mononuclear Cells

1. Withdraw blood (generally ~60 mL) from the umbilical cord using a 20-mL plastic syringe attached to a Butterfly-21ST needle (*see* **Note 1**). Transfer the blood immediately to 50-mL Falcon tubes containing 200 IU heparin and mix well by inversion.
2. Dilute blood with 3 volumes of PBS/EDTA (*see* **Note 2**) and mix thoroughly.
3. Carefully layer 35 mL of the diluted blood over 15 mL Ficoll-paque™ PLUS in a 50-mL Falcon tube (ensure that the Ficoll is at room temperature). Fill as many tubes as necessary to process the entire blood sample.
4. Centrifuge at 400*g* for 35 min in a benchtop centrifuge equipped with a swinging-bucket rotor. Ensure that the centrifuge brake is off.
5. The mononuclear cells settle in a band at the interface between the Ficoll and plasma. Remove the upper plasma layer without disturbing the mononuclear cells, then transfer these, with as little Ficoll as possible, to two fresh 50-mL centrifuge tubes (*see* **Note 3**).
6. Top off the tubes containing the mononuclear cells with PBS/EDTA and centrifuge at 300*g* for 10 min.
7. Carefully transfer supernatants into fresh tubes and centrifuge again as in **step 6** above (*see* **Note 4**).
8. Combine the cell pellets from **steps 6** and **7** into one tube by resuspending in a total volume of 30 mL PBS/EDTA (*see* **Note 3**) and centrifuge as in **step 6**.
9. Aspirate supernatant and resuspend cell pellet in a final volume of 0.3 mL PBS/EDTA/BSA (*see* **Note 3**).

3.1.2. Magnetic Labeling and Separation of CD34⁺ Cells

The steps described below are carried out using a commercially available kit, essentially as described by the manufacturers (*see* **Note 5**). The method involves labeling the cells with a hapten-conjugated primary antibody against CD34 (QBEND/10), followed by an anti-hapten antibody coupled to colloidal super-paramagnetic microbeads. The magnetically labeled cells are subsequently loaded onto a separation column under a magnetic field. Under the action of this field the labeled cells are trapped in the column, whereas the unlabeled cells are removed by washing with a buffer solution. The positively labeled cells are then recovered from the column by eluting with buffer once the magnetic field is removed. Finally the eluted cells are loaded into a new column and the magnetic purification step is repeated in order to improve cell purity.

1. To 0.3 mL mononuclear cell suspension (*see* **step 9** in **Subheading 3.1.1.**), add 0.1 mL FcR-blocking reagent and 0.1 mL hapten-conjugated anti-CD34 antibody, mix well, and incubate for 15 min at 6–12°C.
2. Wash the cells with 10 mL PBS/EDTA/BSA, centrifuge at 300g for 10 min at 4°C, and carefully aspirate the supernatant.
3. Resuspend the cell pellet in 0.4 mL PBS/EDTA/BSA, add 0.1 mL anti-hapten microbeads, mix well, and incubate for 15 min at 6–12°C.
4. Wash the cells as described in **step 2** above and resuspend the cell pellet in 0.5 mL ice-cold PBS/EDTA/BSA. Place the cells on ice until further use (*see* **Note 6**).
5. Place the MS MACS separation column in the magnetic field of the MiniMACS separation unit. Rinse the column with cold PBS/EDTA/BSA.
6. Load the cells from **step 4** onto the column; wash the column three times with 0.5 mL cold PBS/EDTA/BSA.
7. Remove the column from the MiniMACS separation unit, place it over a 15-mL centrifuge tube, add 1 mL cold PBS/EDTA/BSA, and elute the retained cells. Keep the cells on ice until further use.
8. Apply the eluted cells to a new MS MACS separation column and repeat the magnetic separation as described in **steps 5–7**, with the exception that the cells are eluted with 1 mL MKBM.
9. Check the purity of the eluted cells. For this purpose, aliquot a sample of 10 μL into a 5-mL tube containing 40 μL PBS/BSA and 5 μL FITC-conjugated anti-HPCA-2 antibody (this reagent binds to an epitope of CD34 distinct from that recognized by QBEND/10). Incubate the cells for 15 min in the dark at 6–12°C and then wash with 1 mL PBS. Finally, resuspend the cells in 0.5 mL PBS and determine the percentage of CD34$^+$ cells by flow cytometry. A sample containing the unfractionated cells (*see* **Note 6**) is labeled and analyzed in parallel (*see* **Note 7**).

3.2. Culture of CD34$^+$ Cells

1. Sample an aliquot of 10 μL CD34$^+$ cell suspension into an equal volume of 0.4% Trypan blue solution and count the live cells (those excluding Trypan blue) with a hemocytometer.
2. Dilute the cell suspension to a density of 1.5×10^5 cells/mL in MKBM freshly supplemented with 40 ng/mL TPO and 10% umbilical cord blood plasma (*see* **Note 8**).
3. Dispense the cells into a 24-well tissue culture plate (1 mL per well) and place in a humidified incubator at 37°C under 5% CO_2.
4. After 4 days of incubation transfer the nonadherent cells to a 50-mL tube and count the cells. Then dilute (approximately threefold) the cell suspension to a density of 1.5×10^5 cells/mL by addition of fresh MKBM supplemented with 10% umbilical cord blood plasma (*see* **Note 9**).
5. Following dilution, replate the nonadherent cells into fresh culture wells as described in **step 3** and return to the incubator.

Table 1
Fluorescence Labeling for Analysis of Megakaryocytic Differentiation by Flow Cytometry

Tube #	Fluorescent label	PBS/BSA	Control Ab	Y2/51 Ab
1	Nonspecific	95 µL	5 µL	–
2	Fluorescein	95 µL	–	5 µL
3	PI	100 µL	–	–
4	Fluorescein/PI	95 µL	–	5 µL

Combinations refer to **Subheading 3.3.1., step 2**.

6. After 12 d of culture harvest the nonadherent cells, measure the cell concentration, and then follow the procedures described below to assess megakaryocytic differentiation (*see* **Note 10**).

3.3. Analysis of Megakaryocytic Differentiation by Flow Cytometry

In this procedure a FITC-conjugated antibody against CD61 recognizes megakaryocytic cells, while PI stains the nuclear DNA. Cells are then analyzed by flow cytometry to estimate the percentage of megakaryocytic cells present in the culture and simultaneously assess their ploidy distribution. Flow cytometry may also be used to obtain a qualitative estimation of the change in cell size (*see* **Subheading 3.4.**).

3.3.1. Fluorescent Labeling

The following steps are carried out at 4°C. Incubations are performed in the dark.

1. Transfer 0.5-mL aliquots of the cell suspension ($5–7.5 \times 10^5$ cells) into four 15-mL centrifuge tubes, add 5 mL PBS/BSA (*see* **Note 11**), centrifuge at 300*g* for 10 min, and then carefully aspirate the supernatants.
2. Resuspend cell pellets by adding PBS/BSA and FITC-conjugated antibodies as described in **Table 1** (*see* **Note 12**).
3. Mix well and incubate for 1 h on ice.
4. Wash the cells with 5 mL PBS, centrifuge at 300*g* for 10 min, and carefully aspirate the supernatants.
5. Resuspend cell pellets in 0.5 mL PBS, then slowly add 0.5 mL 1% paraformaldehyde and leave on ice for 45 min (*see* **Note 13**).
6. Wash the cells as described in **step 4** and then resuspend pellets in 1 mL DNA staining solution (*see* **Note 14**), omitting the PI in tubes 1 and 2.
7. Stain cells overnight and then analyze by flow cytometry (*see* **Note 15**).

3.3.2. Cytofluorimetric Analysis

The instructions given in this section are intended for workers with some experience in flow cytometry. Chapters 19 and 20, vol. 1 give further details of flow-cytometric techniques. A Becton Dickinson FACScan™ flow cytometer connected to an Apple computer system is used in this protocol. Data are recorded and analyzed using the

Table 2
Flow Cytometer Settings for Analysis of Cultured Megakaryocytes

	FSC	SSC	FL1	FL2
Detectors	E-1	325 V	519 V	257 V
Amplifier gains	7.5	2.94	log	log

Settings refer to a Becton Dickinson FACScan™.
FSC: forward scatter; SSC: side scatter; FL1: fluorescein fluorescence; FL2: PI fluorescence.

CELLQUEST software program. FACSflow is used to purge the apparatus prior to analysis. The detailed running of the instrument is beyond the scope of this chapter. Equivalent instruments with a wide-diameter nozzle are equally appropriate.

1. Set up the instrument for acquisition. Adjust photomultiplier settings and gains to record forward scatter (FSC), side scatter (SSC), fluorescein fluorescence (FL1), and PI fluorescence (FL2) of each cell (*see* **Note 16**). Set the fluidics flow rate to "low." **Table 2** shows the initial settings routinely used with our instrument to analyze cultured MKs.
2. Run tube no. 1 in set-up mode. Using a dot plot of FSC vs SSC, adjust the analyzer threshold on the FSC channel to exclude small debris (*see* **Note 17**).
3. Continue to run tube no. 1; using a dot-plot display of FL1 vs FL2, adjust the FL1 and FL2 channel voltages so that all events fall within the first decade of the corresponding logarithmic scales (*see* **Note 18**).
4. Run tube no. 2 in set-up mode; using a dot plot of FL1 vs FL2, correct electronically (compensation) for spillage of the green fluorescence signal into the red fluorescence detector.
5. Run tube no. 3 in set-up mode; using a dot plot of FL1 vs FL2, correct electronically for spillage of the red fluorescence signal into the green fluorescence detector. In addition, adjust the FL2 channel voltage so that the 2n cell subpopulation falls within the second decade of the FL2 logarithmic scale.
6. Run tube no. 4 in set-up mode and quickly perform the following adjustments:
   a. Check that the sample flow rate falls within 750–2000 cells/s. If necessary adjust the cell concentration by diluting the sample with PBS.
   b. Using a dot plot of FL1 vs FL2, check again for spillage of the green fluorescence signal into the red fluorescence detector. If required, adjust the electronic compensation (*see* **Note 19**).
7. Switch the instrument to acquisition mode. Run the remainder of tube no. 4, collecting at least 10,000 events.
8. Following acquisition of the data determine the percentage of megakaryocytic cells, their relative level of CD61 expression, and the frequency of cells in each ploidy class, using the software analysis tools (*see* **Note 20**).

3.4. Determination of MK Size

MK diameter can be determined using commercially available particle analyzers such as a Multiziser 3 (Beckman Coulter) or Sysmex CDA-500 (Malvern Instruments), both of which are based on measurements of changes in impedance. In addition,

MK size can be estimated by flow cytometry using the forward scatter parameter, a measure that is also related to particle size. In this case latex particles of known size (Fluospheres, Molecular Probes, Oregon) are used to calibrate the forward scatter channel of the flow cytometer. This technique has the added advantage of allowing determination of MK size within heterogeneous cell populations as well as the estimation of relative differences in cell size between MK ploidy subclasses.

4. Notes

1. Umbilical cord blood may be donated by women giving birth by Caesarian section, who have no previous history of hematological disease or transmissible infections. The blood sample must be obtained not later than 10 min after the placenta has been removed from the womb. Sample volume (40–100 mL) may vary according to the size and state of the placenta and umbilical cord. In the United Kingdom collection of blood for research purposes requires the patient's informed written consent and hospital ethics committee approval.

2. When preparing plasma, centrifuge the unprocessed blood sample (without dilution) at 1800g for 20 min at 4°C. Then, transfer the supernatant (plasma) into a new 50-mL centrifuge tube and repeat the centrifugation step to remove residual blood cells. The cell pellet may be then diluted with PBS/EDTA in the usual way to purify mononuclear cells.

3. If the initial blood volume is larger than 80 mL, the number of tubes and volumes of buffers should be doubled.

4. Recentrifugation of the first wash supernatant increases the yield of mononuclear cells by approx 25%.

5. The reagents and method apply to a two-step isolation procedure; Miltenyi Biotec also offers a one-step CD34$^+$ progenitor cell isolation kit, which gives comparable results.

6. Before magnetic separation an aliquot of 5 μL from the labeled cell suspension may be sampled into a 5-mL tube containing 45 μL PBS/BSA and kept on ice to check the efficiency of the isolation procedure at a later stage.

7. The frequency of CD34$^+$ cells in umbilical cord blood is less than 0.5%. An average sample of cord blood (60 mL) usually yields ~1.5 × 10^6 cells (range = 0.9 to 2.5 × 10^6 cells) with a purity exceeding 90%.

8. Alternatively MKs may be grown from CD34$^+$ cells in plasma-free media *(27–29)*. We and others have obtained good results growing these cells in ready-made commercially available media such as X-vivo 20 (Biowhittacker, Maryland) or Stemspan$^{™}$ (Stem Cell Technologies Inc.), supplemented with TPO, either in the presence or in the absence of other proliferation-inducing factors such as IL-3 and SCF. However, in our hands, the highest levels of MK differentiation (particularly polyploidization) are observed when cultures are grown in umbilical-cord plasma-containing media.

9. At this step TPO is purposely omitted from the feeding medium. If TPO is also added the final cell count will be higher but the percentage of polyploid cells will be reduced.

10. Cultures may be harvested at any time to follow the evolution of the differentiation process. The frequency of CD61$^+$ cells reaches a maximum after 7–8 d of culture (*see* **Fig. 3B**) and this level is maintained for up to 2 wk, when the culture begins to lose viability. The total number of cells, the frequency of MKs, and their ploidy status may vary somewhat from culture to culture. For example a representative set of results from eight separate consecutive donors demonstrated a 17- to 36-fold increase (mean = 26.6 ± 7.2) in cell number after 12 d in culture. The percentage of CD61$^+$ cells found within these cultures

ranged from 58% to 81% (mean = $72 \pm 9\%$). We have also found such a degree of variability when cells were grown in plasma-free media. Since the experimental conditions are standardized, these differences can only be attributed to the initial characteristics of the CD34$^+$ cells from different donors. Due to this natural variability comparisons should be made only using cells from the same donor (e.g., when testing the activity of pharmacological agents).

11. During the labeling procedure care should be taken to perform all cell resuspensions and washing steps with ice-cold solutions. It is also important to filter solutions through a 0.2-μm pore filter to remove any insoluble material. This latter procedure greatly improves the quality of the flow cytometric analysis.

12. When only levels of CD61 expression are to be determined, tubes no. 3 and no. 4 are not required.

13. Mild fixation with paraformaldehyde is included to prevent washing off the antibody during the subsequent incubation in DNA staining solution. This step may be omitted when levels of CD61 expression alone are to be determined (i.e., when ploidy analysis is not required). In that case cells may be resuspended in PBS and analyzed immediately by flow cytometry.

14. DNA staining is carried out in the presence of the detergent saponin, which allows complete permeabilization of the plasma and nuclear membrane to PI while maintaining sufficient integrity to enable cellular discrimination on the basis of morphological parameters. RNAse A may be omitted from the staining solution without significantly affecting the quality of the results.

15. Cells should be left in staining solution for at least 4 h but for not more than 72 h. Staining times outside these boundaries affect the quality of the results. The use of a fluorescence microscope may help to assess the success of the staining procedure prior to analysis by flow cytometry. Mature MKs are easily identified as large cells displaying a diffuse green fluorescence on the cell surface and a strong red fluorescence in the nucleus, which may appear as a multilobed compartment. This protocol can be used to label MKs from bone marrow suspensions, in which case the initial cell density should be adjusted to at least 1×10^7 cells/mL.

16. PI fluorescence may also be acquired on the FL3 channel of the FACScan™.

17. Debris may be also excluded by running tube #3 in set-up mode and adjusting the analyzer threshold on the FL2 channel so that only events with a fluorescence corresponding to a DNA content of 2n or greater are included in the acquisition of the data (see the example shown in **Fig. 2**). While this alternative procedure is suitable in most cases, it is not appropriate when the presence of late apoptotic cells (i.e., cells having a sub-diploid DNA content) is to be assessed.

18. If a bone marrow sample is analyzed, set up a live gate that excludes all the nonspecific green fluorescence. This is necessary to avoid saturating the analyzer with nonmegakaryocytic cells.

19. A typical dot-plot display of FL1 vs FL2 **(Fig. 2)** shows the presence of individual "streaks" representing the different ploidy subsets. This "streaky" appearance is due to the fact that within each ploidy subset cells display varying levels of green fluorescence. Adequate electronic compensation of the fluorescein fluorescence signal is achieved when these "streaks" become aligned parallel to the FL1 axis.

20. The acquired data can be analyzed using different setups. For example, a green-fluorescence histogram can be used to determine the percentage of cells expressing CD61, as shown in **Fig. 3A**. This type of analysis can be used to follow the differentiation of the system over the culture period, as shown in **Fig. 3B**. To establish the DNA ploidy distri-

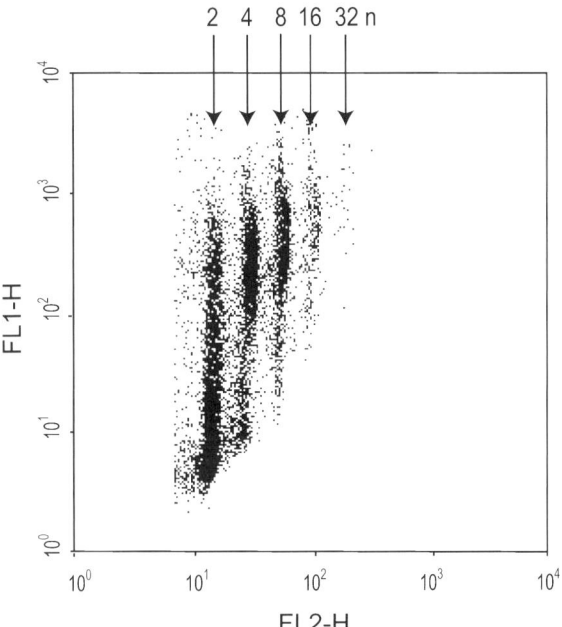

Fig. 2. Flow-cytometric dot plot of CD61 expression (FL1-H) vs DNA content (FL2-H) in cultured megakaryocytes. Cells were double-labeled with FITC-conjugated Y2/51 antibody and PI. Note that in this example the analyzer threshold has been adjusted on the FL2 channel. The different ploidy subclasses are indicated (*see* **Notes 17** and **19**).

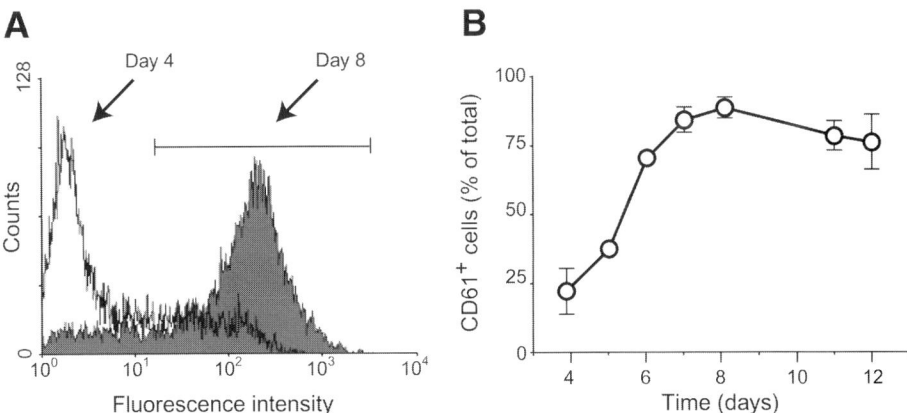

Fig. 3. Time course of megakaryocytopoiesis in culture as assessed by flow-cytometric analysis of CD61 expression. (**A**) Green-fluorescence histograms of cells stained with FITC-labeled Y2/51 antibody after 4 (open tracing) and 8 (shadowed tracing) d of culture; the marker encompasses the CD61$^+$ cells. (**B**) Percentage of cells ± SD (pooled data from six donors) expressing CD61 as a function of time in culture.

A

B

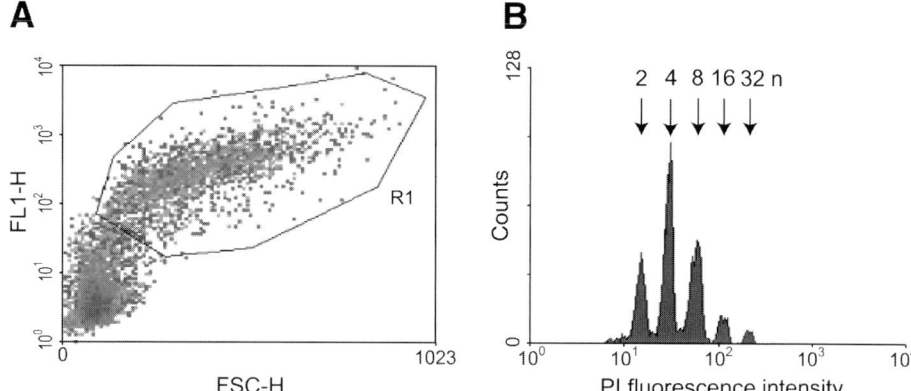

Fig. 4. Flow-cytometric analysis of the ploidy distribution of megakaryocytes grown in culture from CD34⁺ cells. After 12 d of culture cells were double-labeled with FITC-conjugated Y2/51 antibody and PI. **(A)** Density plot of forward scatter (FSC) vs CD61 expression (FL1-H) showing an analysis region (R1) drawn around the subpopulation representing MKs. **(B)** PI fluorescence histogram of cells found within R1 in panel A. The different ploidy subclasses are indicated.

bution, a two-parameter display of FSC vs FL1 can be used to identify the MK population **(Fig. 4A)**. In this display, MKs appear as a distinct subset comprising the most fluorescent cells. An analysis region is set around this cell population (R1 in **Fig. 4A**), and all the cells within this region are depicted in a DNA histogram **(Fig. 4B)**. The histogram is then divided into compartments that correspond to the different ploidy classes. Ploidy classes are identified using as a reference the position of the 2n peak in a sample of human peripheral blood mononuclear cells or isolated CD34⁺ cells which may be run in parallel (in these samples the majority of cells are 2n). Boundaries of ploidy compartments are determined manually by setting markers at the nadirs between peaks. The frequency of cells in each ploidy compartment is calculated by dividing the number of cells in the compartment by the total number of cells in the histogram.

Acknowledgments

This work has been generously supported by a Programme Grant (RG/98011) awarded by the British Heart Foundation.

References

1. Mazur, E. M. (1987) Megakaryocytopoiesis and platelet production: a review. *Exp. Hematol.* **15,** 340–350.
2. Kaushansky, K. (1995) Thrombopoietin: the primary regulator of megakaryocyte and platelet production. *Blood* **86,** 419–431.
3. Hoffman, R. (1989) Regulation of megakaryocytopoiesis. *Blood* **74,** 1196–1212.
4. Long, M. W. (1993) Population heterogeneity among cells of the megakaryocyte lineage. *Stem Cells* **11,** 33–40.

5. Long, M. W., Williams, N., and McDonald, T. P. (1982) Immature megakaryocytes in the mouse: in vitro relationship to megakaryocyte progenitor cells and mature megakaryocytes. *J. Cell Physiol.* **112,** 339–344.

6. Italiano, J. E., Jr., Lecine, P., Shivdasani, R. A., and Hartwig, J. H. (1999) Blood platelets are assembled principally at the ends of proplatelet processes produced by differentiated megakaryocytes. *J. Cell Biol.* **147,** 1299–1312.

7. Gordon, M. S. and Hoffman, R. (1992) Growth factors affecting human thrombocytopoiesis: potential agents for the treatment of thrombocytopenia. *Blood* **80,** 302–307.

8. Debili, N., Masse, J. M., Katz, A., Guichard, J., Breton-Gorius, J., and Vainchenker, W. (1993) Effects of the recombinant hematopoietic growth factors interleukin-3, interleukin-6, stem cell factor, and leukemia inhibitory factor on the megakaryocytic differentiation of CD34+ cells. *Blood* **82,** 84–95.

9. Guerriero, R., Mattia, G., Testa, U., Chelucci, C., Macioce, G., Casella, I., et al. (2001) Stromal cell-derived factor 1alpha increases polyploidization of megakaryocytes generated by human hematopoietic progenitor cells. *Blood* **97,** 2587–2595.

10. Vainchenker, W. and Kieffer, N. (1988) Human megakaryocytopoiesis: in vitro regulation and characterization of megakaryocytic precursor cells by differentiation markers. *Blood Rev.* **2,** 102–107.

11. Phillips, D. R., Charo, I. F., Parise, L. V., and Fitzgerald, L. A. (1988) The platelet membrane glycoprotein IIb-IIIa complex. *Blood* **71,** 831–843.

12. Levene, R. B., Leung, L. L., and Nachman, R. L. (1981) Human megakaryocytes. II. Expression of platelet proteins in early marrow megakaryocytes. *J. Exp. Med.* **154,** 88–100.

13. Levene, R. B., Lamaziere, J. M., Broxmeyer, H. E., Lu, L., and Rabellino, E. M. (1985) Human megakaryocytes. V. Changes in the phenotypic profile of differentiating megakaryocytes. *J. Exp. Med.* **161,** 457–474.

14. Kieffer, N. and Phillips, D. R. (1990) Platelet membrane glycoproteins: functions in cellular interactions. *Annu. Rev. Cell Biol.* **6,** 329–357.

15. Tomer, A., Harker, L. A., and Burstein, S. A. (1988) Flow cytometric analysis of normal human megakaryocytes. *Blood* **71,** 1244–1252.

16. Isenberg, W. M., Bainton, D. F., and Newman, P. J. (1990) Monoclonal antibodies bound to subunits of the integrin GPIIb-IIIa are internalized and interfere with filopodia formation and platelet aggregation. *Blood* **76,** 1564–1571.

17. Nurden, A. T., Macchi, L., Bihour, C., Durrieu, C., Besse, P., and Nurden, P. (1994) Markers of platelet activation in coronary heart disease patients. *Eur. J. Clin. Invest.* **24(Suppl. 1),** 42–45.

18. Vainchenker, W., Deschamps, J. F., Bastin, J. M., Guichard, J., Titeux, M., Breton-Gorius, J., et al. (1982) Two monoclonal antiplatelet antibodies as markers of human megakaryocyte maturation: immunofluorescent staining and platelet peroxidase detection in megakaryocyte colonies and in vivo cells from normal and leukemic patients. *Blood* **59,** 514–521.

19. Erusalimsky, J. D. and Martin, J. F. (1996) Cellular model systems to study megakaryocyte differentiation, in *Platelets: A Practical Approach* (Watson, S. P. and Authi, K. S., eds.), Oxford University Press, New York, pp. 27–46.

20. Bobik, R., Hong, Y., Breier, G., Martin, J. F., and Erusalimsky, J. D. (1998) Thrombopoietin stimulates VEGF release from c-Mpl-expressing cell lines and haematopoietic progenitors. *FEBS Lett.* **423,** 10–14.

21. Mathur, A., Hong, Y., Martin, J., and Erusalimsky, J. (2001) Megakaryocytic differentiation is accompanied by a reduction in cell migratory potential. *Br. J. Haematol.* **112,** 459–465.

22. Zucker-Franklin, D., Yang, J. S., and Grusky, G. (1992) Characterization of glycoprotein IIb/IIIa-positive cells in human umbilical cord blood: their potential usefulness as mega-karyocyte progenitors. *Blood* **79,** 347–355.

23. Nichol, J. L., Hornkohl, A. C., Choi, E. S., Hokom, M. M., Ponting, I., Schuening, F. W., et al. (1994) Enrichment and characterization of peripheral blood-derived megakaryocyte progenitors that mature in short-term liquid culture. *Stem Cells* **12,** 494–505.

24. Miyazaki, R., Ogata, H., Iguchi, T., Sogo, S., Kushida, T., Ito, T., et al. (2000) Comparative analyses of megakaryocytes derived from cord blood and bone marrow. *Br. J. Haematol.* **108,** 602–609.

25. Civin, C. I., Strauss, L. C., Brovall, C., Fackler, M. J., Schwartz, J. F., and Shaper, J. H. (1984) Antigenic analysis of hematopoiesis. III. A hematopoietic progenitor cell surface antigen defined by a monoclonal antibody raised against KG-1a cells. *J. Immunol.* **133,** 157–165.

26. Caux, C., Favre, C., Saeland, S., Duvert, V., Mannoni, P., Durand, I., et al. (1989) Sequential loss of CD34 and class II MHC antigens on purified cord blood hematopoietic progenitors cultured with IL-3: characterization of CD34-, HLA-DR+ cells. *Blood* **74,** 1287–1294.

27. Norol, F., Vitrat, N., Cramer, E., Guichard, J., Burstein, S. A., Vainchenker, W., et al. (1998) Effects of cytokines on platelet production from blood and marrow CD34+ cells. *Blood* **91,** 830–843.

28. Hamada, T., Mohle, R., Hesselgesser, J., Hoxie, J., Nachman, R.L., Moore, M. A., et al. (1998) Transendothelial migration of megakaryocytes in response to stromal cell-derived factor 1 (SDF-1) enhances platelet formation. *J. Exp. Med.* **188,** 539–548.

29. Kie, J. H., Yang, W. I., Lee, M. K., Kwon, T. J., Min, Y. H., Kim, H. O., et al. (2002) Decrease in apoptosis and increase in polyploidization of megakaryocytes by stem cell factor during ex vivo expansion of human cord blood CD34+ cells using thrombopoietin. *Stem Cells* **20,** 73–79.

25

Assays of Megakaryocyte Development

Cytoplasm, Storage Granules, and Demarcation Membranes

Arnaud Drouin, Gulie Alimardani, and Elisabeth M. Cramer

1. Introduction
1.1. General Background

Megakaryocytes (MKs), the bone-marrow precursors of platelets, are remarkable cells because of their rarity among hematopoietic cells, their exceptionally large size, and their polylobulated, polyploid nuclei. In order to accurately assay the precise stage of MK cytoplasmic differentiation, a large array of morphological techniques can be used, depending on the type of information required.

Light microscopic examination using standard optical staining techniques is easy to perform and provides information on the general richness of the lineage, size, and number of various cellular elements. Immunofluorescence, immunocytochemistry, and immunohistochemistry are complementary approaches that allow one to study the progressive appearance of membrane receptors and secretory proteins. Electron microscopy (EM) is performed for detailed subcellular and organelle examination, e.g., demarcation membrane system development and storage granule formation. Immuno-EM allows analysis of the pattern of intracellular protein trafficking at various steps of cytoplasmic maturation. These techniques can be applied to MKs from bone marrow; however, the discovery of thrombopoietin (TPO) and its availability for experimental purposes has led to the study of cultured MKs as a useful alternative *(1,2)*. MKs can be cultured from precursors obtained from bone marrow, neonatal cord blood, or adult peripheral blood *(3,4)* (*see also* Chapter 23, vol. 1).

The hematopoietic marrow is located within flat bones and long bone diaphyses, between adipose tissue. A good way to evaluate the megakaryocytic lineage is to perform a bone-marrow biopsy, which, in contrast to aspirated marrow, removes a sample of intact marrow and thus allows examination of MKs in their topographical natural environment. Histological study allows accurate evaluation of the richness of the MK lineage among other hematopoietic cell lines, the distribution of the cellular elements,

From: *Methods in Molecular Biology, vol. 272:*
Platelets and Megakaryocytes, Vol. 1: Functional Assays
Edited by: J. M. Gibbins and M. P. Mahaut-Smith © Humana Press Inc., Totowa, NJ

either isolated or grouped in clusters, and the pattern of maturation of the MK cells. It also allows studies of the marrow microenvironment, such as reticulin and collagen fibers and vascular sinusoids. Normal MKs are typically located close to a vascular sinusoid and are gathered in small groups *(5)*. In myeloproliferative syndromes they appear in large clusters. Close intercellular interactions may also exist between marrow MKs and other hematopoietic cells, which can drive through the MK cytoplasm, without harm for both host and passenger, in order to reach the vessel lumen (emperipolesis).

1.2. Transmission Electron Microscopy

The major advances in our understanding of MK ultrastructure using electron microscopy (EM) have resulted from transmission EM (TEM) rather than scanning EM (SEM). TEM allows examination of cell sections and therefore investigations of the intracellular compartments of MKs. TEM has provided many seminal observations on MK structure and the mechanisms and kinetic of appearance of MK-specific organelles, secretion granules and demarcation membranes. It has demonstrated that the demarcation membrane system originates from plasma membrane invagination and that its channels always remain connected to the extracellular space *(6)*. MKs contain a range of cytoplasmic structures that can be classified according to their ultrastructural features (density, content, aspect). MK cytoplasmic differentiation is characterized by the presence of several Golgi complexes and centrioles, the demarcation membrane system (DMS), and the formation of specific granules. These include alpha and dense granules that are used during exocytosis in the future platelet and nonspecific granules, lysosomes, and peroxisomes *(7,8)*.

The process of platelet production during culture of human MKs has also been visualized, which has demonstrated the important step of proplatelet extension and the determinant role of microtubules in platelet formation and shedding *(9)*. Subtle differences between the ultrastructures of mouse and human platelet production have recently been shown, which might also explain many previous debates and divergent hypotheses concerning the presumed mechanisms of platelet shedding by MKs published in the literature. The flow model implies proplatelet formation and may be close to what happens in humans. The static model implies dilation of the demarcation membrane system and may reflect the observation made in the mouse *(10)*.

1.2. Immuno-EM Examination

Since the pionieer works of Coons 60 years ago, immunocytochemistry has become a key technique for cell biologists. The increased commercial availability of monoclonal antibodies has significantly advanced the potential of immunolabeling. Its adaptation to EM studies has allowed high-resolution ultrastructural observations of the location of various proteins in the MK *(8,11,12)*. Indeed, identification of various proteins during MK maturation, characterisation of their trafficking pattern, storage, or excretion are of major importance in the study of MK lineage.

Successful immuno-EM depends on achieving the correct balance between preserving ultrastructural features and retaining optimal antigen structure to allow sufficient levels of immunoreactivity. Preservation of cell structures when less-drastic

EM techniques are used for protein antigenicity conservation can remain one of the last problems to solve, especially when sections obtained from cryomethods are used. The basic process proposed here must be modulated for each type of experiments. Prior to immuno-EM, preliminary studies using a standard immunofluorescence approach are useful for assessing the quality and concentration requirements of each primary antibody and evaluating the overall subcellular pattern of localization of the protein studied. Immuno-EM is a quite recent improvement of classic immunological techniques to EM. Antigens are detected by the use of antibodies coupled to a range of 5- to 20-nm gold particles, which are highly electrondense. Immuno-EM techniques also allow the use of double labeling with gold particles of different diameters selected by their reactivity to the species of the primary antibodies.

Two types of immuno-EM techniques can be used: preembedding and postembedding. Preembedding techniques can be used on small specimens or isolated cells. This requires permeabilization with detergents to facilitate the penetration of antibodies and electrondense tracers, although it is extremely difficult to utilize permeabilizing agents gently enough to allow membrane penetration at the same time as preserving recognizable cell ultrastructure. An alternative method, postembedding immuno-EM techniques on ultrathin sections, was developed during the early 1980s and has considerably increased the field of ultrastructural exploration. Cells or tissues are fixed, embedded, and sectioned so that intracellular antigens exposed on the surface of the section can be reached by specific antibodies. Intracellular antigens can be visualized and intracellular trafficking of proteins studied.

Several embedding media are available. Hydrosoluble plastics are the embedding media of choice, as they minimize the use of organic solvents that are deleterious to antigens: glycol methacrylate (GMA), lowikryl, and LR white are the most frequently employed media. Ultrathin cryosectioning, after sucrose infiltration, is tricky to perform however is an ideal tool for immunological detection of intracellular antigens requiring only gentle fixation with no embedding. This results in minimal chemical deformation of intracellular antigens, although the ultrastructure is not well preserved.

Double labeling on sections is rendered possible by the combined use of polyclonal and monoclonal antibodies from different species, followed by specific antiglobulins coupled to gold particles of different size *(13,14)*. Both sides of the section can be used, with one type of immunological reaction on each side, and a quenching fixation in between. This has allowed simultaneous detection of antigens with different localizations, such as membrane receptor GPIb and its intragranular ligand, von Willebrand factor *(15)*. Immuno-EM can also be used with enzyme cytochemistry for localizing intracellular proteins and their enzymatic activity, such as peroxidase *(16)*.

2. Materials

2.1. Cytological Examination of Marrow Smears

1. Marrow can be obtained by aspiration from the sternum or posterior iliac crest. Local ethical guidelines for obtaining and using human tissue samples must be followed at all times.
2. Phosphate buffer, pH 7.0: 3.54 g KH_2PO_4 and 7.75 g $Na_2HPO_4\cdot2H_2O$ in 1 L of distilled water. Adjust pH with HCl or NaOH.

3. Solutions for Romanovsky staining: May-Grunwald and Giemsa solutions are purchased from Biolyon (Lyon, France). Filter the May-Grunwald solution (0.2-μm pore) before use and dilute the Giemsa (1 part Giemsa + 9 parts phosphate buffer).
4. Glass slides and coverslips.
5. For morphometric evaluation of nuclear perimeter, cell area, and nuclear area, a computer software package can be used (Samba 2005, Alcatel, France) *(17)*.

2.2. Immunohistochemical Analysis of Marrow Samples Using Alkaline Phosphatase Anti-Alkaline Phosphatase (APAAP) (18,19)

The procedure can be performed on marrow smears from aspirates or from biopsy samples. **Items 2–3** are required for marrow biopsy samples and **items 4–10** for smears.

1. Bone marrow biopsy sample: for example, after hip (iliac crest) biopsy (or aspirate, *see* **Subheading 2.1.**). Local ethical guidelines must be followed at all times.
2. Fixative for biopsies: Bouin's fluid (Labonord, Villeneuve d'Ascq, France).
3. Decalcification mix TBD-1 (Shandon, Inc., Pittsburgh, PA) *(20)*: 50 mL for 20 mg of marrow sample.
4. Methanol.
5. Paraformaldehyde (PFA), 16% solution (EMS, Washington, PA).
6. PBS, pH 7. 2 (X10 solution, GIBCO, Paisley, UK).
7. Fixative solution for marrow smears: 1% PFA in PBS (or 100% methanol) at 22°C.
8. Paraffin.
9. Xylene or chloroform.
10. Rehydration medium.
11. Reagents for APAAP *(18)*.

2.3. Immunofluorescence (21,22)

1. Marrow smears (*see* **Subheading 3.1.**) or cytospin preparations on slides.
2. *N*-2-Hydroxyethylpiperazine-*N*-2-ethanesulfonic acid (HEPES)-buffered saline or PBS.
3. PFA solution: 2% (w/v) PFA in HEPES-buffered saline or PBS. To dissolve the PFA, warm the saline to about 60°C. Ready-to-use paraformaldehyde solution 16% can also be purchased from EM Sciences (Washington, PA).
4. 0.1% (w/v) Triton X-100.
5. Glass slides.
6. Hydrophobic Dako® pen.
7. Primary antibody against species from which marrow is obtained (unconjugated).
8. Secondary antibody against species used to generate the primary antibody, conjugated to fluorophore of choice.
9. Mounting medium (e.g., Vectashield) (Vector Lab, Burlingame, CA).
10. Coverslip glass.
11. Nail polish.
12. Fluorescence microscope or confocal fluorescence microscope.

2.4. Transmission Electron Microscopy (TEM)

2.4.1. Fixation

1. 0.2 *M* phosphate buffer, pH 7.3: prepared by mixing 0.2 *M* monosodium phosphate (NaH_2PO_4) and disodium phosphate (0.2 *M* Na_2HPO_4) in an 11:39 proportion.

2. 0.1 *M* phosphate buffer is prepared immediately before use by diluting 0.2 *M* phosphate buffer with distilled water.
3. Sodium heparinate (Sanofi-Synthelabo, Paris, France) (final concentration: 10 U/mL of blood or HBSS for bone-marrow harvesting.
4. Hank's balanced salt solution (HBSS) without calcium and magnesium (Mediatch, Fischer Scientific, Philadelphia, PA).
5. 6% glutaraldehyde fixative solution in 0.1 *M* phosphate buffer. This is made from EM-grade glutaraldehyde, 25% solution in distilled water, from TAAB, Berks, UK.
6. Osmium tetroxide (OsO_4): 1% solution made by combining 1 part 2% (w/v) OsO_4 in distilled water and 1 part 0.2 *M* phosphate buffer (*see* **Note 1**).

2.4.2. Dehydration

70%, 90%, and 100% ethanol (v/v in distilled water).

2.4.3. Epon Embedding and Sectioning *(23)*

1. Erlenmeyer flask (or conical flask). Use 90% ethanol to clean the Erlenmeyer flask.
2. Propylene oxide (epoxy 1–2 propane) (*see* **Note 2**).
3. Epon embedding solution (*see* **Note 3**): Epikote 812 (88 mL), dodecenyl succinic anhydride (DDSA; 30 mL), MNA (60.3 mL), 2,4,6-Tri(dimethylaminomethyl) phenol (DMP-30; 2.7 mL). It is a fluid at room temperature, which then polymerizes and thus solidifies upon heating.
4. Gelatin capsules (no. 4) (EM Sciences, Washington, PA) or BEEM capsules (EM Sciences). These are used as the "container" in which the embedding solution is placed prior to insertion of the sample, capping, and poymerization.
5. Large (75 mesh) copper grids from TAAB Laboratory Equipments Ltd., UK. Grids are cleaned with acetone, then heated at 37°C and protected from dust (*see* **Note 4**).
6. Ultramicrotome (Reichert) equipped with diamond (Drukker, Cuijk, The Netherlands) rather than glass (Reichert ultracut) knives.

2.4.4. Sectioning of Samples Embedded in Epon: Toluidine Blue Staining to Identify Tissue in Section

1. 0.2 *M* Tris-HCl buffer, pH 8.5 (stock solution): 25 mL 0.2 *M* Tris-HCl, 15 mL 0.2 *M* HCl and 60 mL H_2O.
2. Toluidine blue staining solution: 1% (w/v) in 0.2 *M* Tris-HCl buffer, pH 8.5.

2.4.5. Contrast Enhancement

1. Saturated aqueous uranyl acetate (Merck, Darmstadt, Germany). Uranyl acetate is a radioactive product and must be handled following all security and safety guidelines for radiation protection.
2. 0.2-μm pore filters.
3. Parafilm® (Pechiney P.P., Chicago, IL).
4. 1 *M* lead citrate (2 mL 1 *M* lead nitrate + 3 mL 1 *M* sodium citrate + 4 mL 1 *M* NaOH + 16 mL distilled H_2O) *(24)*.
5. 1 *M* NaOH.

2.5. Immuno-EM

2.5.1. Fixation

1. Glutaraldehyde: 1% to 1.5% in phosphate buffer 0.1 *M*, pH 7.2 (*see* **Note 5**).
2. HEPES or PBS.

2.5.2. Glycol Methacrylate (GMA) Embedding (25)

1. 2-Hydroxyethyl-methacrylate 80% in distilled water (freshly prepared).
2. 2-Hydroxyethyl-methacrylate 97% in distilled water (freshly prepared).
3. Embedding medium: a mixture of 2-hydroxyethyl-methacrylate 97% (7 volumes), *n*-butyl-methacrylate (3 volumes) and benzoyl peroxide (1% or 2%). It can be stored for 1 wk at 4°C.
4. Pre-polymerized solution: to prepare, gently heat embedding medium over a Bunsen burner until the solution becomes yellowish and viscous, then rapidly cool the solution on ice. Can be stored for about 6 mo at –20°C.
5. UV light source: Type A lamp 405 L Allen Serlabo and 2 lamps Philips, 9 in, 6-volt fluorescent tubes, color 05, from TL6 W/05.
6. Ultramicrotome with diamond (Drukker, Cuijk, The Netherlands) or glass knives (Reichert).
7. Large (75) mesh nickel grids, formvar coated (TAAB Laboratory Equipments Ltd). Nickel grids are used because of long incubation times in solution in order to prevent grid oxidation.

2.5.3. Cryomethod (26,27)

1. Gelatin 10%: add 10 g gelatin powder (Merck 4078) to 100 mL 0.1 *M* phosphate buffer plus 200 µL azide and place, covered with a Petri dish, in an oven at 60°C for 4 h (or until dissolved) or in a water bath if you need it quickly. Stir to produce a homogenous solution before pouring into small tubes and storing in the refrigerator for as long as 1 yr.
2. Gelatin 2% may be obtained in the same way as 10% gelatin using only 2 g gelatin powder instead of 10 g and leaving for a shorter time in the oven (15 min can be long enough). The solution is mixed well, then poured into small Petri dishes.
3. Formvar-carbon coated grids: 75 mesh for megakaryocytes. These coated grids provide a thin support for sections on the mesh grid. Pre-prepared Formvar-coated grids can be prepared in-house or purchased from TAAB Laboratories Equipment Ltd, UK or EM Sciences. *In-house preparation:* Rinse a 250-mL conical flask with glass stopper with acetone followed by chloroform and then leave it to dry in an oven. In this flask add 1.2 g Formvar powder (Formvar 15/95E Sigma F-6146) to 100 mL chloroform (Merck 2447) and stir until dissolved. This solution can be stored for 1 yr in a dark place at room temperature. For preparation of the Formvar film, clean a microscope slide thoroughly. Place the Formvar solution in a glass dish (pre-rinsed with acetone and chloroform), dip the slide, and remove slowly over a period of 12–15 s. This will leave a thin film of Formvar on the slide. Dry for 5 min, then cut the film by scoring around the edges with a razor blade. Gently introduce the slide at a shallow angle into a trough filled with distilled water. This allows the film to be released from the slide and to float on the water surface. The thickness of the film can be judged by its color, which should be gray. Place the grids, previously cleaned with acetone and dried in an oven at 37°C, on the film. Remove the grids from the water by covering them with a sheet of unused newsprint-type paper (an absorbent medium, but not excessively so), then lift off the water surface and invert to dry, or use parafilm. The sheet of paper covered with grids must be dried carefully before it can be supplemented with a carbon layer by carbon vaporation.

4. PVP-sucrose: For 20 mL 15% PVP (polyvinylpyrolidone), add 3 g PVP (MW 10,000) to 0.6 mL 1.1 M Na_2CO_3 and 17 mL 2 M sucrose in phosphate buffer. Stir until all the PVP is dissolved, then let stand until the bubbles have disapeared. Do not leave the PVP-sucrose vials with specimens open for very long, as the mixture tends to thicken rapidly to more than 15% PVP.

5. Knives: Cryosectioning can be performed with either a diamond or a glass knife.

6. Wooden stick with mounted eyelash on top for section guiding.

7. Stainless-steel loop 2–2.5-mm diameter, for section retrieval.

2.5.4. Immunogold Labeling (GMA-Embedded Samples)

1. Parafilm®.
2. 10% H_2O_2 in distilled water.
3. Tris-HCl buffer saline (TBS), pH 8.2.
4. Bovine serum albumin (BSA).
5. Normal goat serum.
6. TBS, 0.1% BSA.
7. TBS, 0.1% BSA, 4% goat serum.
8. TBS, 1% BSA.
9. Unconjugated primary antibody against protein of interest.
10. Secondary antibody coupled to gold particles (5–20 nm diameter) (British Biocell, Cardiff, UK).
11. 1% glutaraldehyde in distilled water.

2.5.5. Immunolabeling of Cryosections

1. Parafilm®.
2. PBS, pH 7.2.
3. 0.1% BSA in PBS.
4. 1% BSA in PBS.
5. 0.15% glycine, 0.1% BSA, in PBS.
6. 0.15% glycine, 0.1% BSA, 10% normal goat serum, in PBS.
7. 1% glutaraldehyde in distilled water 3 min.
8. Methylcellulose-uranyl acetate: 4 drops of saturated uranyl acetate (Merck, Darmstadt, Germany) in 1 mL of 2% methyl cellulose 25 centipoises (Sigma) in 0.1 M phosphate buffer, pH 7.2.
9. Stainless-steel loop, 2–2.5 mm for section retrieval.
10. Blotting paper.
11. Immuno-EM controls: Control antigenic peptide and/or nonimmune normal serum from the same animal origin as the secondary antibody *(28)*.

2.5.6. Silver Intensification of Immunogold Labeling *(29)*

1. Citrate buffer: a mix of 2.3 M citric acid (10 parts) and 1.6 M sodium citrate dihydrate (4 parts), adjusted to pH 3.6 with HCl.
2. Gum arabic 50% (w/v) (*see* **Note 6**).
3. Hydroquinone 56% (w/v).
4. Intensification mixture: a mix of citrate buffer (0.5 mL), gum arabic (3 mL), and hydroquinone (0.5 mL).

5. Complete intensification solution: dissolve 0.055 g silver lactate in 2.5 mL of distilled water and add 0.75 mL to the intensification mixture. Use immediately (*see* **Note 7**).
6. Rapid fix® from Kodak. Dilute 1:4 in distilled water.

2.6. Special EM Methods

2.6.1. Horseradish Peroxidase as an Extracellular Tracer

1. 0.5% horseradish peroxidase (Sigma, St. Louis, MO).
2. 1.5% glutaraldehyde.
3. Diaminobenzidine (DAB) solution (*see* **Note 8**): 20 mg 3-3′ diaminobenzidine tetra HCl in 10 mL of 0.05 *M* Tris-HCl buffer, pH 7.6.
4. Osmium tetroxide (OsO_4): 1% solution made by combining 1 part 2% (w/v) OsO_4 solution in distilled water and 1 part 0.2 *M* phosphate buffer (*see* **Note 1**).
5. Dehydration alcohols.
6. Epon embedding.

2.6.2. Lanthanum Nitrate as an Extracellular Tracer *(30)*

1. 1–4% PFA in phosphate buffer (PB).
2. 0.2 *M* phosphate buffer.
3. 0.2 *M* S-collidine-HCl, pH 7.2.
4. 0.2 *M* 4% lanthanum nitrate in S-collidine-HCl (adjusted to pH 7.8 with 0.1 *N* NaOH).
5. 2% (w/v) OsO_4 solution in distilled water.
6. Dehydration alcohols.

2.6.3. Platelet Peroxidase Activity *(31)*

1. Gey's buffer stock solution A: 7g NaCl, 0.37 g KCl, 0.225 g $Na_2HPO_4 \cdot 7H_2O$, 0.0237 g KH_2PO_4, 1 g glucose, 0.005 g phenol red in 100 mL distilled water. This can be stored at 4°C.
2. Gey's buffer stock solution B: 10 mL Gey's buffer stock solution A, 83 mL H_2O, 5 mL 0.1 *M* Tris hydroxymethylaminomethane and 2 mL 0.1 *M* $MgCl_2$.
3. Gey's buffer: 49 mL Gey's stock solution B, 1 mL EGTA, pH 6.9. Adjust to pH 7.2 and store at 4°C.
4. Diaminobenzidine (DAB) solution (*see* **Subheading 2.6.1.**). Before use add 100 µL of H_2O_2 1% (*see* **Note 9**).
5. 1.25% glutaraldehyde in Gey's buffer, pH 7.3.
6. 0.1 *M* phosphate buffer, pH 7.3.
7. Osmium tetroxide (OsO_4): 1% solution made by combining 1 part 2% (w/v) OsO_4 solution in distilled water and 1 part 0.2 *M* phosphate buffer (*see* **Note 1**).
8. Dehydration series of alcohols.

3. Methods

3.1. Cytological Examination of Marrow Smears

MKs can be distinguished from other bone marrow cells by morphological examination as a consequence of their relatively large size and polylobulated nuclei. Good-quality smears allow cytoplasmic examination, nucleocytoplasmic ratio and nuclear lobularity estimation.

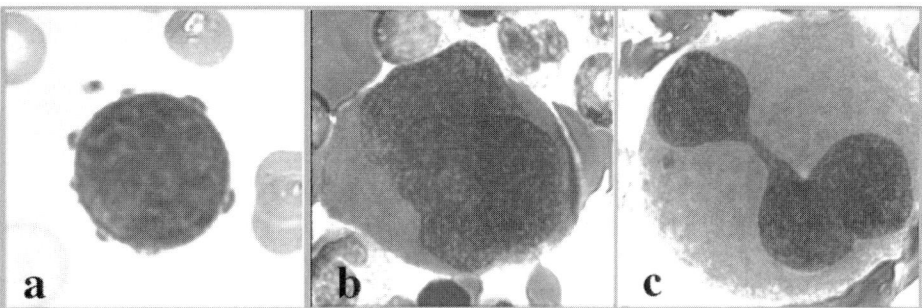

Fig. 1. Light microscopic appearance of MKs from a normal bone marrow smear, stained by the Romanovski technique. The 3 sequential maturation stages are represented: **(A)** Immature MK or megakaryoblast: the relatively large size of this otherwise poorly differentiated hemoblast (high nucleus:cytoplasm ratio, thin chromatin, basophilic cytoplasm) allows it to be assigned to the MK lineage. **(B)** MK of an intermediate maturation: large size, convoluted large polyploid nucleus, surrounded by a uniformly basophilic cytoplasm; some azurophilic granules appear toward the cell center. **(C)** Mature MK: Large cell with a polylobulated nucleus, and a large uniformly granular and azurophilic cytoplasm. See color insert following p. 44.

1. After bone marrow aspiration, gently spread the aspirate on a glass slide. Alternatively, squash small clumps of bone marrow on the glass slide with a cover slip. We prefer the spreading (smearing) technique, as the morphology looks better.
2. Cover the slides with filtered May-Grunwald solution for 4 min.
3. Remove May-Grunwald solution and cover the slides with diluted Giemsa solution for 10 min.
4. Rinse with distilled water.
5. Examine the slide under the microscope using ×10 to 100 magnification. MKs can be identified according to the following classification (*see* **Note 10**). Since MKs are large cells, their distribution on the bone marrow smear is not homogeneous; they are frequently concentrated at the edges of the smear.
   a. *Immature MKs:* larger cell size (>14 μm in diameter) and perimeter than other bone marrow diploid cells, a high nucleocytoplasmic ratio, a large nucleus with thin chromatin and sometimes apparent nucleolus, a basophilic cytoplasm, and frequent cytoplasmic blebs **(Fig. 1A)**.
   b. *Intermediate MKs:* 15–40 μm diameter, medium nucleocytoplasmic ratio, polylobulated nucleus with deep-blue cytoplasm due to the richness in RNA **(Fig. 1B)**.
   c. *Mature MKs:* large diameters (>40 μm) and perimeters, low nucleocytoplasmic ratio, and high lobularity, purple nucleus surrounded by a large uniformly granular and mauve cytoplasm **(Fig. 1C)**.

3.2. Immunohistochemical Studies of Marrow Samples Using Alkaline Phosphatase Anti-Alkaline Phosphatase (APAAP) (18)

Immunohistochemistry allows one to ascertain the MK lineage among bone marrow cells. The APAAP technique is a method of choice for bone marrow immunohisto-

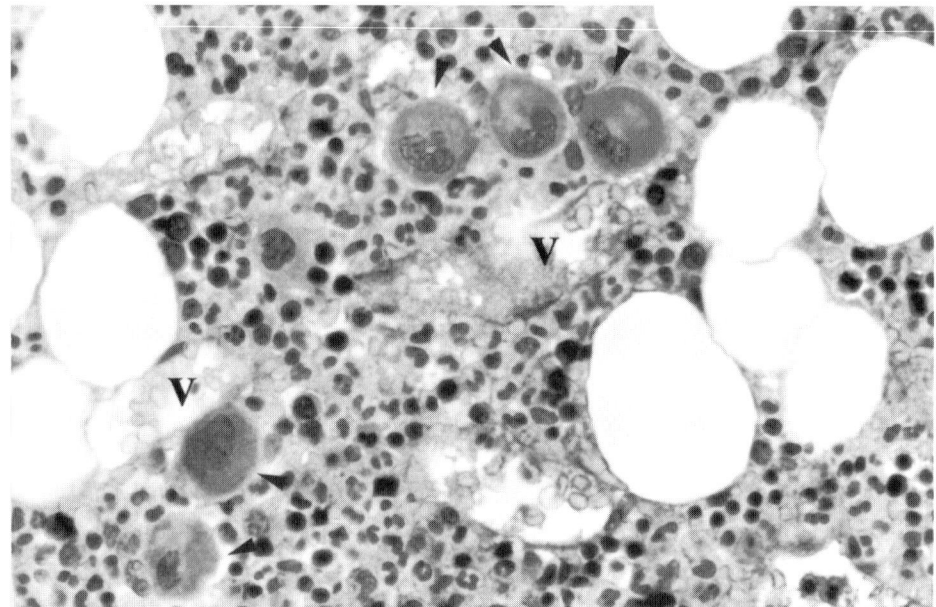

Fig. 2. Human normal bone marrow biopsy immunostained for fibrinogen by the APAAP technique. MKs are frequently grouped and located along a vascular sinusoid (v). Fibrinogen displays peripheral staining in mature MK (arrowheads). The staining intensity is weak in the small immature MK while it is maximal in the large mature MK. The cell periphery is intensely stained, and the juxta nuclear region appears to be weakly labeled. This staining pattern is typical of an alpha-granule protein endocytosed from the extracellular medium. See color insert following p. 44.

chemistry; it is preferable to immunoperoxidase because endogenous peroxidase is massively present in the granulocytic cells and is able to interfere with the reaction if not properly inhibited. APAAP can also be used with smears or cytospun preparations. The pattern of staining in the cytoplasm for secretory proteins appears different according to the origin of the proteins, peripheral for endocytosed proteins and central for endogenously synthesized proteins. It allows one to specifically identify MK cells on a bone marrow section among other hematopoietic cells **(Fig. 2)**.

1. Fix marrow-biopsy samples immediately in Bouin's fluid for 4–8 h. Smears from aspirated marrow should be fixed with 1% PFA in PBS, pH 7.2, or with methanol at 22°C for 5 min. Proceed to **step 8** for smears.
2. Immerse in decalcification medium, 50 mL of decalcification mix for 20 mg of sample.
3. Leave under constant gentle stirring .t room temperature for >30 min, but no more than 3 h in order to avoid alteration of ιne antigenic epitopes.
4. Wash several times with distilled water.
5. Embed in paraffin.
6. Cut 4-µm sections and leave for 24 h at 37°C.

7. Deparaffinize with xylene or chloroform and rehydrate the tissue using distilled water.
8. Perform immunohistochemistry with the alkaline phosphatase anti-alkaline phosphatase (APAAP) method revealed by fast red TR salt as described in **ref. 18**. All incubations are carried out at 22°C. Controls are replacement of primary antibodies by nonimmune serum, by an irrelevant antibody from the same species, or by omission of the primary antibody.

3.3. Immunofluorescence

Immunofluorescence (IF) allows the sensitive and specific staining of MKs using primary antibodies directed against either cytoplasmic antigens or membrane receptors.

1. Fix marrow smears or cytospun preparations of MKs by immersion in 2% PFA for 5 min.
2. Permeabilize with 0.1% triton for 3 min.
3. Draw a circle on the glass slide around the sample with an hydrophobic Dako pen, in order to minimize antibody usage in the following steps.
4. Incubate with primary antibody diluted in PBS, pH 7.2, in a humid chamber for 30 min at 22°C.
5. Wash in PBS and incubate in a dark container with secondary fluorophore-coupled antibody diluted in PBS pH 7.2.
6. Wash with PBS and mount the slide in a mounting medium (e.g., Vectashield with DAPI for nuclear staining) under a cover slip.
7. Seal the cover slip to the glass slide with nail polish to prevent the sample from drying.
8. Store at 4°C in the dark prior to examination on a fluorescence microscope (*see* **Note 11**). Due to the large size of the MK, it may be preferable to use a confocal microscope to improve contrast due to out-of-focus fluorescence.

3.4. Transmission Electron Microscopy (TEM)

TEM is able to yield magnifications up to 10^5 and a resolution of 0.2 nm. For examination, samples must be processed through successive steps of fixation, dehydration, hardening of the sample by inclusion in a resin (embedding), ultrathin sectioning, collection on copper grids, and eventually contrast enhancing with heavy-metal staining. A beam of electrons is passed through the ultrathin sample and focused onto a high-resolution photographic plate to create an image of the sample **(Figs. 3, 4)**.

3.4.1. Fixation (see **Note 12**)

3.4.1.1. MKs Cultured in Liquid Medium Suspension (*see* **Note 13**)

1. To 1 volume of medium with cells in flask, add 1 volume of 6% glutaraldehyde (*see* **Note 14**) fixative solution in 0.1 *M* phosphate buffer to reach a final 3% concentration of glutaraldehyde.
2. Leave for 60 min at room temperature.
3. Recover the cells by centrifugation, then wash three times in 0.1 *M* phosphate buffer. The minimal cell number for EM processing is 2×10^5 to 10^6 cells, roughly the amount obtained in a visible cell pellet.

3.4.1.2. Aspirated Marrow

Harvest one drop of concentrated marrow on culture medium (e.g., HBSS without calcium and magnesium) containing lithium heparinate (10 U/mL).

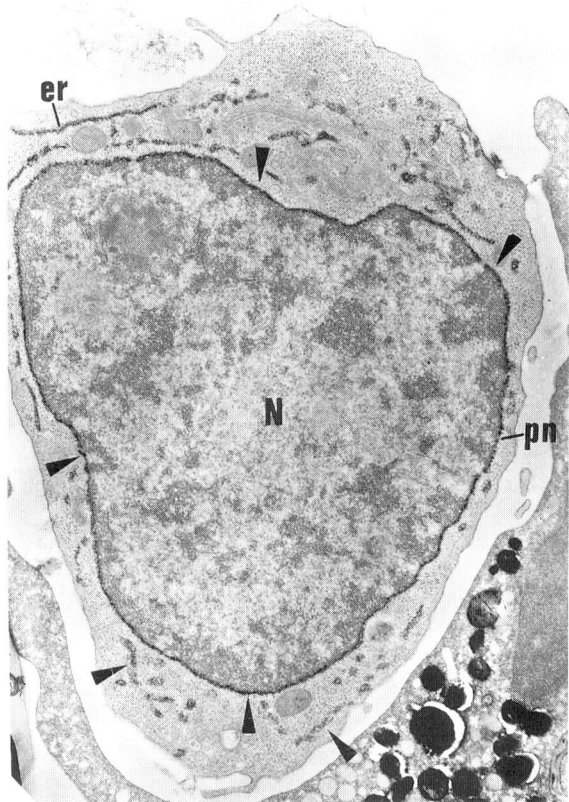

Fig. 3. Ultrastructural demonstration of platelet peroxidase in poorly differentiated MK precursors by a cytochemical reaction based on Graham and Karnovsky's technique. The diploid MK precursor, which lacks distinctive morphological features, can be identified based on its content of peroxidase activity revealed by a cytochemical reaction (arrowheads), which opacifies and thus darkens the structures in which it is contained: the perinuclear cisternae (pn) and endoplasmic reticulum (er). Golgi complex (Go) (apart from an occasional cisternae) and the rare secretion granules are consistently negative. N: nucleus. (Original magnification ×10,000).

3.4.1.3. MARROW FRAGMENTS

1. Pick out the fragments of marrow one after another and drop into fixative solution (usually 1.5–3% glutaraldehyde in phosphate buffer).
2. After 30 min fixation, wash the fragments three times, leaving in wash solution for 5 min each, and process as described for other samples.

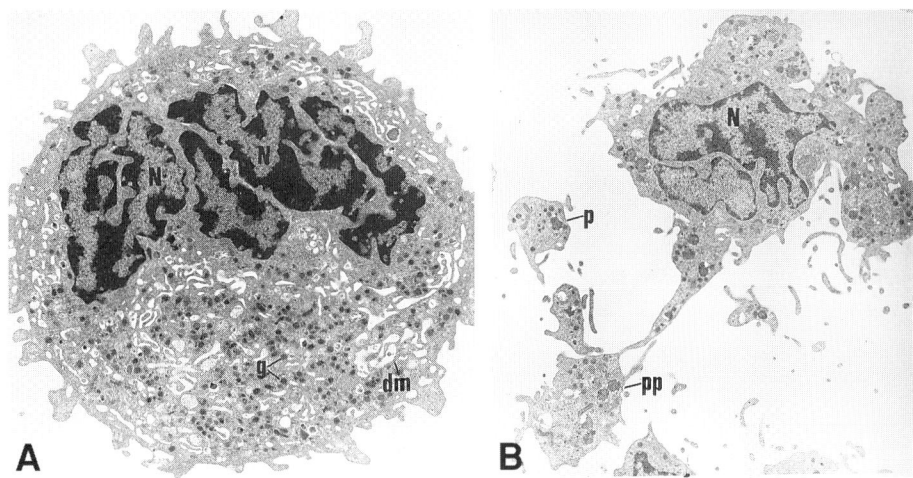

Fig. 4. Electron microscopic appearence of human MKs before and during platelet production. **(A)** Mature MK, characterized by its large size and multilobed nucleus. It contains specific organelles, i.e., numerous alpha-granules (g) and a well-developed demarcation membrane system (dm) regularly scattered throughout the cytoplasm. This system is formed by invagination of the plasma membrane, develops extremely rapidly, and is the precursor of the platelet membrane system (plasma membrane and surface-connected canalicular system). N: nucleus. (Original magnification × 5940). **(B)** After reaching full maturation, MKs display alignment and dilation of some peripheral demarcation membranes, creating an outer ring of cytoplasm. The peripheral layer of cytoplasm extends away from the core of the mother cell, forming a proplatelet (pp). Newly formed platelets (p) have detached from its tip. N: nucleus. (Original magnification ×5000).

3.4.1.4. POST-FIXATION

Post-fixation improves visualization of ultrastructure and is necessary only prior to Epon embedding.

1. Post-fix with 1% osmium tetroxide (OsO_4) for 30 min at 4°C (prepare 2% $OsSO_4$ [Euromedex, Souffelweyersheim, France] in distilled water and mix v/v with 0.1 M phosphate buffer, pH 7.2).
2. Wash three times in phosphate buffer.

3.4.2. Sample Dehydration

Dehydration is necessary only prior to embedding in non hydrophilic resin (Epon). At 22°C, immerse the sample in increasing concentrations of ethanol: 70% and 90% for 15 min each, then two times in pure absolute ethanol for 15 min. This can be modified depending on the thickness of the sample (reduce dehydration times for a cell suspension, and increase for bone-marrow tissue).

3.4.3. Embedding in Epon and Sectioning

Epon is a fluid mix at room temperature; like other epoxy resins, it polymerizes and hardens when exposed to heat. Two steps are required: first, sample impregnation in Epon/propylene oxide then pure Epon, and second, heat polymerization of resin. Epon is a hydrophobic resin, soluble in ethanol, acetone, and epoxy 1–2 propane. Its volume is unchanged after polymerization, it has good sectioning quality, and is stable even when exposed to a high-voltage electron beam. Epon embedding produces little distortion and is especially recommended for ultrastructural observations.

1. After alcohol dehydration, immerse the sample in propylene oxide (epoxy 1–2 propane) for 1 min.
2. Immerse the sample in a mixture of 1 volume epoxy 1–2 propane and 1 volume of Epon embedding solution for 15 min.
3. Transfer the sample to a gelatin capsule containing Epon embedding solution. Leave in contact for 10 min.
4. Polymerize the embedding solution by heating in a 60°C oven for 12–24 h (*see* **Note 15**).
5. Section on an ultramicrotome onto a water surface using a diamond knife and collect on copper grids. Sectioning speed can be low (1 mm/s).
6. Dry sections and store in a dust-free environment.

3.4.3.1. STAINING OF SEMI-THIN SECTIONS EMBEDDED IN EPON WITH TOLUIDINE BLUE

During the sectioning procedure above, it is useful to initially cut and examine semi-thin sections stained with toluidine blue. Once it is clear that you are cutting at the correct level of the tissue, ultrathin sectioning can commence.

1. Attach samples on glass slides using heat (100°C) on a hot plate for 1 min.
2. Cover with toluidine blue staining solution for 3 min.
3. Wash with distilled water.
4. Examine the staining to check that the sample has been reached within the Epon block and that the cells are located centrally and at an adequate frequency, before progressing onto thin sections.

3.4.4. Contrast Enhancement With Uranyl Acetate:Lead (16)

1. Prepare fresh saturated aqueous uranyl acetate solution and filter through 0.22-μm pores.
2. Incubate the grid for 10 min at room temperature on a drop of uranyl acetate solution on a sheet of Parafilm.
3. Wash with distilled water three times for 5 min.
4. To 16 mL H_2O add 3 mL 1 *M* lead nitrate solution, 3 mL 1 *M* lead citrate, and 4 mL 1 *M* NaOH. Store this lead solution away from air contact and light exposure.
5. Filter the above solution through 0.2-μm pore filters before use.
6. Immerse the grid in a drop of lead solution on a Parafilm sheet for 4–5 s; then jet-wash with distilled water.

3.5. Immuno-EM Examination

Samples for immuno-EM can be fixed and then embedded in GMA as described in **Subheading 3.5.1.–3.5.3,** *(24,25)* (*see* **Note 16**). Alternatively, they can be fixed, supported in a gelatin-based medium, infiltrated with sucrose antifreeze, and frozen (*see* **Subheading 3.5.3.**).

3.5.1. Fixation

1. Fix with 1% to 1.5% glutaraldehyde in 0.1 *M* phosphate buffer, pH 7.2, for 60 min at room temperature (*see* **Note 17**).
2. Wash three times in buffer (HEPES or PBS).

3.5.2. GMA Method

We refer here to the method of Leduc and Bernhard *(25)*. Work under a fume hood.

1. Immerse the sample sequentially in the following solutions, each for 20 min:
    a. 80% 2-hydroxyethyl-methacrylate.
    b. 97% 2-hydroxyethyl-methacrylate.
    c. A 1:1 mixture of 2-hydroxyethyl-methacrylate and embedding medium.
2. Immerse the sample in the pre-polymer solution overnight at 4°C.
3. Place the sample at the bottom of a gelatin capsule, fill with pre-polymerized GMA solution, and expose to UV light at 4°C for at least 24 h to cause polymerization.
4. *Sectioning:* GMA sectioning requires precautions, especially because of its hydrophilic nature. Clean and well-trimmed blocks are necessary, with a perfectly shaped pyramid. Semi-thin sections can be either stained with toluidine blue or observed directly on the glass slide, under phase-contrast microscopy. Speed for ultrathin sectioning must be high (2.6 mm/s) and the section thickness 90–100 nm (white-grey). Sectioning is performed on an ultramicrotome with diamond or glass knives.

3.5.3. Cryomethod *(22,25,26)*

The main concern in freezing samples is to prevent the formation of ice crystals within the cell, which is achieved by the use of sucrose as a cryoprotectant. Cells in suspension, or even solid tissue, require support during the freezing procedure. The most commonly used embedding medium is 10% gelatin in buffer. Due to its molecular size, gelatin does not enter the cells.

3.5.3.1. PROCESSING OF CELLS IN SUSPENSION

1. Pellet the fixed cells in an Eppendorf centrifuge at 200*g*.
2. Remove the supernatant and resuspend the pellet in 1 mL 10% gelatin.
3. After 10 min at 37°C, pellet the cells and remove the excess gelatin.
4. Resuspend the pellet in the remaining gelatin, then solidify it by placing the suspension between two glass slides covered with parafilm and separated with spacers, on ice.
5. After solidification cut the gelatin containing the cells into small blocks. Transfer the blocks to small vials containing PVP-sucrose and store at 4°C for at least 24 h before freezing.

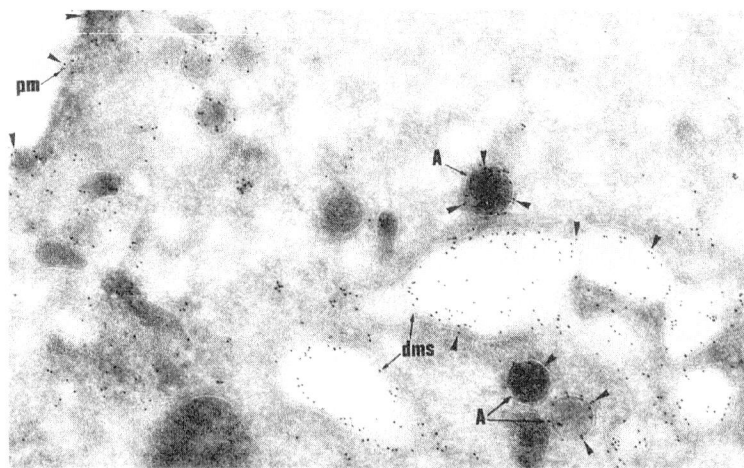

Fig. 5. Immunoelectron microscopic visualization of the GPIIb-IIIa repartition in MKs with immunogold. In MKs, GPIIb-IIIa receptors (immunolabeled with gold particles, which appear as black dots [arrowheads]), are expressed on the plasma membrane (pm), and evenly distributed along the luminal surface of the demarcation membrane system (dms) and at the inner surface of alpha-granule (A) membranes (Original magnification ×46,000).

3.5.3.2. Processing of Tissue

Cut small blocks (<1 mm^3) of tissue fixed as described in **Subheading 3.5.1.** and transfer them to vials containing PVP-sucrose and store at 4°C for at least 24 h before freezing.

3.5.3.3. Freezing in Liquid Nitrogen

Under a binocular microscope place a sample block on top of the specimen holder then plunge specimen and holder in the liquid nitrogen.

3.5.3.4. Cryosectioning and Recovery of Cryosections

The shape of the block is important and in contrast to plastics, which are usually pyramidal, should ideally be rectangular.

1. Flatten the front of the specimen by sectioning at a relatively high temperature (knife, specimen, and chamber at –95 to –110°C). The first sections will have a "snowy" appearance and consist mostly of plain sucrose. When shiny colored sections appear, the actual tissue is being sectioned. Do not allow any snowy spot in the semi-thin section.
2. After cutting, guide the sections using an eyelash mounted on a wooden stick so they can be retrieved with the stainless-steel loop dipped in the PVP-sucrose. The sections will stick to the almost-frozen droplet. Melt the droplet by pushing it, with the sections facing downward, onto a microscope slide at room temperature. The sections will remain on the slide and can be stained with 1% toluidine blue in water to monitor the specimen. The sections can be apposed on the carbon-Formvar-coated grids by the same procedure.

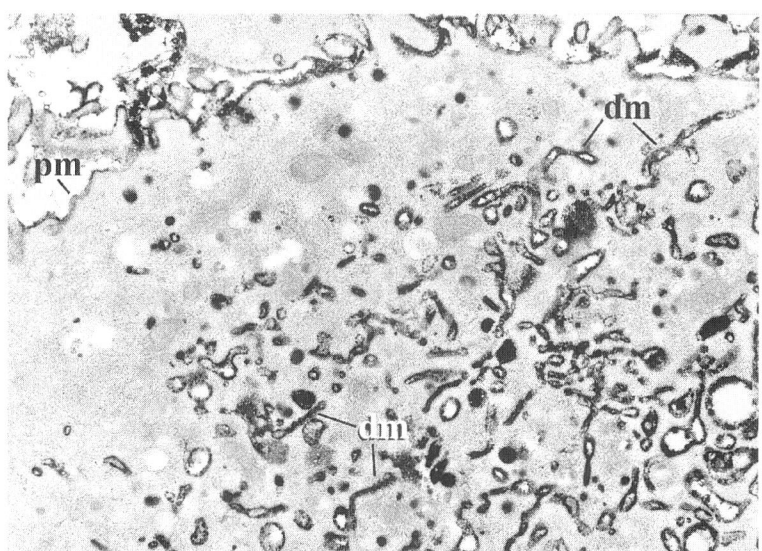

Fig. 6. Staining of the demarcation membrane system by an electron dense tracer. When a mature MK incubated with horseradish peroxidase in the extracellular culture medium, the tracer penetrates the numerous cisternae of the demarcation membrane system (dm), demonstrating that it is connected with the surface. pm = plasma membrane (Original magnification ×20,000).

3. The grids are put in a small Petri dish containing 2% gelatin, sections facing downward, at 4°C for a maximum 24 h before labeling.

3.5.4. Sample Immunolabeling

Most immuno-EM techniques label antigens with specific antibodies coupled to gold particles (direct labeling). Specific primary antibodies (e.g., raised in rabbits) can be labeled by a secondary one (e.g., anti-rabbit) coupled to electron-dense gold particles (indirect labeling). Amplification of the diameter of gold particles (silver enhancing) can be performed, but false-positive labeling can be very hard to differentiate from true labeling. Other detector molecules allow a certain amount of labeling amplification, e.g., horseradish peroxidase/DAB. Prior to immuno-EM, antibodies must be tested to ascertain optimal dilution and preservation of antigenicity during fixation.

3.5.4.1. PROCESSING FOR IMMUNOLABELING ON GMA

1. The grids are processed by placing on top of drops of the following solutions on a parafilm sheet. Protect from dust deposition throughout the procedure.
2. Incubate on 10% H_2O_2 for 10 min (the grids should not sink in but should stay on the surface).
3. Drop wash on distilled water 1 min, three times.
4. Incubate on first antibody in TBS, 0.1% BSA, 4% normal goat serum for 2 h at 22°C.

5. Wash twice on TBS, 0.1% BSA; 15 min then 5 min.
6. Incubate on secondary antibody coupled to gold particles diluted in TBS, containing 1% BSA, for 1 h at 22°C.
7. Drop-wash twice with TBS, 0.1% BSA; 5 min each.
8. Incubate on 1% glutaraldehyde in distilled water for 3 min.
9. Drop-wash in distilled water 1 min, 3 times.
10. Contrast enhance with uranyl acetate (10 min) and lead citrate (5 s) (see **Subheading 3.4.4.**).

3.5.4.2. IMMUNOLABELING OF CRYOSECTIONS (FIG. 5)

1. Put the Petri dishes containing the grids for 10 min in the oven at 37°C. The grids will centralize. Process grids on drops of solutions on a parafilm surface as described in the following steps, protecting from dust deposition.
2. PBS, pH 7.2, 0.15% glycine three times for 5 min.
3. PBS, 0.15% glycine, 0.1% BSA, 5 min.
4. PBS, 0.15% glycine, 0.1% BSA, 10% normal goat serum, 15 min
5. Incubate on the first antibody in PBS, 0.1% BSA, 4% normal goat serum for 30 min up to 2 h at 22°C (incubation time should be adjusted for each antibody).
6. Wash 3 times on PBS, 0.1% BSA, each for 5 min.
7. Incubate on secondary antibody coupled to gold particles diluted in PBS, containing 1% BSA, for 30 min to 1 h at 22°C.
8. Drop-wash twice with PBS, 5 min each.
9. Incubate on 1% glutaraldehyde in distilled water for 3 min.
10. Drop-wash with distilled water three times, each for 1 min.
11. Incubate on methylcellulose-uranyl acetate for a few seconds. Then stain for 10 min with methylcellulose-uranyl acetate on ice.
12. Recover the grids with the stainless-steel loop.
13. Remove the excess methylcellulose by touching the grid edge to filter paper and allow to dry for at least 20 min before EM examination.

3.5.5. Immuno-EM Controls

To demonstrate the specificity of the labeling, several controls can be processed. Absorption of the antiserum with an excess of antigen preliminary to incubation on the sample is the ideal control *(28)*. Other controls include omission of the primary antibody and first incubation in nonimmune normal serum from the same animal origin as the secondary antibody, or replacement of the primary antibody by nonimmune serum.

3.5.6. Silver Intensification of Immunogold Labeling *(29)*

Silver intensification increases the diameter of gold particles 2 to 10 times. Strict controls are required with the second antibody alone and another reaction without any antibody because the process of silver enhancing generates multiple artifacts.

1. Place grids with sections to be processed on drops of freshly made complete intensification solution on a Parafilm sheet. The procedure should be carried out in a light-tight box, protecting from dust deposition throughout.
2. Allow the reaction to proceed for 5 to 30 min. Silver intensification is proportional to the time spent in the developing solution.

3. At the end of incubation, transfer grids to developer drops (Rapid fix® from Kodak), diluted 1:4 with distilled water. The Rapid fix stops the silver intensification reaction.
4. Wash on drops of distilled water, initially several quick washes and then a wash of 15 min or more, to remove the gum arabic.
5. Counterstain with uranyl acetate and lead citrate as described in **Subheading 3.4.4.**

3.6. Special Methods in EM

3.6.1. Use of Electron-Dense Tracer

The demarcation membrane system (DMS) is a major element of the MK cytoplasmic maturation process. It forms a network of smooth membrane channels and is derived from multiple invaginations of the MK plasma membrane. In some models of thrombopoiesis, the DMS is believed to delimit future platelet territories. Since the membranes of the DMS are connected with the extracellular medium at all stages of development, electron-dense tracers can freely diffuse into the channels formed by the DMS. Therefore these tracers allow one to monitor the expansion of the DMS through the cytoplasm and to estimate the degree of MK cytoplasmic maturity.

3.6.1.1. HORSERADISH PEROXIDASE

Live cells are incubated with horseradish peroxidase, an enzyme that permeates the DMS without crossing the cell membrane and can be revealed with diaminobenzidine (DAB).

1. Incubate live cells in cell-culture medium with 0.5% horseradish peroxidase for 10 to 30 min at 37°C.
2. Fix in 1.5% glutaraldehyde then wash three times in 0.1 M phosphate buffer, pH 7.2.
3. Incubate in DAB solution at room temperature and in the dark for 30 min.
4. Wash three times in phosphate buffer.
5. Post-fix with 1% OsO_4, dehydrate in an alcohol series and embed in Epon (*see* **Subheadings 3.4.1.4.** and **3.4.3.**).

3.6.1.2. LANTHANUM NITRATE *(30)*

1. Fix the cells in 1–4% PFA in phosphate buffer (PB).
2. Wash five times for 20 min each in 0.2 M phosphate buffer.
3. Wash two times for 10 min each in 0.2 M S-collidine-HCl, pH 7.2.
4. Post-fix two h at RT in a 1:1 (v/v) mix of 4% lanthane-nitrate in 0.2 M S-collidine-HCl (adjusted to pH 7.8 with 0.1 N NaOH) and 2% OsO_4.
5. Rapidly dehydrate using an alcohol series (70, 90, and 100%, 3 min maximum in each) prior to Epon embedding.
6. Contrast-enhance by incubation in with lead citrate for 10 to 30 s.

3.6.2. Ultrastructural Detection of Platelet Peroxidase Activity

EM studies after cytochemical reaction processing for myeloperoxidase (MPO) and subsequent embedding in Epon are used to detect peroxidase activity of cyclooxygenase (COX). COX is part of the enzymatic set that will allow future platelets to produce prostaglandin metabolites. This activity can be used to identify the MK hematopoietic lineage as a result of its specificity, its particular localization in the perinuclear cisternae and in the lumen of the endoplasmic reticulum but not in the Golgi complexes and the granules **(Fig. 3)**. Platelet peroxidase activity is detectable in certain leukemic cells with MK differentiation, in the early progenitors of the MK lineage and remains at all more mature stages *(31,32)*.

1. MKs are fixed in 1.25% glutaraldehyde in Gey's buffer, pH 7.3, for 60 min at room temperature and washed three times in Gey's buffer. Store at 4°C.
2. Incubate the cell pellet for 30 min in DAB solution at room temperature and in the dark.
3. Wash twice in 0.1 M phosphate buffer.
4. Post-fix in OsO_4 as described in **Subheading 3.4.1.4.** before Epon embedding (*see* **Subheading 3.4.3.**).

4. Notes

1. OsO_4 vapor is extremely toxic and post-fixation must be performed under a chemical fume hood. OsO_4 is an oxidative fixative with very slow penetrative ability. It reacts with proteins, nonsaturated lipids (cell membranes), triglycerides, and glycogen (if used in phosphate buffer). It is used as a fixative and as a staining agent that increases the contrast of subcelluar structures and especially of lipid membranes. Post-fixation with OsO_4 preserves the membranous structures by interacting with lipids. It is normally used for one hour, and the time of OsO_4 post-fixation must be strictly observed.
2. Use glass test tubes (plastic should not be used as it melts in contact with propylene oxide).
3. All products are highly toxic (cutaneous allergenic), and must be stored at 4°C. Avoid humidity contact when restored to room temperature before use.
4. Use good-quality sharp and clean forceps to pick up the grids carefully and safely. Store the grids vertically in plastic boxes. Large-mesh grids (75 mesh) are used for MK examination; tight-mesh grids (200 mesh) are used for examination of platelets.
5. Glutaraldehyde is toxic and must be handled with gloves, eye protection, and masks. Glutaraldehyde is stable at 4°C for several months.
6. Gum arabic is very sticky and samples need to be abundantly washed after silver intensification reaction.
7. The complete intensification solution with silver lactate is light-sensitive and must be prepared immediately before use in a light-tight box.
8. DAB is highly carcinogenic; commercially available pre-prepared aliquots are the safest to work with.
9. The enzymatic activity of platelet peroxidase is labile and sensitive to fixation.
10. Some cytoplasmic fragments and naked nuclei may also be seen on bone marrow smears but they are usually artifactual, the cells being broken during spreading.
11. Several different fluorescence patterns can be observed: *Juxtanuclear* coincides with the Golgi complex; *diffuse intracytoplasmic* often reflects protein synthesis within the widely distributed endoplasmic reticulum; *granular staining* corresponds to alpha-granule storage and localization; and *peripheral reinforcement* indicates plasma-membrane-associated antigens.
12. The ideal, and so far unsurpassed, fixative for EM is glutaraldehyde. It can be mixed in various proportions with PFA, depending on the requirements. Enzyme activity and immuno-reactivity are reduced less by PFA than by glutaraldehyde; thus the concentration of the latter should be kept to a minimum. In our hands, we have experienced no differences as far as sensitivity of immunolabeling is concerned and glutaraldehyde consistently yielded

the best ultrastructural result. Optimal ultrastructure is obtained with a 3% glutaraldehyde concentration and optimal post-embedding immunolabeling with 1% glutaraldehyde.

13. MKs in culture are large cells that are easily activated and should thus be manipulated with great care. This is achieved by performing fixation in the flask directly in the culture medium.

14. Glutaraldehyde is an aldhehyde that reacts with the lysine residues of proteins and creates inter- and intra-chemical bridges that stabilize the quaternary structure. This fixation also modifies the antigenicity of the protein and is not reversible. Glutaraldehyde fixation is relatively slow and its penetration rate is limited (1 mm/h); thus the thickness of the sample should not exceed 1 mm and the duration of exposure should not exceed more than 1 h. Glutaraldehyde preserves the morphology of cells very well and is used in the range of 0.5–3%. For cytochemistry and immuno-EM the usual concentration is 1–1.5%. 3% glutaraldehyde is better for ultrastructure studies since granules and mitochondria are better preserved.

15. Use capsules without sample to test the hardening of Epon.

16. Like other methacrylate resins, GMA is hydrosoluble. It has a low viscosity, which may cause changes of volume during polymerization, and is fragile under the electron beam. GMA, as other methacrylate-type resins, polymerizes and hardens when exposed to UV light. The main advantages of GMA are that it is hydrosoluble and still permeable after polymerization; it allows good preservation of protein-antigenic epitopes because of its hydrophilic nature, which prevents passage through organic solvents, and because of its ability to polymerize at low temperature. Glycolmethacrylate is a toxic, corrosive, and allergenic chemical compound that must be handled with care, especially during pre-polymer preparation. It must be handled under a chemical fume hood with mask and gloves.

17. This is our current fixative for immuno-EM studies. If it inactivates antigenicity, try 1–4% PFA + 0.1–0.5% glutaraldehyde in HEPES buffer, pH 7.2, or PBS at room temperature for 1–4 h. PFA possesses one aldehyde group that reacts with proteins in order to form methylene bridges. PFA diffuses rapidly and fixation is slow and reversible. PFA is generally considered as a relatively weak fixative that preserves enzyme activity and protein antigenicity; adequate preservation of cell morphology requires prolonged fixation of 8–72 h.

References

1. Kaushansky, K., Lok, S., Holly, R. D., Broudy, V. C., Lin, N., Bailey, M. C., et al. (1994) Promotion of megakaryocyte progenitor expansion and differentiation by the c-Mpl ligand thrombopoietin. *Nature* **369**, 568–571.

2. Choi, E. S., Nichol, J. L., Hokom, M. M., Hornkoh, A. C., and Hunt, P. (1995) Platelets generated in vitro from proplatelet-displaying human megakaryoyctes are functional. *Blood* **85**, 402–413.

3. Norol, F., Vitrat, N., Cramer, E., Guichard, J., Burstein, S. A., Vainchenker, W., et al. (1998) Effects of cytokines on platelet production from blood and marrow CD34+ cells. *Blood* **91**, 830–843.

4. Drouin, A., Favier, R., Massé, J. M., Debili, N., Schmitt, A., Elbim, C., et al. (2001) Newly recognized cellular abnormalities in the gray platelet syndrome. *Blood* **98**, 1382–1391.

5. Lichtman, M. A., Chamberlain, J. K., Simon, W., and Santillo, P. A. (1978) Parasinusoidal location of megakaryocytes in marrow: a determinant of platelet release. *Am. J. Hematol.* **4**, 303–312.

6. Behnke, O. (1968) An electron microscope study of megakaryocytes of rat bone marrow. I. The development of the demarcation membrane system and the platelet surface coat. *J. Ultrastructural Res.* **24**, 412–433.

 7. Breton-Gorius, J. and Vainchenker, W. (1986) Expression of platelet proteins during the in vitro and in vivo differentiation of megakaryocytes and morphological aspects of their maturation. *Semin. Hematol.* **23,** 43–67.

 8. Cramer, E. M., Debili, N., Martin, J. F., Gladwin, A. M., Breton-Gorius, J., Harrison, P., et al. (1989) Uncoordinated expression of fibrinogen compared with thrombospondin and von Willebrand factor in maturing human megakaryocytes. *Blood* **73,** 1123–1129.

 9. Cramer, E. M., Norol, F., Guichard, J., Breton-Gorius, J., Vainchenker, W., Massé, J. M., et al. (1997) Ultrastructure of platelet formation by human megakaryocytes cultured with the Mpl ligand. *Blood* **89,** 2336–2346.

10. Schmitt, A., Guichard, J., Masse, J. M., Debili, N., and Cramer, E. M. (2001) Of mice and men: comparison of the ultrastructure of megakaryocytes and platelets. *Exp. Hematol.* **29,** 1295–1302.

11. Cramer, E. M., Vainchenker, W., Vinci, G., Guichard, J., and Breton-Gorius, J. (1985) Gray platelet syndrome: immunoelectron microscopic localization of fibrinogen and von Willebrand factor in platelets and megakaryocytes. *Blood* **66,** 1309–1316.

12. Cramer, E. M., Meyer, D., le Menn, R., and Breton-Gorius, J. (1985) Eccentric localization of von Willebrand factor in an internal structure of platelet alpha-granule resembling that of Weibel-Palade bodies. *Blood* **66,** 710–713.

13. Bendayan, M. and Zollinger, M. (1983) Ultrastructural localization of antigenic sites on osmium-fixed tissues applying the protein A-gold technique. *J. Histochem. Cytochem.* **31,** 101–109.

14. Tapia, F. J., Varndell, I. M., Probert, L., De Mey, J., and Polak, J. M. (1983) Double immunogold staining method for the simultaneous ultrastructural localization of regulatory peptides. *J. Histochem. Cytochem.* **31,** 977–981.

15. Berger, G., Massé, J. M., and Cramer, E. M. (1996) Alpha-granule membrane mirrors the platelet plasma membrane and contains the glycoproteins Ib, IX, and V. *Blood* **87,** 1385–1395.

16. Cramer, E., Pryzwansky, K. B., Villeval, J. L., Testa, U., and Breton-Gorius, J. (1985) Ultrastructural localization of lactoferrin and myeloperoxidase in human neutrophils by immunogold methods. *Blood* **65,** 423–432.

17. Nafe, R., Georgii, A., Kaloutsi, V., Fritsch, R. S., and Choritz, H. (1991) Planimetric analysis of megakaryocytes in the four main groups of chronic myeloproliferative disorders. *Virchows Arch. B. Cell. Pathol. Incl. Mol. Pathol.* **61,** 111–116.

18. Cordell, J. L., Fallimi, B., Erber, W. N., Ghosh, A., Abdulaziz, Z., McDonald, S., et al. (1984) Immunoenzymatic labeling of monoclonal antibodies using immune complexes of alkaline phosphatase and monoclonal anti-alkaline phosphatase (APAAP complexes). *J. Histochem. Cytochem.* **32,** 219–229.

19. de Larouzière, V., Brouland, J. P., Souni, F., Drouet, L., and Cramer, E. (1998) Inverse immunostaining pattern for synthesized versus endocytosed alpha-granule proteins in human bone marrow megakaryocytes. *Brit. J. Haematol.* **101,** 618–625.

20. Dietrich, H. F. and Fontaine, A. R. (1975) A decalification method for ultrastructure of echinoderm tissues. *Staining Technology* **50,** 351–354.

21. Vinci, G., Tabilio, A., Deschamps, J. F., Van Haecke, D., Henri, A., Guichard, J., et al. (1984) Immunological study of in vitro maturation of human megakaryocytes. *Brit. J. Haematol.* **56,** 589–605.

22. Drouin, A., Schmitt, A., Massé, J. M., Cieutat, A. M., Fichelson, S., and Cramer, E. M. (2001) Identification of PML oncogenic domains (PODs) in human megakaryocytes. *Exp. Cell Res.* **271,** 277–285.

23. Luft, J. H. (1961) Improvement in epoxy resin embedding methods. *J. Biophys. Biochem. Cytol.* **9,** 409–411.

24. Reynolds, E. S. (1963) The use of lead citrate at high pH as an electron opaque stain in electron microscopy. *J. Cell Biol.* **17,** 208–212

25. Leduc, E. H. and Bernhard, W. (1967) Recent modification of the glycol methacrylate embedding procedure. *J. Ultrastructural Res.* **10,** 196–199.

26. Sander, H. J., Slot, J. W., Bouma, B. N., Bolhuis, P. A., Pepper, D. S., and Sixma, J. J. (1983) Immunocytochemical localization of fibrinogen, platelet factor 4, and b-thromboglobulin in thin frozen section of human blood platelets. *J. Clin. Invest.* **72,** 1277–1287.

27. Roth, J., Bendayan, M., and Orci, L. (1978) Ultrastructural localization of intracellular antigens by the use of protein A gold complex. *J. Histochem. Cytochem.* **26,** 1074–1081.

28. Meyer, D., Zimmerman, T. S., Obert, B., and Edgington, T. S. (1984) Hybridoma antibodies to human von Willebrand factor. I. Characterization of seven clones. *Br. J. Haematol.* **57,** 597–608.

29. Lah, J. J., Hayes, D. M., and Burry, R. W. (1990) A neutral pH silver development method for the visualization of 1-nanometer gold particles in pre-embedding electron microscopic immunocytochemistry. *J. Histochem. Cytochem.* **38,** 503–508.

30. Revel, J. P. and Karnovsky, M. J. (1967) Hexagonal array of subunits in intercellular junctions of the mouse heart and liver. *J. Cell Biol.* **33,** C12.

31. Breton-Gorius, J. and Guichard, J. (1972) Ultrastructural localization of peroxidase activity in human platelets and megakaryocytes. *Am. J. Pathol.* **66,** 277–293.

32. Bentfeld-Barker, M. E. and Bainton, D. F. (1982) Identification of primary lysosomes in human megakaryocytes and platelets. *Blood* **59,** 472–481.

33. Graham, R. C., Jr. and Karnovsky, M. J. (1965) The histochemical demonstration of monoamineoxidase activity by coupled peroxidatic oxidation. *Histochem. Cytochem.* **13,** 604–605.

26

Thrombopoietin Bioassay

Warren S. Alexander and Craig Hyland

1. Introduction

The production of megakaryocytes (MKs) and platelets is a finely controlled process that maintains circulating platelet numbers within a narrow range in normal individuals while providing sufficient reserve capacity for rapid production in emergencies such as bleeding. Forty years ago, it was recognized that a humoral regulator circulating in thrombocytopenic animals was able to stimulate platelet production in normal recipients *(1)*. Termed *thrombopoietin* (TPO), the properties of this activity were defined over subsequent years but only in the early 1990s was the cDNA encoding TPO cloned *(2–5)*. The availability of recombinant TPO allowed precise analysis of the properties of this cytokine in vitro and in vivo. These analyses, coupled with studies in mice lacking the genes for TPO or its receptor, c-Mpl, conclusively demonstrated that TPO is the major physiological regulator of steady-state platelet production *(6,7)*. It is anticipated that the potent capacity of TPO to stimulate platelet production in vivo will allow improved clinical management of thrombocytopenia *(8)*. Accordingly, TPO and related c-Mpl ligands are currently being evaluated as clinical reagents for the stimulation of platelets in thrombocytopenic patients, particularly following cytotoxic cancer treatment.

The gene encoding TPO is located on chromosome 3q26-27 in humans and the proximal part of chromosome 16 in the mouse *(9,10)*. TPO is produced by hepatocytes in the liver, in the proximal tubules of the kidney, and within the bone marrow and spleen, primarily by stromal cells *(11,12)*. The mature, secreted protein contains 332 amino acids and appears to consist of two distinct domains (**Fig. 1**). The N-terminal domain is predicted to fold with 4-α-helical bundle tertiary structure, a topology typical of many hematopoietic cytokines. Engineered forms of TPO consisting solely of the N-terminal domain retain potency, consistent with this domain containing the receptor-binding moieties and biological activity *(13)*. The C-terminal domain shares no significant homology with known proteins, but contains several predicted *N*-linked glycosylation sites and is significantly glycosylated in vivo *(14,15)*. The function of this domain appears to be to assist appropriate protein folding and secretion, and may also

From: *Methods in Molecular Biology, vol. 272:*
Platelets and Megakaryocytes, Vol. 1: Functional Assays
Edited by: J. M. Gibbins and M. P. Mahaut-Smith © Humana Press Inc., Totowa, NJ

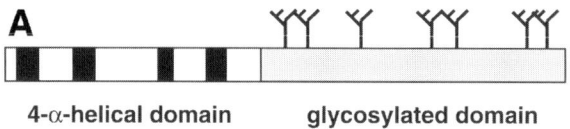

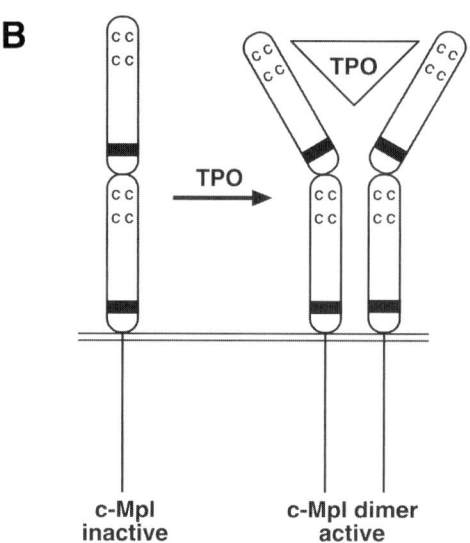

Fig. 1. Structure of TPO and its receptor, c-Mpl. (**A**) Dual domain structure of TPO. The N-terminal domain is predicted to assume a 4-α helical bundle conformation similar to many other hematopoietic cytokines. The C-terminal domain bears no homology to known proteins but contains several potential *N*-linked glycosylation sites. (**B**) The c-Mpl protein is the specific cell surface receptor for TPO. TPO induces homodimerisation of inactive receptor monomers leading to receptor activation and signal transduction. The receptor extracellular domains contain conserved cysteine pairs (C C) and the hallmark WSXWS pentapeptide motif (shaded) typical of the hematopoietin receptor family.

enhance the in vivo half-life of circulating TPO (*16,17*). The levels of circulating TPO are low in normal individuals but become significantly elevated if platelet levels fall. Transcription of the gene encoding TPO at the major sites of cytokine production appears not to significantly alter during thrombocytopenia (*18*). Rather, the weight of evidence supports a model in which the level of circulating TPO is controlled by receptor-mediated internalization and degradation by megakaryocytes and platelets (*19–21*).

A key discovery in the ultimate purification of TPO and the cloning of its cDNA was the realisation that the cellular homolog of v-Mpl, the viral oncoprotein encoded by the myeloproliferative leukemia virus, was the specific cell surface receptor for

TPO *(22)*. c-Mpl, the TPO receptor, is an integral transmembrane protein that contains the extracellular motifs typical of the hemopoietin family of cell-surface receptors (**Fig. 1**). The specific binding of TPO to c-Mpl at the surface of target cells leads to receptor aggregation and phosphorylation, recruitment and activation of signal transduction molecules, and ultimately the alterations in gene expression that drive the biological actions of TPO *(7)*.

The discovery of c-Mpl allowed the development of specific bioassays for TPO that provided the means for sensitive detection of the cytokine in complex biological mixtures and accelerated the purification and cloning of the TPO cDNA *(4,5)*. Typically these bioassays exploit growth-factor-dependent cell lines in which the c-Mpl receptor is exogenously expressed. The addition of TPO can be assayed by withdrawal of the cytokine that usually supports the cells followed by the measurement of proliferation induced by the specific interaction of TPO with c-Mpl. This chapter describes the methodology for assembling and using a typical TPO bioassay based on exogenous expression of the murine c-Mpl receptor in Ba/F3 cells, a murine pro-B cell line. Alternative assays for TPO, most commonly based on the use of specific anti-TPO antibodies in enzyme-linked immunosorbent assays (ELISA), have also been developed and have proven to be highly effective (*see* **Subheading 5.**).

2. Materials

1. Ba/F3 cells.
2. Ba/F3 cell growth medium: Dulbecco's modified Eagle's medium (DMEM) containing 3.4 g/L NaHCO$_3$, 0.1 g/L penicillin, 0.1 g/L streptomycin, 10% fetal calf serum (FCS), and either interleukin-3 (1.25×10^2 U/mL recombinant murine IL-3) or 10% WEHI3B cell-conditioned medium.
3. cDNA plasmid encoding FLAG®-tagged murine c-Mpl receptor and conferring G418-resistance (*see* **Subheading 3.1.** for further details).
4. Electroporation cuvets, 0.4-cm gap (Bio-Rad, Hercules, CA).
5. Electroporator (Gene Pulser, Bio-Rad).
6. 48-well tissue culture plate (Becton Dickinson Labware, Franklin Lakes, NJ).
7. G418 (Geneticin, Life Technologies, Rockville, MD).
8. Phosphate-buffered saline (PBS): 0.016 *M* Na$_2$HPO$_4$, 0.004 *M* NaH$_2$PO$_4$, 0.149 *M* NaCl, pH 7.3.
9. Propidium iodide (Sigma, St. Louis, MO).
10. Unconjugated M2 anti-FLAG® mouse monoclonal antibody (Sigma).
11. Goat anti-mouse Ig-FITC (BD Pharmingen, San Diego, CA).
12. Flow cytometer, e.g., FACStar Plus (Becton-Dickinson, San Jose, CA).
13. Bioassay medium (DMEM + 10% FCS).
14. 96-well microtiter plate, flat-bottomed (Becton Dickinson Labware, Franklin Lakes, NJ).
15. 60-well microwell tissue culture tray (Sarstedt Australia, Technology Park, SA).
16. Recombinant murine TPO.

3. Methods

The TPO bioassay described below is based on exogenous expression of c-Mpl, the TPO receptor, in factor-dependent Ba/F3 cells *(23)*. Although a number of factor-dependent cells have proven useful in generating TPO bioassays, the responsiveness of

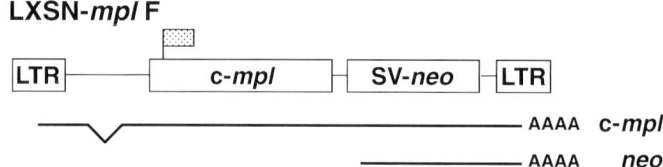

Fig. 2. c-Mpl expression plasmid. The cDNA encoding c-Mpl was engineered to include an eight-amino-acid FLAG epitope tag at the N-terminus of the mature receptor. This sequence was then incorporated into the LSXN retroviral vector. c-Mpl is expressed from a transcript initiated within the retroviral long-terminal repeat (LTR) and the selectable neo marker is expressed from an internal SV40 promoter *(29)*.

Ba/F3 cells to very few cytokines affords significant advantages (*see* **Subheading 5.**); these cells have also been exploited to establish bioassays for a number of other cytokines *(24)*. The methods outlined below describe (1) the plasmid for c-Mpl expression, (2) transfection of Ba/F3 cells for expression of exogenous c-Mpl, (3) screening Ba/F3 transfectants for c-Mpl expression by flow cytometry, and (4) using c-Mpl-expressing Ba/F3 cells for TPO bioassay.

3.1. c-Mpl Expression Plasmid

The cDNA encoding the murine c-Mpl receptor was isolated from a spleen cDNA library using standard molecular biological techniques *(25,26)*. In vitro mutagenesis or overlap polymerase chain reaction techniques *(27,28)* were used to incorporate the sequence encoding the 8 amino acid FLAG epitope such that this peptide is incorporated at the N-terminus of the mature c-Mpl receptor (*see* **Note 1**). The cDNA encoding the full-length, epitope tagged c-Mpl receptor was ligated into the LXSN retroviral vector *(29)*. In this vector, receptor expression is driven by the Moloney murine leukemia virus (Mo-MLV) long-terminal repeat, which performs efficiently in many cell types (*see* **Note 2**). The vector also includes an internal SV40 promoter-controlled *neo*® gene, which confers resistance to the cytotoxic drug G418, allowing selection for cells transfected with this vector (**Fig. 2**). The retroviral expression plasmid can be directly transfected into cells, as described below, or used to make murine ecotropic retrovirus for infecting cells (*see* **Note 3**).

3.2. Transfection of Ba/F3 Cells by Electroporation for Expression of Exogenous c-Mpl

Ba/F3 is an IL-3-dependent pro-B cell line established from the bone marrow of Balb/c mice (23) that is maintained as a nonadherent suspension cell line. Ba/F3 cells are strictly dependent on IL-3 for survival and proliferation and die rapidly in the absence of cytokine. The cells can be maintained in standard media, usually Dulbecco's modified Eagles medium (DMEM) containing 10% FCS and IL-3 (1.25×10^2 U/mL recombinant murine IL-3 or 10% WEHI3B cell-conditioned medium, an alternative source of IL-3 *[30]*). Ba/F3 cells proliferate rapidly, doubling within 24 h, and can be maintained up to a density of 10^6 cells/mL. Parental Ba/F3 cells respond to very few cytokines other than IL-3; a weak response to IL-2 has been reported, but the cells responded to no other cytokines tested *(31)*. However, Ba/F3 cells have the capacity to proliferate in response to a wide variety of cytokines, including TPO *(27)*, upon exogenous expression of their specific receptors *(31)*.

The process of transfecting Ba/F3 cells by electroporation has proven effective in our laboratory, and will be described in detail here. The method is based on exposure of cells to electrical impulses, the characteristics of which induce transient changes in the structure of lipid bilayer membranes resulting in reversible pore formation that allows flow of extracellular material into the cells *(32)*.

1. Collect parental Ba/F3 cells by centrifugation at 500*g* for 5 min; wash the cells once by resuspending in PBS. Count the cells and resuspend at 5×10^6 cells/mL in PBS.
2. Add 15–20 µg of c-Mpl expression plasmid, sterilized by ethanol precipitation, dissolved in water or PBS, and preferably linearized (*see* **Note 4**), to a 0.4-cm gap electroporation cuvet, followed by 800 µL of the suspension of washed Ba/F3 cells (4×10^6 cells in total).
3. Electroporate according to instrument directions at 0.27 kV and 960 µFD. A time constant for electroporation of 11–12 ms should be observed.
4. Incubate electroporated cells at room temperature for 10 min and then add 1 mL of growth medium to the cuvet, mix gently and layer over 2 mL of FCS in a 10-mL centrifuge tube.
5. Centrifuge at 500*g* for 5 min, remove medium, and resuspend the cells in 25 mL growth medium. Dispense 0.25 mL into each well of two 48-well plates.
6. After 36–48 h, commence selection by allowing cells to settle to bottom of well, and then aspirating most of the medium and replacing with growth medium supplemented with 1 mg/mL G418. Expect the majority of cells to die within 2 to 3 d and for resistant cells to emerge over the subsequent 7 to 10 d. Change medium in this way every 3 to 4 d.

3.3. Screening Ba/F3 Transfectants for FLAG-Tagged c-Mpl Receptor Expression Using Flow Cytometry

Effective expression of c-Mpl will result in the presence of cell-surface receptor protein; therefore flow cytometry using antibodies specific to the transfected receptor is a rapid and efficient method of screening Ba/F3 transfectants for receptor expression. The method described here outlines the use of antibodies to the FLAG epitope tag that was incorporated into the c-*mpl* cDNA in the expression vector, but antibodies to the untagged receptor can be used equally effectively.

1. When proliferating well, remove approximately half the electroporated and G418-selected cells from each 48-well plate, centrifuge at 500*g* for 5 min, and wash the cells once by resuspending in PBS.
2. Centrifuge as above and resuspend the cells in 50–100 µL of M2 anti-FLAG monoclonal antibody (diluted to 40 µg/mL in PBS containing 2% FCS (PBS/FCS)) and incubate on ice for 20–30 min.
3. Wash away excess M2 antibody by adding 3 mL PBS/FCS.
4. Centrifuge as above, add 50 µL goat anti-mouse Ig-FITC (diluted to 20 µg/mL in PBS/FCS) and incubate on ice for 20–30 min.
5. Wash away excess antibody by adding 3 mL PBS/FCS.

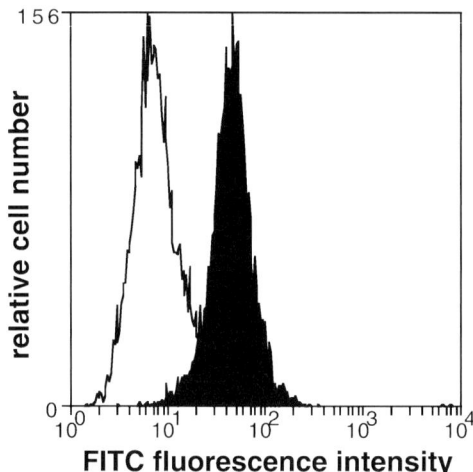

Fig. 3. Identification of Ba/F3 cells expressing cell-surface c-Mpl by flow cytometry. Cell-surface expression of c-Mpl in a transfected Ba/F3 cell clone stained with the M2 anti-FLAG antibody (shaded peak). As a negative control, the same cell clone was stained with an isotype-matched control antibody of irrelevant specificity (open peak).

6. Centrifuge as above, resuspend in 100 μL PBS/FCS, and just prior to analysis, add 50 μL of a 1 μg/mL solution of propidium iodide.
7. Analyze cells for c-Mpl expression (FITC-positive) on a suitable flow cytometer using propidium iodide staining to exclude fluorescence from dead cells (*see* **Fig. 3** and **Note 5**).
8. Clone cells from those wells containing c-Mpl-expressing cells by limit dilution or culture in semisolid medium using standard techniques (*see* **Note 6**).
9. Assay TPO responsiveness of selected c-Mpl-expressing clones using recombinant TPO as outlined in **Subheading 3.4.** and choose the most sensitive clone for maintenance as standard assay line (*see* **Note 7**).

3.4. TPO Bioassay Using c-Mpl-Expressing Ba/F3 Cells

The presence of TPO is assayed by determining whether samples stimulate proliferation of the c-Mpl-expressing Ba/F3 cells. The concentration of bioactive TPO can be determined by reference to a standard curve constructed from a dilution series of a solution of recombinant TPO of known concentration. In all assays, but particularly when assaying complex biological materials such as serum, it is advisable to duplicate the assay using parental Ba/F3 cells. In this way, activity in samples detected using c-Mpl-expressing Ba/F3 cells can be specifically attributed to TPO (*see* **Note 8**).

1. Harvest healthy, proliferating c-Mpl-expressing and parental Ba/F3 cells and wash four times by successively centrifuging at 500*g* and gently resuspending in 10 mL of bioassay medium. After the final wash, count the cells and resuspend at 2×10^4 cells/mL in bioassay medium.

2. Prepare a serial twofold dilution series (undiluted, 1/2, 1/4, etc. to 1/2048) in bioassay medium of (a) each sample to be assayed, (b) recombinant TPO (typically starting with 500 ng/mL as undiluted) and (c) recombinant IL-3 (typically starting at 100 U/mL as undiluted). This is most easily performed in a flat-bottomed 96-well microtiter plate.

3. Aliquot 5 μL of each dilution of either the sample, the recombinant TPO, or recombinant IL-3 into the wells of a 60-well microwell tray. It is advisable to leave the outer lane of each tray empty to prevent samples in these wells from drying out.

4. Prepare all of the plates in **step 3** in duplicate. One set is used with c-Mpl expressing BaF3 cells and the other with parental BaF3 cells as a specificity control to ensure that stimulation of the c-Mpl-expressing BaF3 cells by the sample can be conclusively attributed to TPO.

5. From the 2×10^4 cell/mL stock, aliquot 10 μL of *either* the c-Mpl-expressing Ba/F3 cells *or* parental Ba/F3 cells into each well (a total of 200 cells).

6. Close lids over trays and incubate at 37°C in a humidified atmosphere of 10% CO_2 in air for 48 h.

7. Score the number of viable cells per well using a standard inverted microscope. These can be identified clearly as refractile, healthy cells. Plot viable cell number, calculated as the average of the duplicate determinations, as a function of sample dilution **(Fig. 4)**. By convention, wells containing more than 200 cells are scored as >200. By reference to the standard curve constructed from the recombinant TPO dilution series, the concentration of TPO in the original sample can be calculated **(Fig. 4)**. If sufficient sample is available, it is advisable to repeat the assay independently to confirm the initial assay.

4. Notes

1. The incorporation of an epitope tag is a convenient method of allowing rapid detection of expression of cell surface receptors with well-defined, readily available antibodies and can easily be incorporated into expression plasmids using routine PCR techniques. This is most valuable when antibodies to the native receptor extracellular domain are not available or are unsuitable for use in flow cytometry. As observed with the c-Mpl receptor, in most cases the presence of the epitope tag has no detectable effect on receptor function, although rare examples have been cited in which the tag impairs receptor activity (33).

2. Retroviral vectors afford reliable expression in most somatic tissues and cell lines. Nevertheless, many other expression systems perform equally effectively in Ba/F3 cells and, for the purposes of receptor expression, could be substituted without loss of efficiency. For example, in addition to retroviral vectors, our laboratory has had particular success expressing receptor proteins using vectors based on the EF-BOS plasmid *(34)*, in which the receptor is expressed from the human elongation factor 1α promoter *(31)*.

3. Retroviral expression plasmids have the flexibility of being able to be directly transfected into cells, or used to make murine ecotropic retrovirus that can be used to infect cells for expression of incorporated cDNAs. While the latter method is valuable for expressing genes of interest in primary cells, which are generally refractory to standard transfection techniques, simple transfection is equally effective for expression of receptors in Ba/F3 and other cells lines.

4. The use of plasmid DNA that has been pre-linearized using a restriction endonuclease that does not disrupt the expression cassette—for example, within the plasmid backbone—may improve efficiency of transfection. This is thought to promote insertion of intact expression vector into the cellular chromosomal DNA.

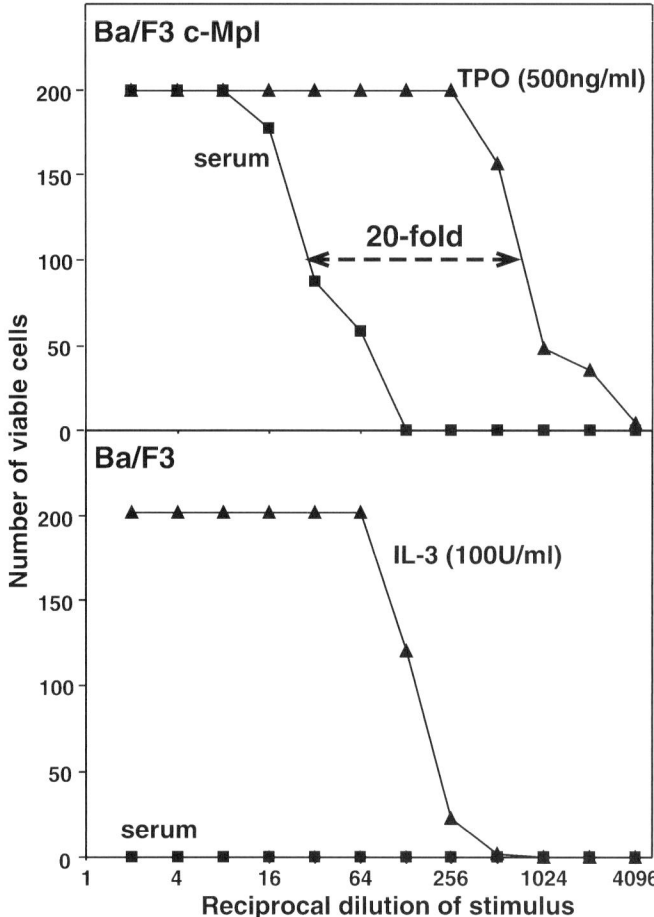

Fig. 4. TPO bioassay using c-Mpl-expressing Ba/F3 cells. The number of viable cells scored 48 h after initiating microwell cultures with 200 Ba/F3 c-Mpl (upper panel) or parental (lower panel) Ba/F3 cells is plotted against the dilution of stimulus added. In the example shown, serum from a thrombocytopenic mouse has been assayed. Any well showing more than 200 cells is scored as >200. By comparison with the standard curve generated by the dilution series initiated with 500 ng/mL recombinant TPO, the serum sample exhibited approx 20-fold lower stimulatory activity on BaF/3 c-Mpl cells. Thus the serum sample contains 25 ng/mL TPO. The absence of activity in the serum on parental Ba/F3 cells in the absence of added cytokines (lower panel) is an important specificity control, confirming that the activity assayed against the Ba/F3 c-Mpl cells is TPO and not any alternative Ba/F3 stimulus.

5. The strength of FITC signal is proportional to the level of receptor expression on the surface of the Ba/F3 cells. It is advisable to select 10–12 of the c-Mpl-expressing cell populations, clone them, and then to test each empirically in the bioassay to select the most TPO-sensitive line for routine assay use. If sterile flow-cytometric sorting facilities are available, an alternative method is to select transfected Ba/F3 cells in G418 in bulk culture, rather than 48-well format, and then to sort and collect the highest expressing Ba/F3 c-Mpl population (e.g., those with highest FITC fluorescence intensity, *see* **Fig. 3**) for cloning and testing in the bioassay.

6. It is important to clone cells from wells containing c-Mpl-expressing Ba/F3 cells, even if the expression profile suggests that a single receptor-expressing population is present. On occasion, sub-populations of low- or non-expressing cells may be present and these can rapidly overgrow the higher-expressing population.

7. Once c-Mpl-expressing Ba/F3 cells have been identified, cloned and tested in the bioassay, they can be maintained in growth medium that includes TPO rather than IL-3. This is advisable, since in our experience, in the absence of selection for receptor expression itself, cell surface c-Mpl expression is readily lost by culture in IL-3 alone, even if G418 is routinely included.

8. Complex biological mixtures such as serum or organ-conditioned medium can also contain toxic components inhibitory to Ba/F3 cell survival or proliferation, even in the presence of added cytokine. This is usually recognisable by the altered appearance of the cells, even in comparison to cells dying simply due to the absence of cytokine. While toxicity may be overcome by dilution, care must be taken in these cases to avoid concluding that TPO is absent, when its proliferative effects may simply be masked by the influence of toxic sample components *(24)*.

5. Discussion

The utility of assays for TPO has rapidly extended beyond their original use in the cloning of the cDNA encoding this cytokine. These assays are essential in the production and quality control of the recombinant TPO used in the laboratory research and clinical trials that have defined the biological actions and potential clinical uses of the cytokine. In addition TPO assays have provided the methodology for myriad studies examining the concentration of circulating TPO in health and disease, comparisons that are hoped to assist in better understanding and clinical management of a variety of diseases *(35,36)*.

The bioassay outlined here utilizes ectopic expression of the murine TPO receptor in Ba/F3 cells. The TPO/c-Mpl system exhibits cross-species specificity such that cells expressing the murine receptor can also be used in bioassays of the human cytokine, although human recombinant TPO must be used as the standard in the assay *(5)*. Alternatively, the expression of human c-Mpl in Ba/F3 cells has also been evaluated and shown to perform well in bioassays of human material *(37)*. Several other factor-dependent cell lines expressing c-Mpl endogenously or from exogenous expression vectors have also proven effective for detection and bioassay of TPO (for example, *see* **refs. 5,38–41**). While some of these cell lines allow examination of a greater variety of biological responses to TPO, such as cellular differentiation, in general these other cell lines exhibit responses to multiple cytokines. The inability of parental Ba/F3 cells to respond significantly to stimuli other than IL-3 *(31)* affords a considerable advantage for routine detection and quantitation of TPO by avoiding interference from other cytokines that may be present, particularly in complex biological mixtures. Routine duplication of assays using parental Ba/F3 cells is used to ensure that activity detected by c-Mpl-expressing Ba/F3 cells can be attributed specifically to TPO.

While the bioassay method outlined here recommends manual microscopic scoring of viable cells following incubation of c-Mpl-expressing Ba/F3 cells with assay material, alternatives such as incorporation of tritiated thymidine for quantitation of TPO-induced DNA synthesis *(39)* or MTT assays for TPO-induced metabolic activity *(42)* are routine techniques that can used as effective alternatives. However, manual inspection of the cultures allows more rapid evaluation of potential technical errors and, particularly where complex biological samples are being assayed, has the advantage of allowing rapid recognition of situations where the assay is inhibited by toxic components in the sample.

Upon the availability of recombinant TPO, cytokine-specific antibodies were rapidly developed and incorporated into antibody-based assays for TPO detection and quantitation. Thus, in addition to the use of bioassays such as that described here, enzyme-linked immunosorbent assays (ELISA) have been widely employed. A typical format for these assays involves coating plastic microtiter plates with TPO-specific monoclonal or polyclonal antibodies and then incubating with assay samples followed by detection with a second anti-TPO antibody conjugated with biotin. The assay is then developed with streptavidin conjugated to the enzyme horseradish peroxidase, which can be readily detected and quantitated colorimetrically (for example, *see* **refs.** *43,44*). Commercially available kits for the detection and quantitation of TPO are now available. These ELISA formats are highly specific and generally are at least as sensitive as cell-based bioassays. In many instances either assay format is appropriate. However, it is noteworthy that the bioassay specifically detects biologically active cytokine, while ELISA formats may not necessarily be able to distinguish active from inactive material. This bears particular consideration in contexts where it is important to define the biological activity of TPO, for example during the production of recombinant material where active TPO may be mixed with denatured or misfolded cytokine.

Acknowledgments

The authors' work is supported by the National Health and Medical Research Council, Canberra, Australia, the National Institutes of Health, Bethesda, Grant No HL62275, and the Australian Government Cooperative Research Centres Program.

References

1. Kelemen, E., Cserhati, B., and Tanos, B. (1958) Demonstration and some properties of human thrombopoietin in thrombocytopenic serum. *Acta Hematol.* **20,** 350–353.
2. Kuter, D. J., Beeler, D. L., and Rosenberg, R. D. (1994) The purification of megapoietin: a physiological regulator of megakaryocyte growth and platelet production. *Proc. Natl. Acad. Sci. USA* **91,** 11,104–11,108.

3. Lok, S. and Foster, D. C. (1994) The structure, biology and potential therapeutic applications of recombinant thrombopoietin. *Stem Cells* **12,** 586–598.

4. de Sauvage, F. J., Hass, P. E., Spencer, S. D., Malloy, B. E., Gurney, A. L., Spencer, S. A., et al. (1994) Stimulation of megakaryocytopoiesis and thrombopoiesis by the c-Mpl ligand. *Nature* **369,** 533–538.

5. Bartley, T. D., Bogenberger, J., Hunt, P., Li, Y. S., Lu, H. S., Martin, F., et al. (1994) Identification and cloning of a megakaryocyte growth and development factor that is a ligand for the cytokine receptor Mpl. *Cell* **77,** 1117–1124.

6. Alexander, W. S. (1999) Thrombopoietin and the c-Mpl receptor: insights from gene targeting. *Int. J. Biochem. Cell Biol.* **31,** 1027–1035.

7. Alexander, W. S. (1999) Thrombopoietin. *Growth Factors* **17,** 13–24.

8. Kuter, D. J. (2000) Future directions with platelet growth factors. *Semin. Hematol.* **37,** 41–49.

9. Foster, D. C., Sprecher, C. A., Grant, F. J., Kramer, J. M., Kuijper, J. L., Holly, R. D., et al. (1994) Human thrombopoietin: gene structure, cDNA sequence, expression, and chromosomal localization. *Proc. Natl. Acad. Sci. USA* **91,** 13,023–13,027.

10. Chang, M. S., Hsu, R. Y., McNinch, J., Copeland, N. G., and Jenkins, N. A. (1995a) The gene for murine megakaryocyte growth and development factor (thrombopoietin, Thpo) is located on mouse chromosome 16. *Genomics* **26,** 636–637.

11. Sungaran, R., Markovic, B., and Chong, B. H. (1997) Localization and regulation of thrombopoietin mRNA expression in human kidney, liver, bone marrow, and spleen using in situ hybridization. *Blood* **89,** 101–107.

12. Nagahisa, H., Nagata, Y., Ohnuki, T., Osada, M., Nagasawa, T., Abe, T., and Todokoro, K. (1996) Bone marrow stromal cells produce thrombopoietin and stimulate megakaryocyte growth and maturation but suppress proplatelet formation. *Blood* **87,** 1309–1316.

13. Hunt, P. (1995) The physiologic role and therapeutic potential of the Mpl-ligand in thrombopoiesis. *Stem Cells* **13,** 579–587.

14. Hunt, P., Li, Y. S., Nichol, J. L., Hokom, M. M., Bogenberger, J. M., Swift, S. E., et al. (1995) Purification and biologic characterization of plasma-derived megakaryocyte growth and development factor. *Blood* **86,** 540–547.

15. Kato, T., Ogami, K., Shimada, Y., Iwamatsu, A., Sohma, Y., Akahori, H., et al. (1995) Purification and characterization of thrombopoietin. *J. Biochem.* **118,** 229–236.

16. Linden, H. M. and Kaushansky, K. (2000) The glycan domain of thrombopoietin enhances its secretion. *Biochemistry* **39,** 3044–3051.

17. Muto, T., Feese, M. D., Shimada, Y., Kudou, Y., Okamoto, T., Ozawa, T., et al. (2000) Functional analysis of the C-terminal region of recombinant human thrombopoietin. C-terminal region of thrombopoietin is a "shuttle" peptide to help secretion. *J. Biol. Chem.* **275,** 12,090–12,094.

18. Stoffel, R., Wiestner, A., and Skoda, R. C. (1996) Thrombopoietin in thrombocytopenic mice: evidence against regulation at the mRNA level and for a direct regulatory role of platelets. *Blood* **87,** 567–573.

19. Stefanich, E., Senn, T., Widmer, R., Fratino, C., Keller, G. A., and Fielder, P. J. (1997) Metabolism of thrombopoietin (TPO) in vivo: determination of the binding dynamics for TPO in mice. *Blood* **89,** 4063–4070.

20. Broudy, V. C., Lin, N. L., Sabath, D. F., Papayannopoulou, T., and Kaushansky, K. (1997) Human platelets display high-affinity receptors for thrombopoietin. *Blood* **89,** 1896–1904.

21. Fielder, P. J., Hass, P., Nagel, M., Stefanich, E., Widmer, R., Bennett, G. L., et al. (1997) Human platelets as a model for the binding and degradation of thrombopoietin. *Blood* **89,** 2782–2788.

22. Souyri, M. (1998) Mpl: from an acute myeloproliferative virus to the isolation of the long sought thrombopoietin. *Semin. Hematol.* **35,** 222–231.

23. Palacios, R. and Steinmetz, M. (1985) IL-3-dependent mouse clones that express B-220 surface antigen, contain Ig genes in germ-line configuration, and generate B lymphocytes in vivo. *Cell* **41,** 727–734.

24. Metcalf, D., Willson, T. A., Hilton, D. J., Di Rago, L., and Mifsud, S. (1995) Production of hematopoietic regulatory factors in cultures of adult and fetal mouse organs: measurement by specific bioassays. *Leukemia* **9,** 1556–1564.

25. Sambrook, J., Fritsch, E. F., and Maniatis, T. (1989) Molecular Cloning, A Laboratory Manual. Cold Spring Harbor Laboratory Press, Cold Spring Harbor, NY.

26. Alexander, W. S. and Dunn, A. R. (1995) Structure and transcription of the genomic locus encoding murine c-Mpl, a receptor for thrombopoietin. *Oncogene* **10,** 795–803.

27. Alexander, W. S., Maurer, A. B., Novak, U., and Harrison-Smith, M. (1996) Tyrosine-599 of the c-Mpl receptor is required for Shc phosphorylation and the induction of cellular differentiation. *Embo. J.* **15,** 6531–6540.

28. Kunkel, T. A. (1985) Rapid and efficient site-specific mutagenesis without phenotypic selection. *Proc. Natl. Acad. Sci. USA* **82,** 488–492.

29. Miller, A. D. and Rosman, G. J. (1989) Improved retroviral vectors for gene transfer and expression. *Biotechniques* **7,** 980–982, 984–986, 989–990.

30. Metcalf, D. (1984) *Hemopoietic Colony-stimulating Factors.* Elsevier, Amsterdam.

31. Metcalf, D., Willson, T., Rossner, M. and Lock, P. (1994) Receptor insertion into factor-dependent murine cell lines to develop specific bioassays for murine G-CSF and M-CSF and human GM-CSF. *Growth Factors* **11,** 145–152.

32. Sugar, I. P. and Neumann, E. (1984) Stochastic model for electric field-induced membrane pores. Electroporation. *Biophys. Chem.* **19,** 211–225.

33. Moritz, R. L., Ward, L. D., Tu, G. F., Fabri, L. J., Ji, H., Yasukawa, K., et al. (1999) The N-terminus of gp130 is critical for the formation of the high-affinity interleukin-6 receptor complex. *Growth Factors* **16,** 265–278.

34. Mizushima, S. and Nagata, S. (1990) pEF-BOS, a powerful mammalian expression vector. *Nucleic Acids Res.* **18,** 5322.

35. Nichol, J. L. (1998) Thrombopoietin levels after chemotherapy and in naturally occurring human diseases. *Curr. Opin. Hematol.* **5,** 203–208.

36. Verbeek, W., Faulhaber, M., Griesinger, F., and Brittinger, G. (2000) Measurement of thrombo-poietic levels: clinical and biological relationships. *Curr. Opin. Hematol.* **7,** 143–149.

37. Park, H. and Hong, H. J. (1997) Development of an in vitro bioassay system for human thrombopoietin by constructing a recombinant murine cell line expressing human thrombo-poietin receptor. *Mol. Cells* **7,** 699–704.

38. Alexander, W. S., Metcalf, D., and Dunn, A. R. (1995) Point mutations within a dimer inter-face homology domain of c-Mpl induce constitutive receptor activity and tumorigenicity. *Embo. J.* **14,** 5569–5578.

39. Page, L. A., Thorpe, R., and Mire-Sluis, A. R. (1996) A sensitive human cell line based bioassay for megakaryocyte growth and development factor or thrombopoietin. *Cytokine* **8,** 66–69.

40. Komatsu, N., Kunitama, M., Yamada, M., Hagiwara, T., Kato, T., Miyazaki, H., et al. (1996) Establishment and characterization of the thrombopoietin-dependent megakaryocytic cell line, UT-7/TPO. *Blood* **87,** 4552–4560.

41. Matsumura, I., Nakajima, K., Wakao, H., Hattori, S., Hashimoto, K., Sugahara, H., et al. (1998) Involvement of prolonged ras activation in thrombopoietin-induced megakaryocytic

differentiation of a human factor-dependent hematopoietic cell line. *Mol. Cell Biol.* **18,** 4282–4290.

42. Lok, S., Kaushansky, K., Holly, R. D., Kuijper, J. L., Lofton-Day, C. E., Oort, P. J., et al. (1994) Cloning and expression of murine thrombopoietin cDNA and stimulation of platelet production in vivo. *Nature* **369,** 565–568.

43. Tahara, T., Usuki, K., Sato, H., Ohashi, H., Morita, H., Tsumura, H., et al. (1996) A sensitive sandwich ELISA for measuring thrombopoietin in human serum: serum thrombopoietin levels in healthy volunteers and in patients with haemopoietic disorders. *Br. J. Haematol.* **93,** 783–788.

44. Folman, C. C., von dem Borne, A. E., Rensink, I. H., Gerritsen, W., van der Schoot, C. E., de Haas, M., et al. (1997) Sensitive measurement of thrombopoietin by a monoclonal antibody based sandwich enzyme-linked immunosorbent assay. *Thromb. Haemost.* **78,** 1262–1267.

27

Culture of Megakaryocytic Cell Lines

Uses and Limitations

Norio Komatsu

1. Introduction

Megakaryocytes (MKs), the precursors of platelets, constitute only 0.03–0.06% of all nucleated cells in the bone marrow and are therefore difficult to isolate in large numbers. Megakaryocytic cell lines represent an important alternative source of material for the study of megakaryopoiesis and thrombopoiesis in vitro. Over the past 30 yr numerous groups have attempted to purify thrombopoietin (TPO), the major regulator of platelet production. These efforts were historically of limited success because of difficulties in measuring TPO activity and the extremely low level of endogenous TPO in thrombocytopenic plasma or cell-culture media. The discovery of the c-Mpl receptor certainly should be described as a critical breakthrough in the search for TPO. The *c-mpl* proto-oncogene was first identified as the cellular homolog of the viral oncogene *v-mpl* in the myeloproliferative leukemia virus (MPLV) *(1)*. However, based on homology with a member of the cytokine receptor superfamily, the *c-mpl* gene was predicted to encode a receptor for a cytokine *(2–4)*. Indeed, an antisense oligomer against *c-mpl* selectively inhibited megakaryocytic colony formation *(5)*. Moreover, *c-mpl*-deficient mice showed a selective but dramatic decrease in the number of circulating platelets and megakaryocytes in the spleen and bone marrow *(6)*. Collectively, these observations suggested that the c-Mpl ligand is identical to thrombopoietin. Finally, in 1994, several groups purified TPO as the c-Mpl ligand *(7–14)*. In fact, extensive in vitro and in vivo studies have revealed that recombinant TPO alone can support the proliferation and differentiation of megakaryocyte progenitor cells and maturation of megakaryocytes *(12–14)*. Several clinical studies are now in progress in the hematology and oncology fields *(15,16)*.

To date, a number of leukemic cell lines displaying megakaryocytic properties have been established from patients with chronic myelogenous leukemia with blastic crisis, acute megakaryoblastic leukemia with Down syndrome, or *de novo* acute

From: *Methods in Molecular Biology, vol. 272:*
Platelets and Megakaryocytes, Vol. 1: Functional Assays
Edited by: J. M. Gibbins and M. P. Mahaut-Smith © Humana Press Inc., Totowa, NJ

Table 1
Human Leukemia Cell Lines With Megakaryocytic Properties

Cell line	Establisher	Reference	Cell bank	Origin
CHRF-288-11	Fugman, A.	*17*		M7
CMK	Sato, T.	*18,19*	JCRB	M7
CMY	Miura, N.	*20*		M7
EST-IU	Sledge, G. W.	*21*		M7
HEL	Martin, P.	*22*	ATCC	M7
HU-3	Morgan, D. A.	*23*		M7
K562	Lozzio, B. B.	*24*	ATCC	CML-BC
KOPM-28	Tsuda, K.	*25*		CML-BC
KU812	Kishi, K.	*26*	JCRB	CML-BC
LAMA-84	Seigneurin, D.	*27*		CML-BC
M-07	Avanzi, G. C.	*28*		M7
MEG-01	Ogura, M.	*29*	ATCC	CML-BC
OCIM2	Papayanopoulou, T.	*30*		M6
T-33	Tange	*31*	ATCC	CML-BC
UT-7	Komatsu, N.	*32*		M7
UT-7/GM	Komatsu, N.	*33*		UT-7
UT-7/TPO	Komatsu, N.	*34*		UT-7/GM

Abbreviations: ATCC: American Type Culture Collection; JCRB: Japanese Collection of Research Bioresources; CML-BC: chronic myelogenous leukemia-blastic crisis; UT-7 and UT-7/GM: names of cell lines (see introduction for derivation); M7: acute megakaryoblastic leukemia; M6: erythroleukemia.

megakaryoblastic leukemia (*see* **Table 1**) *(17–34)*. However, until recently, a TPO-dependent permanent cell line with mature megakaryocytic features has not been available. Prior to the cloning of TPO, we had established the human leukemia cell line UT-7 from the bone marrow cells of a patient with acute megakaryoblastic leukemia *(32)*. We found that UT-7/GM, a subline isolated after long-term culture of UT-7 with granulocyte-macrophage colony-stimulating factor (GM-CSF), proliferated slightly in response to TPO *(33)*. Therefore, we attempted to establish a UT-7 subline with mature megakaryocytic features from the UT-7/GM and succeeded in isolating a novel subline, designated UT-7/TPO *(34)*. UT-7/TPO cells are absolutely dependent on TPO for growth and survival, and have mature megakaryocytic properties such as polyploidy and demarcation membrane systems. This chapter describes the development, maintenance, and applications of the UT-7/TPO line.

2. Materials

1. Culture medium: Iscove's modified Dulbecco's medium (IMDM; Invitrogen (Carlsbad, CA) Life Technologies) with 100 µg/mL streptomycin and 100 U/mL penicillin G (Invitrogen) (*see* **Note 1**).
2. Fetal calf serum (FCS) (Hyclone Laboratories, Logan, UT).
3. Granulocyte/macrophage colony-stimulating factor (GM-CSF) (Kirin Brewery Co., Tokyo Japan).

4. Human recombinant thrombopoietin (TPO) (Kirin Brewery Co.).
5. 25-cm^2 and 75-cm^2 tissue culture flasks.
6. 24- and 96-well tissue culture plates.
7. FACStar^{plus} flow cytometer equipped with an automatic cloning device (Becton Dickinson Co., Mountain View, CA).
8. Bovine serum albumin (BSA) (Sigma Chemical Co., St. Louis, MO).
9. 0.9% methylcellulose (Dow Chemical, Midland, MI).
10. 35-mm culture dishes (Falcon, Oxnard, CA).
11. Methylcellulose-based culture medium: IMDM containing 0.9% methylcellulose, 30% FCS, 1% BSA, and 10 ng TPO/mL. A premixture of methylcellulose-based medium is also available commercially (e.g., ClonaCell™-TCS Transfected Cell Selection Kit, StemCell Technologies, Vancouver, BC, Canada), although TPO (10 ng/mL) must be added to the medium.
12. Sterilized MTT [3-(4.5-dimethylthiazol-2-yl)-2.5-diphenyltetrazolium bromide]: stock 5 mg/mL (Sigma).
13. Sodium dodecyl sulfate (SDS, Wako Pure Chemical Industries, Osaka, Japan): 20% (w/v) solution in 0.01 N hydrochloric acid solution.
14. Microplate reader (model 3550; Bio-Rad, Richmond, CA).
15. Plasmid DNA with gene of interest in a vector expressing an antibiotic resistance gene (e.g., resistance to Geneticin® (G418 sulfate), Hygromycin B, Zeocin™, or Blastcidin).
16. Saline G: 8.0 g NaCl, 0.4 g KCl, 0.395 g Na$_2$HPO$_4$•12H$_2$O, 0.15 g KH$_2$PO$_4$, 0.1 g MgCl$_2$•6H$_2$O, 0.1 g CaCl$_2$ (anhydrous), 1.1 g glucose, adjusted to pH 7.1–7.2 with NaOH in total volume of 1 L.
17. Electroporator (GenePulser®, Bio-Rad).
18. Electroporation cuvets (Bio-Rad 165-2085).
19. Antibiotics: Geneticin® (Sigma), Hygromycin B (Wako Pure Chemical Industries, Osaka, Japan), Zeocin™ (Invitrogen), and Blastcidin (Kaken Pharmaceutical Co., Tokyo, Japan).
20. Tfx™-20 reagent (Promega, Madison, WI).
21. T-REx™ tetracycline-inducible expression system including vectors, antibiotics, and tetracycline (Invitrogen, Carlsbad, CA).

3. Methods

3.1. Establishing a Megakaryocytic Cell Line: A Historical Account of the Development of UT-7/TPO Cells

To indicate the steps involved in establishing a megakaryocytic cell line, the development of UT-7/TPO cells is outlined below:

1. Bone marrow cells obtained from a patient with acute megakaryoblastic leukemia (M7) were cultured in IMDM containing 10% FCS.
2. Within a week, the majority of the cells died. The few cells that remained alive failed to grow.
3. We had previously reported that GM-CSF is produced from PMA-treated CMK cells, a cell line established from acute megakaryoblastic leukemia with Down syndrome *(35)*. Based on this experience, we added GM-CSF (1 ng/mL) to the culture containing dying cells. Surprisingly, these cells were revived and began to grow soon after the addition of GM-CSF. This appeared to represent an important, novel finding. We designated this cell line UT-7 (Ul̲trase̲ve̲n) *(32)*. ("Ultraseven" is the hero of a popular TV program among Japanese children and means "resuscitation.")

4. This cell line was maintained in liquid culture in IMDM containing 10% FCS and 1 ng/mL GM-CSF. UT-7/GM, a subline of UT-7, was developed from the original UT-7 by long-term exposure of UT-7 cells to GM-CSF (>2 yr) *(33)*.

5. Next, UT-7/GM cells were initially cultured with supernatant containing a lower concentration of recombinant human TPO (crude supernatant from Chinese hamster cells transfected with human TPO cDNA; less than 0.1 ng/mL) in place of GM-CSF. While the majority of the UT-7/GM cells died within a short period, a minor population remained alive (*see* **Note 2**).

6. One month later, cells were growing well in the culture medium. Surprisingly, some of the cells were much larger than the original UT-7/GM cells. The size was identical to that of normal mature megakaryocytes (MKs). These larger cells were subcloned using the following method (**step 7**) and led to the UT-7/TPO cell line, a TPO-"hypersensitive" subclone capable of growing well in the presence of TPO *(34)*. These cells were positive for MK-specific markers, such as glycoprotein IIb/IIIa and platelet peroxidase activity.

7. To obtain a single clone, a colony assay was performed using semisolid methylcellulose culture medium (*see also* Chapter 23, vol. 1 for further details of culturing with methylcellulose medium). In the case of UT-7/TPO, the cells were suspended in methylcellulose-based culture medium with 10 ng TPO/mL. Aliquots of this semisolid culture medium (1 mL) containing 500 cells were cultured in 35-mm culture dishes at 37°C in a 5% CO_2 humidified atmosphere for 10 days, then a single colony containing large cells was picked out under an inverted microscope and transferred to liquid culture medium containing 10 ng/mL of TPO with a sterile microtip or Pasteur pipet. Finally, a TPO-"hypersensitive" subclone, UT-7/TPO, was selected.

3.2. Considerations for Culture of Megakaryocytic Cell Lines

The following are important issues to consider when maintaining megakaryocytic cell lines:

1. One of the most important issues in cell culturing is to select a good-quality FCS for the cell line, because the growth condition usually depends on the batch of FCS. We choose a suitable serum for each cell line, because growth of cells may become remarkably poor due to differences in serum.

2. In addition to standard antibiotics (penicillin and streptomycin, *see* **Note 1**) we pay close attention to the possibility of mycoplasma infection. When infected with a mycoplasma, growth of cells may deteriorate suddenly and the character may change.

3. It is important to determine the character of each cell line, that is the doubling time and the cell density at the peak. For example, UT-7 cells die rapidly when the cell density reaches a plateau at a cell concentration of 5×10^5/mL.

4. Cultivating the cell lines long-term must be avoided, because this may alter the property of the cell lines and clones compared to the original cell line. If the cell line is from the establisher or a cell bank, this must be expanded as soon as possible, then aliquots frozen and preserved in liquid nitrogen.

5. In addition, information about the culture conditions (the type of the culture solution, fetal calf serum, and optimal cell density, etc.) should be obtained from the provider.

3.3. Colorimetric MTT Assay for Cell Proliferation

Cell growth can be examined by a colorimetric assay according to Mosmann with some modifications *(36)*. Several kits are now commercially available. The assay can detect living, but not dead cells and the signal generated is dependent on the degree of activation of the living cells. This method is useful for measuring cytotoxicity and proliferation. The main advantages of the MTT assay are its rapidity and precision, and the lack of any radioisotope.

1. Resuspend cells at a density of 1×10^5/mL in IMDM containing 10% FCS and transfer 100-µL aliquots to the wells of a 96-well plate. Incubate in the absence or presence of various concentrations of TPO (0.01–100 ng/mL).
2. After 72-h culture at 37°C, add 20 µL of sterilized 5 mg/mL MTT to each well.
3. Following a 2-h incubation at 37°C, add 100 µL of 20% SDS to each well to dissolve the dark-blue crystal product.
4. The optical density (OD) is measured at a wavelength of 595 nm using a microplate reader. The values represent the mean +/– SD from at least triplicate cultures and are expressed as a percentage of UT-7/TPO cells cultured in the absence of TPO.

3.4. Generation of Stable Transfectants From UT-7/TPO

Genes of interest can be introduced into the UT-7/TPO cells by several methods, including electroporation and lipofection. Exponentially growing cells must always be used for gene transfection experiments.

3.4.1. Electroporation

1. Linearize 10–50 µg plasmid DNA and perform ethanol precipitation procedure. To obtain ethanol precipitate, add 0.1 volume of 3 M sodium acetate (pH 4.8) and 2.5 volumes of ethanol to the microtube (1.5 mL) containing the DNA solution. To precipitate the DNA, keep the tube at –20°C overnight or –70°C for 30–60 min. Then, centrifuge the tube at 15,000g for 20 min at 4°C. Discard the supernatant.
2. Wash the pellet with 70% ethanol. Aspirate the supernatant and dry the pellet. Then, solubilize the pellet in 0.4 mL sterile saline G.
3. Prepare the cells by harvesting exponentially growing cells and wash once with sterile saline G for 5 min at 400g. Resuspend the cells at a concentration of 1×10^7 cells/mL in sterile saline G.
4. Transfer 0.4 mL cell suspension to an electroporation cuvet and add 0.4 mL of plasmid solution to the cuvet.
5. Stand on ice for 10 min.
6. Pulse (250 V, 960 µFD).
7. Stand on ice for 10 min.
8. Dilute with culture medium (IMDM containing 10% FCS and 10 ng TPO/mL) to 24 mL.
9. Incubate in a 75-cm^2 cell culture flask.
10. 24–48 h later, add the appropriate antibiotics (e.g., 0.8 mg/mL Geneticin; 0.2–0.3 mg/mL Hygromycin B; 0.2 mg/mL Zeocin; 5 µg/mL Blastcidin) to the culture.
11. Dispense into 24-well plates (1 mL/well).
12. Incubate the cells for the next 14 d. If the cells are still growing at the end of this period, the culture can be continued for several days after addition of 0.5–1 mL of fresh selective medium (IMDM containing 10% FCS and 10 ng/mL TPO and the appropriate antibiotics) to the 24-well plate.
13. Monitor the cultures for the formation of cell clusters of surviving cells.

14. Transfer individual cell cluster (aggregation of cells) to 6-well plates and continue to maintain the cultures in medium containing the appropriate antibiotic for the expansion of the cloned cells.
15. Confirm whether the protein encoded by the transfected gene is expressed in the transfectant (e.g., by Western blotting with an antibody against the protein).
16. Continue to maintain the transfectant in medium containing the appropriate antibiotic.
17. Next, stably transfected cells should be cloned by limiting dilution or methylcellulose-based culture (*see* **Subheading 3.1., step 7**). Culture the transfectant in medium with the appropriate antibiotic continuously present.

3.4.2. Lipofection

Products from several companies can be used for lipofection. We have adopted the Tfx-20 reagent for the transfection of UT-7/TPO cells used according to the protocol of the company.

1. Linearize plasmid DNA, precipitate and wash in ethanol as described in **Subheading 3.4.1., steps 1** and **2**, and resuspend in distilled water at 1 µg/µL.
2. Prepare the cells by harvesting exponentially growing cells and wash (5 min at 400g) twice with serum-free IMDM. Resuspend the cells at a concentration of 2×10^6 cells/mL in serum-free IMDM.
3. Prepare the DNA/Tfx-20 reagent mixtures: add serum-free IMDM, prewarmed to 37°C, to the linearized plasmid DNA to make a final volume of 0.5 mL and vortex. Add 4.5 µL Tfx-20 reagent and vortex immediately.
4. Allow the Tfx-20 reagent and DNA mixture to incubate for 10–15 min at room temperature.
5. In the interval, aliquot 0.5 mL of cells (1×10^6 cells) to a 25-cm^2 cell-culture flask.
6. Briefly vortex the Tfx-20 reagent and DNA mixture and add to the cells (0.5 mL/flask). Return the cells to the incubator for 1 h. During the incubation, prewarm complete medium (containing 10% FCS and 10 ng TPO/mL) to 37°C.
7. At the end of the incubation period, add 5 mL of the prewarmed complete medium to the flask. Return the cells to the incubator.
8. Maintain the cells in nonselecting medium for 1 d posttransfection.
9. Add 18 mL of the selective medium (IMDM containing 10% FCS, 10 ng/mL TPO and the appropriate antibiotic (e.g., 0.8 mg/mL Geneticin; 0.2–0.3 mg/mL Hygromycin B; 0.2 mg/mL Zeocin; 5 µg/mL Blasticidin) and transfer the cells to 24-well plates (1 mL/well).
10. Incubate the cells for the next 14 d. Add 0.5–1 mL of the selecting medium to the 24-well plates.
11. Monitor the cultures for the formation of cell clusters of surviving cells and gene expression (*see* **Subheading 3.4.1., steps 14–17**).

3.5. Tetracycline-Inducible Expression System in UT-7/TPO

We have also used an inducible expression system in UT-7/TPO cells, in which transcription of a target cDNA is initiated by tetracycline (Tet) treatment (T-REx) *(37)*. The cells are co-transfected with a regulatory plasmid, encoding the Tet repressor, and an expression plasmid containing the gene of interest. The Tet repressor prevents transcription of the gene of interest until tetracycline treatment.

1. Use lipofection (*see* **Subheading 3.4.2.**) to transfect UT-7/TPO cells with expression vectors for the Tet repressor, pcDNA6/TR, which also expresses the blasticidin resistance gene.
2. Culture with 0.5 μg/mL of blasticidin for 14 d to select the positive clone (designated UT-7/TPO/pcDNA6/TR-2).
3. Use lipofection to transfect this clone with FKHRL1-TM, a mutant of FKHRL1, in the Tet-inducible expression vector, pcDNA4/TO, which also expresses a Zeocin resistance gene. FKHRL1-TM is a human homolog of DAF-16, which is involved in lifespan extension of *Caenorhabditis elegans* and is a potentially important transcription factor in megakaryopoiesis *(37)*.
4. Select FKHRL1-TM-expressing cells with Zeocin at a concentration of 200 μg/mL.
5. Examine the induction levels of the FKHRL1-TM protein before and after 1 μg/mL Tet treatment using Western blot analyses.
6. Isolate subclones of UT-7/TPO/FKHRL1-TM displaying the most efficient induction of target protein following Tet treatment for further studies of this signaling pathway.

3.6. Applications of Megakaryocytic Cell Lines

Permanent cell lines are appropriate systems for the investigation of whether a growth factor is capable of inducing proliferation and differentiation. In particular, unlike other human leukemia cell lines, UT-7/TPO has absolute dependence on TPO. TPO stimulates mature megakaryocytic features within the UT-7/TPO line. Therefore, UT-7/TPO could serve a model system for resolving issues concerning megakaryopoiesis. The following are examples of applications using the UT-7/TPO line.

3.6.1. Discovery of Low-Molecular-Weight Compounds That Mimic Biological Effect of TPO

TPO is the key regulator of platelet production. However, thrombocytopenia occurs unexpectedly after administration of TPO in healthy volunteers and patients receiving chemotherapy. Moreover, Basser et al. *(38)* recently described a case of prolonged pancytopenia associated with the development of neutralizing antibodies against TPO after multicycle chemotherapy supported by TPO. Thus, generation of neutralizing antibodies against TPO is a potential obstacle in the clinical development of this cytokine. Therefore, the development of low-molecular-weight compounds that mimic the biological effect of TPO is of great clinical importance. Indeed, many efforts have been undertaken to identify these compounds using UT-7/TPO cells. Kimura et al. *(39)* identified two benzodiazepinones (TM41) that compete with the binding of TPO to the extracellular region of c-Mpl. These nonpeptide compounds can mimic the effect of thrombopoietin via c-Mpl in that they promote proliferation and activation of Stat5 in UT-7/TPO cells, although a high dosage (more than 30 μM) of TM41 is required for exerting its action on UT-7/TPO cells. Erickson-Miller et al. *(40)* have also identified a selective non-peptidyl TPO receptor agonist SB394725 from a large library of low-molecular-weight compounds. SB394725 supported the proliferation of UT-7/TPO cells without TPO. These results demonstrate the usefulness of UT-7/TPO in the characterization of potent low-molecular-weight compounds with TPO-like activity that could ultimately be developed into orally administered thrombopoietic drugs.

3.6.2. Study of Signal Transduction

The study of the intracellular events provoked by signals from the TPO/c-Mpl receptor system, leading to megakaryocyte maturation and platelet production, has been limited by the difficulty of isolating large numbers of normal MKs from bone marrow. Thus, a TPO-dependent permanent cell line with mature megakaryocytic features, such as the UT-7/TPO cell line described earlier, represents a useful model system. A number of groups, including our own, have been studying signal transduction of TPO using UT-7/TPO and other TPO-responsive cell lines *(41–47)*. The action of cytokines is mediated by the activation of their cognate receptors and downstream signal transduction pathways including protein kinase C, phospholipase C-γ1, phosphatidylinositol 3-kinase (PI3K) Akt, RAS-mitogen-activated protein kinase (MAPK), and Janus tyrosine kinase (Jak)-signal transducer and activator of transcription (Stat) activation pathways. Recent studies have revealed that these signal transduction pathways are actually commonly activated by several cytokines in normal megakaryocytes and play important roles in the regulation of megakaryopoiesis. For example, the constitutive activation of MAPK is required for the maturation of megakaryocytes with an increase of ploidy *(46)*. Protein kinase C-α is involved in pro-platelet formation *(47)*. At present, the precise function of Stat proteins in megakaryopoiesis remains to be elucidated. Among the Stat proteins, normal megakaryocytes predominantly express Stat3 *(48)*. In addition, thrombopoietic cytokines appear to commonly activate Stat3 *(48,49)*. For example, TPO and IL-11 activate Stat3 and Stat5, and Stat3, respectively, in normal MKs, suggesting that Stat3 has an important role in megakaryopoiesis and thrombopoiesis.

Although Stat3 knockout mice have already been established, these mice showed embryonic lethality at E6.5 d before the onset of hematopoiesis *(50)*. Therefore, an alternative approach is required for examining the Stat3 function in in vivo megakaryopoiesis and thrombopoiesis *(51,52)*. To overcome this problem, we used transgenic (Tg) constructs in which the expression of a dominant negative form of Stat3, Stat3F, is controlled by the GATA-1 regulatory gene elements, because GATA-1 expression is restricted to MKs and erythroid cells *(53,54)*. We established Tg mice selectively expressing Stat3F in megakaryocytic lineage cells and demonstrated that Stat3 activation is required for promoting the expansion of megakaryocytic progenitor cells *(55)*. Thus, the data obtained from cell lines will extend to in vivo experiments using the promoter of the megakaryocytic lineage-specific gene including platelet factor 4 *(56)*.

3.6.3. Comparison With Normal Megakaryocytes

It should be noted that megakaryocytic cell lines including UT-7/TPO are originally of leukemic origin. It is therefore important to confirm whether results obtained from the cell line also apply to normal cells using highly purified megakaryocytic populations. MKs are a minor population in bone marrow and several methods have been attempted to obtain a pure population of megakaryocytes. Many of these procedures have included a step in which MKs are separated from other marrow cells based on their larger size using density gradient centrifugation and velocity sedimentation (*see* Chapter 22, vol. 1).

As another method for obtaining a large number of megakaryocytes, ex vivo generation of MKs is available (*see* Chapters 23 and 24, vol. 1). We have generated human megakaryocytic cells ex vivo from CD34+ cells as described previously with minor modifications *(57)*. CD34+ cells are separated from the peripheral blood (PB) of healthy volunteers receiving recombinant human granulocyte colony-stimulating factor as described *(58)*. PB CD34+ cells are isolated using immunomagnetic beads *(59,60)* and can be cryopreserved in liquid nitrogen until required. After thawing, PB CD34+ cells are cultured in the presence of of iron-saturated transferrin, insulin, lipid suspension (oleic acid, L-α-phosphatidylcholine and cholesterol) *(61)*, vitamin B12, folic acid, and TPO (*see* **Note 3**). After culture for 10 d, megakaryocytic lineages are separated immunomagnetically using anti-CD41 or anti-CD42 antibodies (*see* Chapters 23 and 24, vol. 1).

4. Notes

1. Unless otherwise stated, all culture media contain the antibiotics streptomycin (100 µg/mL) and penicillin G (100 U/mL). Ready-made penicillin-streptomycin solution (prepared with 10,000 U/mL penicillin G sodium and 10,000 µg/mL streptomycin sulfate in 0.85% saline) can be purchased from Invitrogen. $NaHCO_3$ (3024 mg/L) and L-glutamine (584 mg/L) are included in ready-made IMDM solution (Invitrogen). Sterile conditions should be observed at all times.

2. At the time of development of the UT-7 and related cell lines, we obtained recombinant human TPO from a pharmaceutical company. It was fortunate that we initially used UT-7/GM but not UT-7 to examine the response to TPO, because we know retrospectively that UT-7/GM cells but not UT-7 cells can respond to TPO.

3. The culture of PB CD34+ cells to generate megakaryocyte-lineage cells is described in detail in Chapter 24 of this book. Conditions we have used are similar. In brief, frozen PB CD34+ cells are thawed, suspended in IMDM containing 30% FCS and 100 U/mL DNase, then centrifuged at 400g for 5 min at 4°C. The cells are washed twice with IMDM containing 0.3% deionized BSA, then resuspended in IMDM containing 0.3% deionized BSA. Next, from 2×10^4 to 4×10^4 cells/mL are suspended in a mixture containing 5% pooled human AB plasma, 1% BSA, 30 mg/mL of iron-saturated transferrin, 10 µg/mL of insulin, lipid suspension (2.8 µg/mL oleic acid, 4.0 µg/mL of L-α-phosphatidylcholine, and 3.9 µg/mL cholesterol; Sigma) *(61)*, vitamin B12 at 10 µg/mL, and folic acid at 15 µg/mL, with TPO at 100 ng/mL, in the presence of 50 µM 2-mercaptoethanol, penicillin at 50 U/mL and streptomycin at 50 µg/mL, and IMDM in a 50-mL polystyrene flask (Corning Coster Corp., Cambridge, MA). After incubation for 10 d (37°C, 5% CO_2), the cells are harvested for isolation of megakaryocytic (CD41+/42+) cells by immunomagnetic separation (see Chapters 23 and 24, vol. 1 for further details).

References

1. Souyri, M., Vigon, I., Penciolelli, J.-F., Heard, J.-M., Tambourin, P., and Wendling, F. (1990) A putative truncated cytokine receptor gene transduced by the myeloproliferative leukemia virus immortalizes hematopoietic progenitors. *Cell* **63,** 1137–1147.
2. Vigon, I., Florindo, C., Fichelson, S., Guenet, J.-L., Mattei, M.-G., Souyri, M., et al. (1993) Characterization of the murine *Mpl* pronto-oncogene, a member of the hematopoietic cytokine receptor family: molecular cloning, chromosomal location and evidence for a function in cell growth. *Oncogene* **8,** 2607–2615.

3. Vigon, I., Mornon, J.-P., Cocault, L., Mitjavila, M.-T., Tambourin, P., Gisselbrecht, S., et al. (1992) Molecular cloning and characterizaion of *MPL*, the human homolog of the v-*mpl* oncogene: Identification of a member of the hematopoietic growth factor receptor superfamily. *Proc. Natl. Acad. Sci. USA* **89,** 5640–5644.

4. Skoda, R. C., Seldin, D. C., Chiang, M.-K., Peichel, C. L., Vogt, T. F., and Leder, P. (1993) Murine c-*mpl:* a member of the hematopoietic growth factor receptor superfamily that transduces a proliferative signal. *Embo. J.* **12,** 2645–2653.

5. Methia, N., Louache, F., Vainchenker, W., and Wendling, F. (1993) Oligodeoxynucleotides antisense to the proto-oncogene c-*mpl* specifically inhibit in vitro megakaryocytopoiesis. *Blood* **82,** 1395–1401.

6. Gurney, A. L., Carver-Moore, K., de Sauvage, F. J., and Moore, M. W. (1994) Thrombocytopenia in c-*mpl*-deficient mice. *Science* **265,** 1445–1447.

7. de Sauvage, F. J., Hass, P. E. Spencer, S. D., Malloy, B. E., Austin, L., Gurney, A. L., et al. (1994) Stimulation of megakaryocytopoiesis and thrombopoiesis by the c-Mpl ligand. *Nature* **369,** 533–538.

8. Lok, S., Kaushansky, K., Holly, R. D., Kuijper, J. L., Lofton-Day, C. E,. Oort. P. J., et al. (1994) Cloning and expression of murine thrombopoietin cDNA and stimulation of platelet production *in vivo. Nature* **369,** 565–568.

9. Bartley, T. D., Bogenberger, J., Hunt, P., Li, Y.-S., Lu, H. S., Martin, F., et al. (1994) Identification and cloning of a megakaryocyte growth and development factor that is a ligand for the cytokine receptor Mpl. *Cell* **77,** 1117–1124.

10. Kuter, D. J., Beeler, D. L., and Rosenberg, R. D. (1994) The purification of megapoietin: A physiological regulator of megakaryocyte growth and platelet production. *Proc. Natl. Acad. Sci. USA* **91,** 11,104–11,108.

11. Kato, T., Ogami, K., Shimada, Y., Iwamatsu, A., Sohma, Y., Akahori, H., et al. (1995) Purification and characterization of thrombopoietin. *J. Biochem.* **118,** 229–236.

12. Kaushansky, K., Lok, S., Holly, R. D., Brondy, V. C., Lin, N., Bailey, M. C., et al. (1994) Promotion of megakaryocyte progenitor expansion and differentiation by the c-Mpl ligand thrombopoietin. *Nature* **369,** 568–571.

13. Wendling, F., Maraskovsky, E., Debili, N., Florindo, C., Teepe, M., Titeux, M., et al. (1994) c-Mpl ligand is a humoral regulator of megakaryocytopoiesis. *Nature* **369,** 571–574.

14. Kaushansky, K., Broudy, V. C., Lin, N., Jorgensen, M. J., McCarty, J., Fox, N., et al. (1995) Thrombopoietin, the Mpl ligand, is essential for full megakaryocyte development. *Proc. Natl. Acad. Sci. USA* **92,** 3234–3238.

15. Komatsu, N., Okamoto, T., Yoshida, T., et al. Pegylated recombinant human megakaryocyte growth and development factor (PEG-rHuMGDF) increased platelet counts in patients with aplastic anemia and myelodysplastic syndrome. *Blood* **96,** 296a.

16. Fanucchi, M., Glaspy, J., Crawford, J., Garst, J., Figlin, R., Sheridan, W., et al. (1997) Effects of polyethylene glycol-conjugated recombinant human megakaryocyte growth and development factor on platelet counts after chemotherapy for lung cancer. *N. Engl. J. Med.* **336,** 404–409.

17. Fugman, D. A., Witte, D. P., Jones, C. L. A., Aronow, B. J., and Lieberman, M. A. (1990) In vitro establishment and characterization of a human megakaryoblastic cell line. *Blood* **75,** 1252–1261.

18. Sato, T., Fuse, A., Eguchi, M., Hayashi, Y., Ryo, R., Adachi, M., et al. (1989) Establishment of a human leukaemic cell line (CMK) with megakaryocytic characteristics from a Down's syndrome patient with acute megakaryoblastic leukaemia. *Brit. J. Haematol.* **72,** 184–190.

19. Komatsu, N., Suda, T., Moroi, M., Tokuyama, N., Sakata, Y., Okada, M., et al. (1989) Growth and differentiation of a human megakaryoblastic cell line, CMK. *Blood* **74,** 42–48.

20. Sato, T., Sekine, H., Kakuda, H., Miura, N., Sunohara, M., and Fuse, A. (2000) HIV infection of megakaryocytic cell lines. *Leukemia and Lymphoma* **36,** 397–404.

21. Sledge, G. W. Jr., Glant, M. Jansen, J., Heereme, N. A., Roth, B. J., Goheen, M., et al. (1986) Establishment in long-term culture of megakaryocytic leukemia cells (EST-IU) from the marrow of a patient with leukemia and a mediastional germ cell neoplasm. *Cancer Res.* **46,** 2155–2159.

22. Martin, P. and Papayannopoulou, T. (1982) HEL cells: a new human erythroleukemia cell line with spontaneous and induced globin expression. *Science* **11,** 1233–1235.

23. Morgan, D., Soslau, G., and Brodsky, I. (1994) Differential effects of thrombopoietin (mpl) on cell lines MB- 02 and HU-3 derived from patients with megakaryoblastic leukemia. *Blood* **84,** 330a (abstract no. 1306).

24. Lozzio, C. B. and Lozzio, B. B. (1975) Human chronic myelogenous leukemia cell-line with positive Philadelphia chromosome. *Blood* **45,** 321–334.

25. Tsuda, H., Sakaguchi, M., Kawakita, M., Nakazawa, S., Mori, T., and Takatsuki, K. (1988) Alterations of cell cycle progression in human leukemia cell line (KOPM-28) induced by 12-O-tetradecanoylphorbol-13-acetate. *Int. J. Cell. Cloning* **6,** 209–220.

26. Nakazawa, M., Mitjavila, M.-T., Debili, N., Casadevall, N., Mayeux, P., Rouyer-Fessard, P., et al. (1989) KU 812: a pluripotent human cell line with spontaneous erythroid terminal maturation. *Blood* **73,** 2003–2013.

27. Seigneurin, D., Champelovier, P., Mouchiroud, G., Berthier, R., Leroux, D., Prenant, M., et al. (1987) Human chronic myeloid leukemia cell line with positive Philadelphia chromosome exhibits megakaryocytic and erythroid characteristics. *Exp. Hematol.* **15,** 822.

28. Avanzi, G. C., Lista, P, Giovinazzo, B., Miniero, R., Saglio, G., Benetton, G., et al. (1988) Selective growth response to IL-3 of a human leukaemic cell line with magakaryoblastic features. *Brit. J. Haematol.* **69,** 359–366.

29. Ogura, M., Morishima, Y., Ohno, R., Kato, Y., Hirabayashi, N., Nagura, H., et al. (1985) Establishment of anovel human megakaryoblastic leukemia cell line, MEG-01, with positive Philadelphia chromosome. *Blood* **66,** 1384–1392.

30. Papayannopoulou, T., Nakamoto, B., Kurachi, S., Tweeddale, M., and Messner, H. (1988) Surface antigenic profile and globin phenotype of two new human erythroleukemia limes: characterization and interpretations. *Blood* **72,** 1029–1038.

31. Tange, T., Nakahara, K., Mitani, K., Yamasaki, I., Yasuda, H., Tanaka, F., et al. (1988) Establishment of a human megakaruoblastic cell line (T-33) from chronic myelogenous leukemia in megakaryoblastic crisis. *Cancer Res.* **48,** 6137–6144.

32. Komatsu, N., Nakauchi, H., Miwa, A., Ishihara, T., Eguchi, M., Moroi, M., et al. (1991) Establishment and characterization of a human leukemic cell line with megakaryocytic features: dependency on granulocyte-macrophage colony stimulating factor, interleukin 3, or erythropoietin for growth and survival. *Cancer Res.* **51,** 341–348.

33. Komatsu, N., Kirito, K., Shimizu, R., Kunitama, M., Yamada, M., Uchida, M., et al. (1997) In vitro development of erythroid and megakaryocytic cells from a UT-7 subline, UT-7/GM. *Blood* **89,** 4021–4033.

34. Komatsu, N., Kunitama, M., Yamada, M., Hagiwara, T., Kato, T., Miyazaki, H., et al. (1996) Establishment and characterization of the thrombopoietin-dependent megakaryocytic cell line, UT-7/TPO. *Blood* **87,** 4552–4560.

35. Komatsu, N., Suda, T., Moroi, M., Tokuyama, N., Sakata, Y., Okada, M., et al. (1989) Growth and differentiation of a human megakaryoblastic cell line, CMK. *Blood* **74,** 42–48.

36. Mosmann, T. (1983) Rapid colorimetric assay for cellular growth and survival: application to proliferation and cytotoxicity assays. *J. Immunol. Methods* **65,** 55–63.

37. Tanaka, M., Kirito, K., Kashii, Y., Uchida, M., Watanabe, T., Endo, H., et al. (2001) Forkhead family transcription factor FKHRL1 is expressed in human megakaryocytes. Regulation of cell cycling as a downstream molecule of thrombopoietin signaling. *J. Biol. Chem.* **276,** 15,082–15,089.

38. Basser, R. L., O'Flaherty, E., Green, M., Edmonds, M., Nichol, J., Menchaca, D. M., et al. (2002) Development of pancytopenia with neutralizing antibodies to thrombopoietin after multicycle chemotherapy supported by megakaryocyte growth and development factor. *Blood* **99,** 2599–2602.

39. Kimura, T., Kaburaki, H., Tsujino, T., Ikeda, Y., Kato, H., and Watanabe, Y. (1998) A non-peptide compound which can mimic the effect of thrombopoietin via c-Mpl. *FEBS Lett.* **428,** 250–254.

40. Erickson-Miller, C. L, Delorme, E., Tian, S.-S., Dillon, S. B., Rosen, J., Luengo, J. I., et al. (2000) Discovery and characterization of a selective, non-peptidyl thromobopoietin receptor agonist. *Blood* **96,** 675a.

41. Miyakawa, Y., Rojnuckarin, P., Habib, T., and Kaushansky, K. (2001) Thrombopoietin induces phosphoinositol 3-kinase activation through SHP2, Gab, and insulin receptor substrate proteins in BAF3 cells and primary murine megakaryocytes. *J. Biol. Chem.* **276,** 2494–2502.

42. Drachman, J., Millett, K. M., and Kaushansky, K. (1999) Thrombopoietin signal transduction requires functional JAK2, not TYK2. *J. Biol. Chem.* **274,** 13,480–13,484.

43. Komatsu, N., Kunitama, M., Yamada, M., Hagiwara, T., Kato, T., Miyazaki, H., et al. (1996) Establishment and characterization of the thrombopoietin-dependent megakaryocytic cell line, UT-7/TPO. *Blood* **87,** 4552–4560.

44. Kunitama, M., Shimizu, R., Yamada, M., Kato, T., Miyazaki, H., Okada, K., et al. (1997) Protein kinase C and c-myc gene activation pathways in thrombopoietin signal transduction. *Biochem. Biophys. Res. Commun.* **231,** 290–294.

45. Yamada, M., Komatsu, N., Okada, K., Kato, T., Miyazki, H., and Miura, Y. (1995) Thrombopoietin induces tyrosine phosphorylation and activation of mitogen-activated protein kinases in a human thrombopoietin-dependent cell line. *Biochem. Biophys. Res. Commun.* **217,** 230–237.

46. Rojnuckarin, P., Drachman, J. G., and Kaushansky, K. (1999) Thrombopoietin-induced activation of the mitogen-activated protein kinase (MAPK) pathway in normal megakaryocytes: role in endomitosis. *Blood* **94,** 1273–1282.

47. Rojnuckarin, P. and Kaushansky, K. (2001) Actin reorganization and proplatelet formation in murine megakaryocytes: the role of protein kinase c alpha. *Blood* **97,** 154–161.

48. Drachman, J. G., Sabath, D. F., Fox, N. E., and Kaushansky, K. (1997) Thrombopoietin signal transduction in purified murine megakaryocytes. *Blood* **89,** 483–492.

49. Weich, N., Wang, A., Fitzgerald, M., Neben, T. Y., Donaldson, D., Giannotti, J., et al. (1997) Recombinant human interleukin-11 directly promotes megakaryocytopoiesis in vitro. *Blood* **90,** 3893–3902.

50. Takeda, K., Noguchi, K., Shi, W., Tanaka, T., Matsumoto, M., Yoshida, N., et al. (1997) Targeted disruption of the mouse Stat3 gene leads to early embryonic lethality. *Proc. Natl. Acad. Sci. USA* **94,** 3801–3804.

51. Akira, S. (2000) Roles of STAT3 defined by tissue-specific gene targeting. *Oncogene* **19,** 2607–2611.

52. Takeda, K., Kaisho, T., Yoshida, N., Takeda, J., Kishimoto, T., and Akira, S. V. (1998) Stat3 activation is responsible for IL-6-dependent T cell proliferation through preventing apoptosis: generation and characterization of T cell-specific Stat3-deficient mice. *J. Immunol.* **161,** 4652–4660.

53. Martin, D., Zon, L. I., Mutter, G., and Orkin, S. H. (1990) Expression of an erythroid transcription factor in megakaryocytic and mast cell lineages. *Nature* **344,** 444–447.

54. Romeo, P., Prandini, M. H., Joulin, V., Mignotte, V., Prenant, M., Vainchenker, W., et al. (1990) Megakaryocytic and erythrocytic lineages share specific transcription factors. *Nature* **344,** 447–449.

55. Kirito, K., Osawa, M., Morita, H., Shimizu, R., Yamamoto, M., Oda, A., et al. (2002) A functional role of Stat3 in in vivo megakaryopoiesis. *Blood* **99,** 3220–3227.

56. Kaluzhny, Y., Yu, G., Sun, S., Toselli, P. A., Nieswandt, B., Jackson, C. W., et al. (2002) BclxL overexpression in megakaryocytes leads to impaired platelet fragmentation. *Blood* **100,** 1670–1678.

57. Koizumi, K., Sawada, K., Yamaguchi, M., Notoya, A., Tarumi, T., Takano, H., et al. (1998) In vitro expansion of CD34+/CD41+ cells from human peripheral blood CD34+/CD41– cells: role of cytokines for in vitro proliferation and differentiation of megakaryocytic progenitors. *Exp. Hematol.* **26,** 1140–1147.

58. Sato. N., Sawada, K., Takahashi, T. A., Mogi, Y., Asano, S., Koike, T., et al. (1994) A time course study for optimal harvest of peripheral blood progenitor cells by granulocyte colony-stimulating factor in healthy volunteers. *Exp. Hematol.* **22,** 973–978.

59. Sawada, K., Krantz, S. B., Dai, C. H., Koury, S. T., Horn, S. T., Glick, A. D., et al. (1990) Purification of human blood burst-forming units-erythroid and demonstration of the evolution of erythropoietin receptors. *J. Cell. Physiol.* **142,** 219–230.

60. Yamaguchi, M., Sawada, K., Sato, N., Koizumi, K., Sekiguchi, S., and Koike, T. (1997) A rapid nylon-fiber syringe system to deplete CD14+ cells for positive selection of human blood CD34+ cells. Use of immunomagnetic microspheres. *Bone Marrow Transplant* **19,** 373–379.

61. Sawada, K., Krantz, S. B., Dessypris, E. N., Koury, S. T., and Sawyer, S. T. (1989) Human colony-forming units-erythroid do not require accessory cells, but do require direct interaction with insulin-like growth factor I and/or insulin for erythroid development. *J. Clin. Invest.* **83,** 1701–1709.

Index